SINGULAR'S

POCKET
DICTIONARY
OF
AUDIOLOGY

SINGULAR'S

POCKET

DICTIONARY

OF

AUDIOLOGY

Lisa Lucks Mendel, Ph.D.
University of Mississippi

Jeffrey L. Danhauer, Ph.D.
University of California Santa Barbara

Sadanand Singh, Ph.D.
San Diego State University

With contributions from
Jennifer Mead and Jennifer Stewart
University of Mississippi

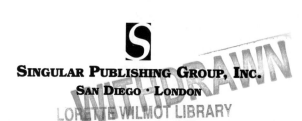

SINGULAR PUBLISHING GROUP, INC.
SAN DIEGO · LONDON

Singular Publishing Group, Inc.
401 West "A" Street, Suite 325
San Diego, California 92101-7904

Singular Publishing Ltd.
19 Compton Terrace
London, N1 2UN, UK

> **Singular Publishing Group, Inc.,** publishes textbooks, clinical manuals, clinical reference
> books, journals, videos, and multimedia materials on speech-language pathology, audiol-
> ogy, otorhinolaryngology, special education, early childhood, aging, occupational therapy,
> physical therapy, rehabilitation, counseling, mental health, and voice. For your conven-
> ience, our entire catalog can be accessed on our website at *http://www.singpub.com*. Our
> mission to provide you with materials to meet the daily challenges of the ever-changing
> health care/educational environment will remain on course if we are in touch with you. In
> that spirit, we welcome your feedback on our products. Please telephone (**1-800-521-8545**),
> fax (**1-800-774-8398**), or e-mail (*singpub@singpub.com*) your comments and requests to us.

© 1999 by Singular Publishing Group, Inc.

Typeset in 8.5/10 Palatino by So Cal Graphics
Printed in the United States of America by Book Crafters

Library of Congress Cataloging-in-Publication Data

Mendel, Lisa Lucks.
    Singular's pocket dictionary of audiology / by Lisa Lucks Mendel,
Jeffrey L. Danhauer, Sadanand Singh : with contributions from
Jennifer Mead and Jennifer Stewart.
    p.   cm.
    This ed. lacks the illustrations of Singular's illustrated
dictionary of audiology
    Includes bibliographical references and index.
    ISBN 0-7693-0042-1 (softcover : alk. paper)
    1. Audiology—Dictionaries.   I. Mendel, Lisa Lucks.   Singular's
illustrated dictionary of audiology.   II. Danhauer, Jeffrey L.
III. Singh, Sadanand.   IV. Title.
RF290 .M4642 1999
617.8'003—dc21   98-55561
                                                                          CIP

Contents

Preface

This dictionary provides comprehensive coverage of over 4,500 terms in the field of audiology and related areas. It is a reference that all students, clinicians, and related professionals should find extremely useful. Terms are defined completely and concisely to provide the reader with sufficient detail for a general overview of the term or topic of interest. In addition, extensive cross-references are included throughout the text to guide the reader to other vocabulary that may be related in some way to the specific item of interest. Many of the definitions provided in this dictionary were adapted from other definitions published in over 60 Singular texts, and a list of all references is provided at the end of the dictionary. Thus, our goal was one of conciseness and completeness, rather than originality.

Obviously, we have not created new terms here; the terms and definitions have evolved along with the rich development of audiology as a field. In compiling the terms and definitions for this text we sought as many definitions as possible from several sources. If the sources disagreed slightly, we included all possibilities for completeness, rather than playing judge as to which was correct. As a result, many terms include more than one definition. In most cases, the terms are defined at length, while in some cases a term may have only a brief definition. In those cases, the reader is often referred to other terms defined within the dictionary that should supplement the reader's understanding of a particular vocabulary item. Thus, when using this dictionary, readers should look up the definitions to additional terms that may be indicated in the "see also" section of the items. Any term listed in boldface type indicates that it is a term defined in the dictionary. If readers want even more detail on a specific term or topic, they are referred to sources such as the *Audiologists' Desk Reference, Volumes I and II,* or many of the other textbooks that deal with specialized topics for more in-depth coverage.

One might ask why the need for another dictionary? There have been others; however, we believe that this text represents a unique and novel compilation of terms that is up-to-date and as complete as possible. The cross-referencing should make it a singular source for audiology. No doubt we have missed a few terms along the way, and needless to say, new terms and acronyms are being generated for our field every day. We encourage comments about the text from our readers and intend to incorporate their feedback to continue to update this text in the future so that it can be the most useful and user-friendly source available.

All terms are listed alphabetically. If the term has a recognized acronym associated with it, that acronym is listed alphabetically and defined within the text of the dictionary. A list of all acronyms can also be found in Appendix A.

Another way to use this dictionary is to identify a topic of interest. Appendix B provides an extensive listing of all terms defined in the dictionary organized by their appropriate categories. Thus, if students wanted to determine all of the terms related to **otoacoustic emissions,** they would turn to the topic listing in Appendix B on otoacoustic emissions. There they would find vocabulary items related to the area of otoacoustic emissions with accompanying page numbers for easy access to the alphabetical definitions of these terms.

This text should be useful to students, clinicians, teachers, researchers, equipment manufacturers, publishers, and others interested in hearing. This dictionary should be invaluable as a quick, complete, and handy reference source to audiologists, otologists, general physicians, speech-language pathologists, and other professionals, as well as lay persons interacting with patients, friends, and relations having interests in the field of hearing.

This work is the result of the combined efforts of an extended academic family: Lisa Lucks Mendel was a doctoral student under Jeffrey Danhauer who was a doctoral student under Sadanand Singh. In addition, significant contributions to this book were made by two of Lisa Lucks Mendel's current master's students, Jennifer Mead and Jennifer Stewart. Thus, it represents (at a minimum) four generations of audiology and hearing science, not to mention the countless contributions from the numerous authors of the other texts from which these terms and definitions were derived. This joint effort speaks to the importance of the lineage of academic teaching and scholarly work. It is our hope that collaborative endeavors such as this one will continue to be contributed to our profession for generations to come.

Special thanks to all those who spent countless hours assisting us while we were writing this text. Without the love, patience, and encouragement of our families, friends, and colleagues, this effort could not have been successful. We thank them for their tireless support of our endeavors. Our most sincere thanks to Maurice Mendel for his persistent patience and steady encouragement of the first author and helping her see this project through completion.

Dedication

To our students
Past, Present, and Future

A

A-weighted scale filter network used by a sound level meter that attenuates low-frequency components of a sound to compensate for less sensitive human hearing for low frequencies; approximates the 40 phon equal loudness contour; measurement is reported in dBA; see also **dBA**

AAA American Academy of Audiology; the professional organization for audiologists that has as its mission "caring for America's hearing;" established in 1988

AABER aided auditory brainstem evoked response; an auditory brainstem response measurement recorded while the patient is wearing hearing aid(s); see also **auditory brainstem response (ABR)**

AABR automated auditory brainstem response audiometry; the use of auditory brainstem response measurement for newborn hearing screening programs; see also **ALGO**

AAO-HNS American Academy of Otolaryngology—Head and Neck Surgery; a professional organization for otolaryngologists

AAS American Auditory Society; an interdisciplinary organization whose primary aims are to increase knowledge and understanding of the ear, hearing, and balance; established in 1974

AB isophonemic word test an open-set monosyllabic word identification task for adults comprised of 15 lists of 10 CVCs each

Abbreviated Profile of Hearing Aid Benefit (APHAB) an assessment scale for hearing aid users that rates patients' perception of hearing aid benefit; part of the Independent Hearing Aid Fitting Forum protocol; see also **Independent Hearing Aid Fitting Forum (IHAFF)**

abducens nerve VIth cranial nerve responsible for control of eye movements

abduction movement of an anatomical structure away from the midline of the body

ABG air-bone gap; difference between hearing threshold levels for air-conducted pure-tone signals and bone-conducted pure-tone signals

ABI (1) auditory behavior index; classification of the type of response and level of adequate stimuli needed to elicit a behavioral response at various ages of normal development for infants and young children; (2) auditory brainstem implant; an implant similar to a cochlear implant that is placed on the cochlear nucleus for individuals with severed VIIIth nerves

ablation the removal of a growth or the excision of any part of the body

ABLB alternate binaural loudness balancing; a traditional diagnostic auditory procedure for detecting loudness recruitment used in differentiating cochlear versus retrocochlear auditory dysfunction in unilateral hearing loss; the task is to balance the sensation of loudness for the better versus the poorer hearing ear

ABONSO automatic brain operated noise suppressor option; acronym coined by Mead Killion to describe how the brain and hearing mechanism should operate for hearing in noise

ABR auditory brainstem response; an objective test that measures the electrical potential produced in response to sound stimuli by the synchronous discharge of the first- through sixth-order neurons in the auditory nerve and brainstem; also known as **brainstem auditory evoked potential (BAEP)** and **brainstem auditory evoked response (BAER)**

abscissa horizontal or x-axis of a graph

absolute bone-conduction test a test of sensorineural function in which a patient's hearing by bone conduction is compared with an examiner's by the use of tuning forks

absolute latency (1) the time in milliseconds from the onset of a stimulus to the onset of the peak of a wave in any electrophysiologic response; (2) an important measurement parameter in the interpretation of the auditory brainstem response; see also **latency**

absolute pitch the ability possessed by certain people to name the musical pitch of a note without the aid of a standard reference

absolute refractory period the time following the excitation of a nerve or muscle fiber during which no new nerve discharge can occur

absolute threshold the minimum stimulus that evokes a response in a specified fraction of trials; the difference between audibility and inaudibility; see also **threshold**

absorption penetration of sound energy through the material of an obstacle when the impedance of the obstacle is not infinite

absorption coefficient the proportion of sound intensity that is absorbed when a sound wave hits a surface

AC (1) air conduction; pure-tone signals presented via earphones to the ear; process by which sound is conducted to the inner ear through the outer and middle ears; (2) alternating current; an electric current that periodically flows in one direction and then the other

Academy of Dispensing Audiologists (ADA) an organization whose primary goal is to represent the interests of audiologists who dispense hearing aids; established in 1979

Academy of Rehabilitative Audiology (ARA) an organization that provides a forum for the exchange of ideas on, knowledge of, and experience with habilitative and rehabilitative programs for persons who are hearing impaired; established in 1966

accelerated speech perception test a task that assesses a patient's ability to perceive temporally degraded speech signals

acceleration the time-rate change in velocity; a vector quantity

accelerometer a device that produces a measurement of/in units of force; the vibrations are then transduced and delivered to a sound level meter for measurement in dB SPL

accessory nerve cranial nerve XI responsible for speech, swallowing, and head and shoulder movements

accommodation making facilities and programs accessible to and usable by persons with disabilities through appropriate modifications, including policy modifications, task restructuring, modified schedules, equipment acquisition or modification, training, or provision of qualified readers or interpreters, and other similar accommodations; see also **Americans with Disabilities Act (ADA)**

ACE Award for Continuing Education; honor presented to individuals who have completed a requisite number of continuing education units; awarded by the American Speech-Language-Hearing Association

acetylcholine (Ach) biochemical that functions as an excitatory neurotransmitter

Ach acetylcholine; biochemical that functions as an excitatory neurotransmitter

achondroplasia an autosomal dominant syndrome characterized by disproportionate short stature, short anterior cranial base, open-bite, maxillary hypoplasia, and occasional hydrocephalus; associated with conductive hearing loss secondary to middle ear disease

acoupedic program developed in 1974 by Doreen Pollack to teach how infants can be educated using aided residual hearing and an aural-oral approach; also known as **auditory-oral approach**; see also **auditory-verbal approach**

acousthesia exceptionally keen sense of hearing

acoustic having to do with sound or sound waves; see also **acoustics**

acoustic admittance (Y) the flow of energy through the middle ear; reciprocal of impedance; Y = G + B, where G = conductance and B = susceptance; expressed in mmhos; also known as **admittance**

acoustic compliance ease with which energy flows through the middle ear system for a given force; the reciprocal of stiffness; see also **compliance**

acoustic conductance ease with which energy flows through the middle ear system for a given force; the reciprocal of resistance; see also **conductance**

acoustic coupler artificial ear used for purposes such as research and measuring hearing aid output; see also **1.5-cc coupler, 2-cc coupler, 6-cc coupler, Zwislocki coupler**

acoustic cue the part of the speech signal that provides auditory information that is necessary for understanding speech and nonspeech sounds

acoustic distortion inaccurate reproduction of a sound signal by modification of the frequency content of the waveform during amplification or transmission; see also **distortion**

acoustic feedback a whistling sound produced by a hearing aid; the return of some of the energy of the output signal from the hearing aid receiver to the input transducer (microphone); see also **feedback**

acoustic gain the difference in dB between the intensity of the input signal to a hearing aid and the intensity of the output signal; see also **2-cc coupler gain, gain**

acoustic immittance general term that indicates either acoustic impedance or acoustic admittance or both; see also **immittance, impedance**

acoustic impedance (Z) the complex quotient of the sound pressure (force per unit area) on that surface by the flux (volume-velocity, or linear velocity multiplied by the area) through the surface; equal to the mechanical

impedance divided by the square of the area of the surface considered; see also **immittance, impedance**

acoustic insulation materials used to absorb sound; useful in sound abatement

acoustic meatus the opening to the external auditory canal; the external auditory canal; see also **external auditory canal, external auditory meatus**

acoustic mmho millimhos; common measurement unit for clinical acoustic admittance measures

acoustic modification modification of earmolds and/or hearing aids in order to enhance the natural acoustics for improvements in amplification

acoustic nerve cranial nerve VIII; consists of two sets of fibers: the anterior branch or cochlear nerve and the posterior branch or vestibular nerve; conducts neural signals from the inner ear to the brain; see also **auditory nerve, auditory-vestibular nerve, VIIIth nerve**

acoustic neuroma benign tumor on the auditory nerve often growing in the internal auditory canal; signs and symptoms produced in cerebellum, lower cranial nerve, and brainstem; can cause tinnitus, progressive hearing loss, headache, dizziness, and unsteady gait, with later stage symptoms of paresis and speaking/swallowing difficulty; also known as **auditory nerve tumor**; see also **acoustic tumor, vestibular schwannoma**

acoustic ohm unit of measurement for both compliant and mass acoustic reactance; equal to 1 dyne per square centimeter producing a volume velocity of 1 cc per second; see also **ohm**

acoustic phonetics the scientific study of speech sounds that focuses on sound patterns that function in language

acoustic radiations flow of information via auditory nerve fibers from the medial geniculate body to the auditory cortex; also known as **auditory radiations**

acoustic reactance (X) the out-of-phase component of impedance that opposes energy flow by storing the energy for a period of time; see also **reactance**

acoustic reflex (AR) response of the middle ear muscles (primarily the stapedius) and the ossicles to intense sound; also known as **acoustic stapedial reflex**

acoustic reflex arc the pathway through the brainstem that is followed when an acoustic reflex occurs; the afferent portion of the arc is cranial nerve VIII, the central portion consists of brainstem centers, and the efferent portion is cranial nerve VII; also known as **reflex arc**

acoustic reflex decay decline in reflex contraction of the stapedius muscle during the presentation of a sustained, acoustic activating signal; indicative of a retrocochlear disorder; also known as **reflex decay, stapedial reflex decay**

acoustic reflex latency the time in milliseconds between the onset of

an auditory stimulus and the identification of an acoustic reflex

acoustic reflex pattern configuration of results obtained from ipsilateral and contralateral acoustic reflexes used to determine the possible site of lesion for an auditory disorder

acoustic reflex threshold (ART) the lowest level of the acoustic activating signal that produces an observable, time-locked change in acoustic immittance; see also **acoustic reflex**

acoustic resistance (R) the in-phase component of impedance; opposition to the flow of energy via dissipation; see also **resistance**

acoustic signature characteristic features that identify a given sound or sound environment as distinct from others

acoustic stria second-order nerve fiber bundles arising from the three cochlear nuclei (dorsal, anterior ventral, and posterior ventral) and projecting to higher brainstem levels

acoustic susceptance component of acoustic admittance that can be divided into two types: compliance and mass; reciprocal of reactance; also known as **susceptance**

acoustic transformer effect for musical instruments, an effect that enhances all frequencies whose one-half wavelength is less than the total length of the tube

acoustic trauma trauma to the auditory system caused by exposure to a very high-intensity, abrupt, or high-impact noise; see also **noise-induced hearing loss (NIHL)**

acoustic tumor a neoplasm arising from cranial nerve VIII (usually the vestibular portion); often referred to as acoustic neuroma; proper term is vestibular schwannoma; also known as acoustic neurilemmoma, acoustic neurinoma, acoustic neurilemma; see also **acoustic neuroma, vestibular schwannoma**

acoustically modified earmolds earmolds that take advantage of venting, sound bore modifications, and tubing adjustments to enhance the natural acoustic amplification features of the device; see also **external ear effects (EEE)**

acoustics the science of the production, control, transmission, reception, and effects of sound and of the phenomenon of hearing

acquired any disease, characteristic, or condition that occurs after birth

acquired hearing loss hearing loss that occurs after speech and language have developed; hearing loss due to nonhereditary factors; also known as **adventitious hearing loss**

acquired immunodeficiency syndrome (AIDS) a syndrome involving a defect in the immune system of the human body; characterized by opportunistic infections; has a long incubation period and a poor prognosis; see also **human immunodeficiency virus (HIV)**

actin protein found in outer hair cells that contributes to their capacity for motility

action potential (AP) (1) gross neural potential; summed or averaged activity of action potentials of cranial nerve VIII in response to acoustic stimulation; (2) in auditory evoked potential measurements, it is the whole-nerve response of cranial nerve VIII; (3) the main component of the electrocochleogram and wave I of the auditory brainstem response; also known as **whole nerve action potential**

active electrode usually refers to the noninverting electrode in auditory evoked potential measurements

acuity (1) the clarity of perception; (2) in acoustics, differential sensitivity to pitch and loudness

acusis normal hearing; see also **audibility, audition**

acute beginning abruptly with marked intensity; a disease process can be classified as being acute

acute labyrinthitis inflammation of the labyrinthine canals of the inner ear resulting in abrupt vertigo with marked intensity; associated with tinnitus and sensorineural hearing loss; see also **labyrinthitis**

acute mastoiditis infection of the mastoid area usually resulting from acute suppurative otitis media; infection may spread to cause facial nerve paralysis, labyrinthitis, and meningitis; see also **mastoiditis**

acute otitis media middle ear inflammation of recent onset accompanied by symptoms and signs of infection; generally lasts 2 to 3 weeks; see also **otitis media (OM)**

acute tympanitis sharp, extreme inflammation of the tympanic membrane often associated with otitis media; also known as acute myringitis

AD right ear; Latin abbreviation for **auris dextra**

ADA (1) Academy of Dispensing Audiologists; an organization whose primary goal is to represent the interests of audiologists who dispense hearing aids; established in 1979; (2) Americans with Disabilities Act; Public Law 101-336 enacted to provide protection from discrimination based on disability; it was modeled after the Rehabilitation Act of 1973 and passed in 1990

adaptation (1) a decrease in the response of sensory receptors with continuous stimulation over time; (2) decline in the sensation of a sustained sound; see also **auditory adaptation, tone decay**

adaptive compression type of compression that has variable release times that change automatically; see also **compression**

adaptive filtering filter characteristics are automatically altered to modify a designated incoming electrical signal optimally with the overall objective of improving the electrical signal-to-noise ratio; nonlinear automatic signal processing used in BILL and TILL circuits; see also **filter, bass increase at low levels (BILL), treble increase at low levels (TILL)**

adaptive frequency response (AFR) the type of hearing aid in which the frequency response changes as input level changes; see also **compression, level dependent frequency response**

adaptive procedure an estimation procedure in which the manner of stimulus change is determined by the listener's response

adaptive signal processing (ASP) an adaptive circuit that reduces background noise interference, primarily by reducing low-frequency amplification, thus making speech easier to hear and understand; also known as **automatic signal processing**; see also **adaptive filtering**

adaptive speech test a speech recognition test that averages the midpoints of several threshold trials

ADC analog to digital converter; an electronic device that converts a continuously varying electrical signal to a series of numeric values, which can then be processed by a computer

ADD attention deficit disorder; a cognitive deficit that limits an individual's ability to pay attention and stay focused on a task; may involve restlessness, distractibility, and hyperactivity; see also **attention deficit hyperactivity disorder (ADHD)**

adenoidectomy surgical procedure performed to remove enlarged adenoids that are causing an obstruction of the nasopharynx

adenoids lymphoid tissue within the nasopharynx

adenoma tumor of glandular tissue causing excess secretion from the gland

ADHD attention deficit and hyperactivity disorder; persistent pattern of inattention and/or hyperactivity-impulsivity that is more frequent and severe than is typically observed in individuals at a comparable level of development; see also **ADD**

adhesion band of scar tissue binding together two anatomical surfaces or structures; can occur in the middle ear (between the ossicles) during adhesive otitis media; see also **adhesive otitis media**

adhesive otitis media condition in which fibrous adhesions are present in the middle ear as a result of previous inflammation; see also **otitis media**

aditus posterior-superior region of the middle ear space containing the head of the malleus and greater part of the incus; communicates upward and backward to the mastoid antrum; also known as the tympanic aditus; see also **antrum, epitympanic recess**

admittance (Y) the flow of energy through the middle ear; reciprocal of impedance; $Y = G + B$, where G = conductance and B = susceptance; expressed in mmhos; also known as **acoustic admittance**

adrenoleukodystrophy (ALS) a demyelinating disease; also known as **Lou Gehrig's disease**; see also **leukodystrophy**

advantage, binaural using two ears in order to improve sound detection, localization, and understanding in noise; see also **binaural hearing**

advantage, right ear (REA) a cerebral dominance phenomenon in which normal right-handed listeners have scores for the right ear that are consistently higher than scores for the left ear for dichotically presented signals

adventitious hearing loss hearing loss that occurs after speech and language have developed; hearing loss due to nonhereditary factors; also known as **acquired hearing loss**

AEP auditory evoked potential; electrical activity evoked by sounds arising from auditory portions of the peripheral or central nervous system traveling from cranial nerve VIII to the cortex; recorded with electrodes; also known as **auditory evoked response (AER)**

AER auditory evoked response; electrical activity evoked by sounds arising from auditory portions of the peripheral or central nervous system traveling from cranial nerve VIII to the cortex; recorded with electrodes; also known as **auditory evoked potential (AEP)**

affective counseling counseling that addresses the patients' emotions and attitudes that result from hearing loss; see also **counseling**

afferent a neural pathway leading from a sense organ (e.g., the ear) to the brain

AFR adaptive frequency response; the type of hearing aid in which the frequency response changes as input level changes

after response a post-stimulus-time histogram response pattern with neural spike activity occurring 15 ms subsequent to the offset of the stimulus

AG Bell Alexander Graham Bell Association for the Deaf; an international organization based in Washington, D.C. dedicated to improving opportunities for people with hearing impairments to speak, speechread, and use their residual hearing to communicate; established in 1890

AGC automatic gain control; a feature in some hearing aids that reduces amplification at high input intensity levels; a nonlinear process in which the gain changes as a function of changing signal levels; see also **compression**

AGC-I automatic gain control-input; type of hearing aid compression circuit in which the volume control setting does not affect the level of the compression threshold; AGC circuit is placed before the volume control in the hearing aid

AGC-O automatic gain control-output; type of hearing aid compression circuit in which the volume control setting affects the level of the compression threshold; AGC circuit is placed after the volume control in the hearing aid

age, chronologic (CA) age of an individual calculated from the date of birth

age, developmental a manifestation of a child's maturational growth based on the acquisition of specific developmental milestones in areas such as speech, language, motor, and social skills

age, gestational the age of a newborn infant, determined by evaluation of physical (specifically neurologic) maturity after birth and comparison to normative data for different ages after birth (usually in weeks)

age, mental (MA) age level at which an individual functions intellectually as determined by standardized psychological tests

ageism view that stigmatizes and discriminates against older individuals based on their chronological age

ageotropic nystagmus type of positional nystagmus that beats away from the ground; if the patient's head is positioned so that the left side is down (toward the ground), then the nystagmus beats away from that side

agnosia partial or total loss of the ability to recognize familiar aspects of the environment through the senses

AI (1) articulation index; (2) audibility index; a number between 0 and 1 that expresses the degree of audibility of a speech signal which is highly correlated with traditional speech intelligibility scores (number of speech items repeated correctly)

aided auditory brainstem evoked response (AABER) an auditory brainstem response measurement recorded while the patient is wearing hearing aid(s); see also **auditory brainstem response (ABR)**

aided thresholds the softest sounds that a person can hear while wearing hearing aid(s); see also **threshold**

AIDS acquired immunodeficiency syndrome; a syndrome involving a defect in the immune system of the human body; characterized by opportunistic infections; has a long incubation period and a poor prognosis

air conduction (AC) pure-tone signals presented via earphones to the ear; process by which sound is conducted to the inner ear through the outer and middle ears; see also **audiometry, pure-tone audiometry**

air-bone gap (ABG) difference between hearing threshold levels for air-conducted pure-tone signals and bone-conducted pure-tone signals

air-conduction audiometry hearing tests that use pure-tone signals presented via earphones to establish thresholds

air-conduction threshold the lowest level that one can hear a pure-tone signal delivered via insert or supra-aural earphones 50% of the time

AJA American Journal of Audiology; clinical audiology journal of the American Speech-Language-Hearing Association

Albers-Schöneberg syndrome an autosomal recessive disease characterized by dense but fragile bone, macrocephaly, cranial nerve palsies, distorted teeth, hydrocephalus; associated with mixed or retrocochlear sensorineural hearing loss

albinism an X-linked recessive disorder characterized by absence of pigment over the entire body except for optic fundi and irises, scanty eyebrows; associated with late onset sensorineural hearing loss

ALD assistive listening device; any of a number of pieces of equipment used to augment hearing or to assist hearing aids in difficult listening situations (e.g., FM, infrared, and induction loop systems)

alerting devices a range of devices for individuals who are hearing impaired that substitute visual or tactile signals for alerting and alarm signals; see also **assistive listening device (ALD)**

Alexander Graham Bell Association for the Deaf (AG Bell) an international organization based in Washington, D.C. dedicated to improving opportunities for people with hearing impairments to speak, speechread, and use their residual hearing to communicate; established in 1890

Alexander's law (1) nystagmus beats most intensely when the eyes are deviated toward the side of the fast phase of the nystagmus; (2) spontaneous ocular square waves, observed during a gaze test, that are caused by lesions of the brainstem or cerebellum

ALGO automated auditory brainstem response screening device that uses click stimuli at 35 dB nHL; used primarily in neonatal screenings; see also **auditory brainstem response (ABR), automated auditory brainstem response audiometry**

algorithm specific mathematical operations performed in a systematic procedure to accomplish a specific task; used in computers and digital hearing aids

aliasing artifactual evoked response waveform components occurring in the waveform after analog-to-digital conversion due to interaction between an inadequately low sampling rate and the frequency of the evoked response activity

allele alternative form of any given gene found at the same locus on homologous chromosomes; only two alleles can exist in any one individual

allogenic indicates tissue that is from an individual or a cell type that belongs to the same species but is genetically different

alpha rhythm electroencephalogram activity within the 8–12 Hz frequency region, normally of high amplitude; sometimes associated with relaxation

Alport syndrome characterized by nephritis, progressive sensorineural hearing loss with variable severity, myopia, stridor, apnea, and dysphagia; delivered either through X-linked dominant or autosomal recessive transmission

ALR auditory late response; electrical activity evoked by sounds that orig-

inates from portions of the auditory cortex, is measured with electrodes placed on the scalp, and occurs within 100–300 ms after the sound is presented

ALS adrenoleukodystrophy; a demyelinating disease; also known as **Lou Gehrig's disease**

Alström syndrome autosomal recessive disorder characterized by obesity, mildly short stature, nystagmus, loss of vision, baldness (males), diabetes mellitus, renal anomalies, and scoliosis; associated with progressive sensorineural hearing loss that is cochlear in origin

alternate binaural bithermal caloric test open-loop caloric irrigation as part of the electronystagmography test battery; each ear is irrigated separately using cool then warm water; the order of irrigation follows right ear cool, left ear cool, right ear warm, left ear warm

alternate binaural loudness balancing (ABLB) a traditional diagnostic auditory procedure for detecting loudness recruitment used in differentiating cochlear versus retrocochlear auditory dysfunction in unilateral hearing loss; the task is to balance the sensation of loudness for the better versus the poorer hearing ear

alternate monaural loudness balancing (AMLB) a diagnostic auditory procedure for detecting loudness recruitment used in differentiating cochlear versus retrocochlear auditory dysfunction in an individual having normal hearing at some frequencies and sensorineural hearing loss at others; the task is to balance the sensation of loudness between the frequencies with better sensitivity versus those with poorer sensitivity

alternating current (AC) an electric current that periodically flows in one direction and then the other

alternating stimulus polarity alternating presentation of rarefaction and condensation polarity stimuli rather than stimuli of all one polarity; often used in evoked potential measurements

Alzheimer's disease dementia characterized by progressive neural degeneration resulting in memory deterioration and failure, confusion, disorientation, and restlessness

AM amplitude modulation; a stimulus type consisting of a carrier sound in which the amplitude is varied (modulated)

AMA American Medical Association; national organization composed of physicians

ambient pertaining to a surrounding area

ambient noise background noise from all sources that are in the test environment

ambient pressure the peak of a tympanogram (0 daPa), which represents the contributions of the ear canal, tympanic membrane, and the entire middle ear system; the point where outer ear pressure is equal to middle ear pressure

ambiguus nucleus one of the cranial motor nuclei of the brainstem with motor neurons that innervates laryngeal, pharyngeal, and esophageal muscles

American Academy of Audiology (AAA) the professional organization for audiologists that has as its mission "caring for America's hearing"; established in 1988

American Academy of Otolaryngology—Head and Neck Surgery (AAO-HNS) a professional organization for otolaryngologists

American Auditory Society (AAS) an interdisciplinary organization whose primary aims are to increase knowledge and understanding of the ear, hearing, and balance; established in 1974

American Journal of Audiology (AJA) clinical audiology journal of the American Speech-Language-Hearing Association

American Medical Association (AMA) national organization composed of physicians

American National Standards Institute (ANSI) a government agency responsible for developing standards for design, construction, and performance of audiologic test equipment; established in 1929

American Sign Language (ASL) a distinct language conveyed as a form of manual communication by some deaf individuals; has its own syntax and language structure; common form of communication among the Deaf community; also known as **AMESLAN**

American Speech-Language-Hearing Association (ASHA) a professional organization for speech-language pathologists and audiologists; formally the American Speech and Hearing Association; established in 1925

American Standards Association (ASA) earlier name for the American National Standards Institute

American Tinnitus Association (ATA) a non-profit, consumer organization for individuals who suffer from tinnitus; established in 1971

Americans with Disabilities Act (ADA) Public Law 101-336 enacted to provide protection from discrimination based on disability; it was modeled after the Rehabilitation Act of 1973 and passed in 1990

AMESLAN another name for **American Sign Language (ASL)**

amikacin aminoglycoside antibiotic derived from kanamycin that is potentially ototoxic and nephrotoxic; vestibular and permanent bilateral auditory ototoxicity can occur in patients with preexisting renal damage

aminoglycosides class of antibiotics effective in treating infections caused by gram-negative aerobic bacteria; are all ototoxic to some degree and are generally the most vestibulotoxic of all ototoxic drugs; includes amikacin, gentamicin, kanamycin, livodomycin, neomycin, netilmicin, sisomycin, streptomycin, and tobramycin

AMLB alternate monaural loudness balancing; a diagnostic auditory procedure for detecting loudness recruitment used in differentiating cochlear versus retrocochlear auditory dysfunction in an individual having normal hearing at some frequencies and sensorineural hearing loss at others; the task is to balance the sensation of loudness between the frequencies with better sensitivity versus those with poorer sensitivity

AMLR auditory middle latency response; an auditory evoked potential occurring between 12 and 80 ms; provides information from the precortical area

ampere (amp) basic unit of electrical current; amount of current 1 volt can send through a resistance of 1 ohm

amplification (1) an increase in the intensity of sounds; (2) collective term used for devices such as hearing aids and auditory trainers

amplification, binaural wearing two hearing aids rather than one to utilize the binaural advantage

amplification, compression a hearing aid or amplification device that reduces the intensity range among audio signals while increasing the overall intensity of all signals; (e.g., automatic gain control, output limiting, wide dynamic range compression)

amplification, linear a hearing aid or amplification device that produces equivalent gain for all input levels up until the maximum output of the device, at which point the signal saturates; see also **peak clipping (PC), linear analog circuitry**

amplification, nonlinear a hearing aid or amplification device that does not provide a one-to-one correspondence between input and output at all input levels

amplification, personal amplification devices that are worn by an individual (e.g., hearing aids) as opposed to by a group (e.g., group auditory trainers)

amplification, sound field electronic equipment that amplifies an entire (class)room through the careful positioning of two to four loudspeakers; the teacher wears an FM microphone/transmitter

amplified speech spectrum frequency range for speech information made audible via amplification

amplifier an electronic device (e.g., hearing aid) for increasing the magnitude of an electrical signal (increasing gain)

amplitude (1) a measure of the size of a signal usually made from either a peak to a preceding or following trough, or from a peak to some index of baseline; expressed in voltage or dB; (2) in auditory evoked potentials it is the magnitude of the response in microvolts

amplitude, peak a measure of amplitude that relates to the peak amount of displacement from either the condensation (positive) component or the rarefaction (negative) component; see also **peak-to-peak amplitude**

amplitude, peak-to-peak a measure of amplitude that relates to the difference between the most positive peak and the most negative trough (i.e., the extremes of the quantity); see also **peak amplitude**

amplitude, RMS a measure of amplitude that uses root mean square to calculate the long-term overall effective level of a signal; the square root of the mean of the squared instantaneous amplitude values of a signal integrated over a time period long enough so that the result is not sensitive to small changes in the integration period

amplitude distortion erroneous reproduction of sound waves in which the output is not linear with respect to the input; often occurs when the system is saturated

amplitude modulation (AM) a stimulus type consisting of a carrier sound in which the amplitude is varied (modulated)

amplitude ratio (1) a calculation of the amplitude of the summating potential (SP) value divided by the amplitude of the action potential (AP) in electrocochleography; (2) a calculation of the amplitude of wave I divided by wave V of the auditory brainstem response

ampulla/ampullae a ciliated enlargement toward the anterior end of each of the three semicircular canals as they communicate with the utricle; each ampulla contains an end organ (crista) for the sense of equilibrium

ampullofugal stimulation stimulation away from the ampulla of the posterior semicircular canal causing nystagmus and excitation of the ipsilateral superior oblique and the contralateral inferior rectus muscles

AN (1) acoustic neuroma; tumor on the auditory nerve; (2) auditory nerve; division of the VIIIth cranial nerve that provides the link between the cochlea and the central auditory system

anacusis complete lack of hearing; deafness

analog a continuously varying signal over time in contrast to a sequence of discrete values or a digital representation of a response

analog hearing aid a hearing aid with conventional circuitry that processes the signal in a continuous fashion in the time domain

analog signal continuous variations in amplitude; the radiated sound-pressure waveform of speech is an analog signal, because its amplitude varies continuously in time; see also **analog**

analog to digital converter (ADC) an electronic device that converts a continuously varying electrical signal to a series of numeric values, which can then be processed by a computer

analysis of variance (ANOVA) a test of statistical analysis to determine if significant differences exist overall in the means of three or more different groups

analysis time the time period after a stimulus is presented during which a response is averaged and analyzed

analytic (1) an instructional method that focuses on the individual components of the signal; used in auditory and speechreading training; (2) a method of scoring speech perception tests that focuses on the correct perception of individual phonemes and awards credit for all parts of the item perceived correctly (e.g., phoneme scoring)

anastomosis surgically joining one nerve to another

anechoic without reverberation or echo

anechoic chamber an echo-free or reflection-free enclosure; a room where propagated sound is completely absorbed

anencephaly absence of brain by congenital deformity; markedly defective development of brain and cranial tissue

anesthesia a condition characterized by the absence of normal sensation; usually induced by certain drugs during medical or surgical procedures to eliminate sensitivity to pain

anesthetic a pharmacological drug used to produce a partial or complete lack of sensation

aneurysm localized dilation of blood vessel walls; can rupture and cause hemorrhaging

angioma growth or tumor composed of blood

angular acceleration (1) placing the head at an angle as in a head turn; (2) used in vestibular assessment to denote head rotation

anhydrosis autosomal dominant disorder characterized by an inability to perspire; salt granules are excreted, not perspiration; results from being dehydrated; accompanied by a progressive sensorineural hearing loss that starts at middle age

ankylosis immobility of a joint due to pathological changes (e.g., immobility of the ossicular chain due to otosclerosis); may be congenital or hereditary or may result from disease; also referred to as stapes fixation; see also **otosclerosis, stapedial ankylosis**

annular ligament thin elastic membrane that attaches the footplate of the stapes to the oval window; see also **stapes, stapes footplate**

annulus fibrous tissue and cartilage that forms the rim of the tympanic membrane

anode positive electrode of an electrode pair; positive part of a battery; see also **cathode**

anomaly an abnormality; a deviation from normal

anotia congenital absence of the ear(s)

anoxia a lack of oxygen in body tissues or systems

ANOVA analysis of variance; a test of statistical analysis to determine if significant differences exist overall in the means of three or more different groups

ANS autonomic nervous system; the part of the nervous system associated with independent or involuntary function

ANSI American National Standards Institute; a government agency responsible for developing standards for design, construction, and performance of audiologic test equipment; established in 1929

anterior referring to structures located forward or toward the front

anterior malleolar ligament one of the ligaments of the middle ear responsible for suspension of the ossicular chain; connects from the anterior process of the malleus to the anterior wall of the tympanic cavity

anterior ventral cochlear nucleus (AVCN) division of the cochlear nucleus; the lower brainstem nucleus into which the auditory nerve terminates

antibiotic an antimicrobial agent used to treat infections; has the ability to destroy or affect the development of a living organism

antibody protein substance normally developed in the body, typically in response to antigens, that provides immunity to diseases

anticoagulant a substance that prevents the blood from forming into a gelatinous mass

antigen a substance that induces the formation of antibodies; may be produced within the body or introduced into the body

antihelix ridge of cartilage on the auricle that is anterior to the helix

antineoplastic drugs class of drugs used in the treatment of cancer and tumors; considered chemotherapeutic agents including cisplatin, carboplatin, and nitrogen mustard; have significant ototoxic potential

antinode the point or line of maximum displacement of a vibrating body or enclosure; see also **node**

antitragus cartilaginous portion of the auricle that is posterior and inferior to the tragus

Antley-Bixler syndrome autosomal recessive disorder characterized by craniosynostosis, malformed ears, arachnodactyly, femoral bowing, digital anomalies, heart anomalies, imperforated anus, kidney anomalies; conductive hearing loss common secondary to middle ear effusion

antrum posterior-superior region of the middle ear space containing the head of the malleus and greater part of the incus; communicates upward and backward to the mastoid antrum

anvil outdated term for the middle ear bone known as the incus; see also **incus**

AP action potential; (1) gross neural potential; summed or averaged activity of action potentials of cranial nerve VIII in response to acoustic stimulation; (2) in auditory evoked potential measurements, it is the whole-nerve response of cranial nerve VIII; the main component of the electrocochleogram and wave I of the auditory brainstem response

aperiodic wave a wave without periodicity; a wave that has no repetition of compression and rarefaction waveforms; completely random activity

Apert syndrome autosomal dominant disorder characterized by syndactyly, short upper arms, hydrocephalus, cognitive impairment, atresia, acne, upper airway obstruction, and occasional cleft palate; associated with conductive hearing loss common secondary to middle ear effusion

apex upper portion of the cochlea; lower-frequency sounds are represented in the apical region of the cochlea

APGAR a tool for evaluating a newborn's condition in the delivery room that is performed at 1 minute and 5 minutes after birth; a rating of 0, 1, or 2 is assigned for each of the following: heart rate, respiratory effort, reflex irritability, muscle tone, and color; named after Virginia Apgar, an American anesthesiologist

APHAB Abbreviated Profile of Hearing Aid Benefit; an assessment scale for hearing aid users that rates patients' perception of hearing aid benefit; part of the Independent Hearing Aid Fitting Forum protocol

aphasia language dysfunction due to damage to certain areas of the cerebral cortex; can result in a receptive disorder in which language cannot be understood or in an expressive disorder in which the words cannot be formulated or produced

aphonia a voice disorder of phonation characterized by a loss of voice; also known as **dysphonia**

apical refers to the apex; at or near the top

aplasia the lack of development of an organ or tissue

apnea absence of respiration

apocrine gland one of the ceruminous glands found in the outer third of the ear canal; produces cerumen along with the sebaceous and ceruminous glands

APR auropalpebral reflex; eye blink reflex associated with stimulation or startle from loud sounds; also known as **cochleopalpebral reflex (CPR)**

apraxia a disorder of voluntary movement affecting the performance of skilled purposeful acts; due to acquired cerebral disease

AR (1) acoustic reflex; response of the middle ear muscles (primarily the stapedius) and the ossicles to intense sound; also known as acoustic stapedial reflex; (2) auditory rehabilitation; aural rehabilitation; intervention aimed at minimizing and alleviating the communication difficulties associated with hearing loss that occurred after speech and language developed; may include diagnosis of hearing loss and communication handicap, amplification, counseling, communication strategies training, speech perception training, speech

and language therapy, and educational management

ARA Academy of Rehabilitative Audiology; an organization that provides a forum for the exchange of ideas on, knowledge of, and experience with habilitative and rehabilitative programs for persons who are hearing impaired; established in 1966

arachnoid membrane surrounding the brain and spinal cord having a spider web appearance

arachnoiditis infection of the arachnoid membrane and subarachnoid space

ARC auditory response cradle; an automatic, microprocessor-based newborn hearing screening system designed to examine several infant motor responses following programmed presentations of auditory stimuli

area-ratio hypothesis the effective vibrating area of the tympanic membrane is greater than that of the stapes footplate resulting in a mechanical advantage for the middle ear transformer action; see also **middle ear transformers**

ARO Association for Research in Otolaryngology; a scientific organization supporting high-quality research in the field of otolaryngology

arousal response a behavioral response represented by an increase in activity after the presentation of an auditory stimulus; characterized by an eye movement and a limb movement occurring within 2.5 sec after the stimulus presentation

ART acoustic reflex threshold; the lowest level of the acoustic activating signal that produces an observable, time-locked change in acoustic immittance

artery blood vessel that carries blood from the heart to organs throughout the body

artery, basilar artery arising from the base of the skull; provides blood supply to the inner ear and brainstem

artery, cochlear artery supplying blood to the majority of the cochlea

artery, internal auditory blood vessel arising from the cerebellar artery that supplies blood to the internal auditory canal; divides into the anterior vestibular artery and the common cochlear artery

articulation (1) the point of union between two structures; (2) movement and positioning of the oral cavity structures, including tongue tip, tongue body, jaw, and lips, during speech production

articulation area the region where auditory (or other) structures meet (or articulate) with other auditory structures

articulation index (AI) a number between 0 and 1 that expresses the degree of audibility of a speech signal which is highly correlated with traditional speech intelligibility scores (number of speech items repeated correctly); also known as the **audibility index (AI)**

artifact any unwanted signal embedded in a recording that is not attributable to the desired neural response

artifact rejection a process during evoked potential measurement for eliminating or reducing the unwanted contamination of the recording by artifact

artificial ear a device for the measurement of earphones that presents an acoustic impedance to the earphone equivalent to the impedance presented by the average human ear; its microphone measures sound pressure developed by the earphone

artificial mastoid device for calibrating bone-conduction oscillators consisting of a resilient surface that simulates the vibrating properties of the mastoid bone of the skull

AS left ear; Latin abbreviation for **auris sinistra**

ASA American Standards Association; earlier name for the **American National Standards Institute (ANSI)**

asepsis the prevention of infection

ASHA American Speech-Language-Hearing Association; professional organization for speech-language pathologists and audiologists; formerly the American Speech and Hearing Association; established 1925

ASL American Sign Language; a distinct language conveyed as a form of manual communication by some deaf individuals; has its on syntax and language structure; common form of communication among the

Deaf community; also known as **AMESLAN**

ASP adaptive signal processing; automatic signal processing; an adaptive circuit that reduces background noise interference, primarily by reducing low-frequency amplification, thus making speech easier to hear and understand

asphyxia impairment of ventilatory exchange of oxygen and carbon dioxide depriving the brain of oxygen

aspirin an analgesic drug that can reduce inflammation; in high doses can cause tinnitus and temporary sensorineural hearing loss; also known as acetylsalicylic acid; see also **salicylates**

ASR automatic speech recognition; sensory aid for discrete word recognition that allows for reasonably accurate recognition of speech for persons who are profoundly hearing impaired

assistive listening device (ALD) any of a number of pieces of equipment used to augment hearing or to assist hearing aids in difficult listening situations (e.g., FM, infrared, and induction loop systems)

Association for Research in Otolaryngology (ARO) a scientific organization supporting high-quality research in the field of otolaryngology

asymmetric peak clipping form of output limiting seen in linear class A amplifiers in hearing aids; the peaks of the positive portion of the waveform are eliminated when the amplifier is saturated; results in significant signal distortion; see also **peak clipping (PC), symmetric peak clipping**

asymmetrical hearing loss bilateral hearing loss with each ear having a different degree and configuration of loss

asymptomatic without symptoms

AT (1) attack time; the onset of the automatic gain control circuit when a sound exceeds the kneepoint; the time between a sudden increase in amplification of input and the stabilization of hearing aid output sound pressure level; (2) auditory trainer; personal or group amplification system used frequently in classroom settings to enhance the signal-to-noise ratio for persons having hearing losses by effectively reducing the distance between the talkers' and listeners' ears

ATA American Tinnitus Association; a non-profit, consumer organization for individuals who suffer from tinnitus; established in 1971

ataxia motor disorder characterized by inability to coordinate muscle activity, causing jerkiness, incoordination, and inefficiency of voluntary movement; most often due to disorders of the cerebellum or the posterior columns of the spinal cord

atelectosis attic retraction pocket in the tympanic membrane; see also **attic retraction pocket**

atoxyl drug used to treat syphilis and other infections; known to be ototoxic causing loss of outer hair cells and degeneration of structures in the organ of Corti

atresia congenital absence or complete closure of a body orifice; in hearing usually affects the ear canal (congenital absence of the external auditory meatus) causing a conductive hearing loss

atropine a drug that blocks the parasympathetic nervous system by raising the response of acetylcholine

attack time (AT) the onset of the automatic gain control circuit when a sound exceeds the kneepoint; the time between a sudden increase in amplification of input and the stabilization of hearing aid output sound pressure level

attention deficit hyperactivity disorder (ADHD) persistent pattern of inattention and/or hyperactivity-impulsivity that is more frequent and severe than is typically observed in individuals at a comparable level of development; see also **attention deficit disorder (ADD)**

attention deficit disorder (ADD) a cognitive deficit that limits an individual's ability to pay attention and stay focused on a task; may involve restlessness, distractibility, and hyperactivity; see also **attention deficit hyperactivity disorder (ADHD)**

attenuation reduction or dampening; in audiology, reduction in magnitude of sound

attenuator a device, usually of variable resistance, used to control the intensity level of an electric signal

attic the superior region of the middle ear space above the superior margin of the tympanic membrane; houses the head of the malleus and the body of the incus; also called the attic of the middle ear; see also **epitympanum**

attic retraction pocket negative pressure in a portion of the tympanic membrane; often occurs in the pars flaccida portion near Prussak's space; also known as **atelectosis, attic perforation**

atticotomy operative opening into the epitympanic recess or attic

AU each ear; both ears together; Latin abbreviation for **aures unitas**

AuD doctor of audiology; an earned postbaccalaureate professional degree primarily designed to prepare audiologists to be competent to perform the wide array of diagnostic, remedial, and other services associated with the current practice of audiology

audibility being able to hear but not necessarily distinguish among speech sounds; see also **acusis**

audibility index (AI) a number between 0 and 1 that expresses the degree of audibility of a speech signal which is highly correlated with traditional speech intelligibility scores (number of speech items repeated correctly); also known as **articulation index (AI)**

audio boot device that connects to a behind-the-ear hearing aid for the use with direct audio input coupling

audiogram a graph expressing hearing loss (hearing sensitivity) as a function of frequency

audiogram, baseline original audiogram used as a reference for comparison of future audiograms; used to monitor hearing and determine any change in hearing sensitivity

audiogram, behavioral audiogram obtained using behavioral hearing tests that involve some form of participation/response from the patient to indicate that a stimulus was heard

audiogram, cookie bite an audiometric configuration characterized by decreased hearing sensitivity in the mid-frequency region only; was often seen in individuals affected by prenatal rubella

audiogram, corner an audiogram configuration that displays a profound hearing loss with thresholds measurable only in the low frequencies; also known as left-corner audiogram

audiogram, flat hearing loss configuration in which the loss of sensitivity is essentially the same as a function of frequency

audiogram, pure-tone a graph expressing hearing loss (hearing sensitivity) as a function of frequency; plot of air- and bone-conduction thresholds in dB HL for the octave frequencies between 250 and 8000 Hz

audiogram, serial an audiogram that is part of a series; used in regular monitoring of hearing sensitivity as part of a hearing conservation program

audiogram tilts audiogram configurations associated with stiffness versus mass controlled middle ear dysfunctions

audiologic evaluation complete battery of tests that assesses hearing sensitivity; see also **audiometric test battery**

audiologist a hearing health care professional who holds a graduate degree and professional certification from an accrediting body in the assessment and management of hearing impairment

audiology the study of normal and disordered hearing as both a scientific discipline and clinical profession; see also **audiometry**

audiology aide nonaudiologist personnel who assists an audiologist under direct supervision in audiology support programs

audiometer an electronic instrument that delivers calibrated pure-tone or speech stimuli for the measurement of sound detection and speech detection, recognition, and identification

audiometer, Békésy hearing measurement instrumentation that allows the patient control of the intensity level of the signal via a push-button attenuation control; used in the method of adjustment; see also **Békésy audiometry**

audiometer, clinical an electronic instrument that delivers calibrated pure-tone, speech, and noise stimuli for the clinical assessment of hearing sensitivity; has broad capabilities to perform routine tests as well as advanced techniques such as masking, special testing, and dual-channel testing

audiometer, high-frequency a clinical audiometer with a wide range of frequencies available, generally above 8000 Hz and ranging as high as 20,000 Hz

audiometer, screening an electronic instrument that delivers calibrated pure-tone stimuli through air conduction only for the purpose of performing pure-tone air-conduction screenings; has limited capabilities for performing extensive clinical assessments of hearing sensitivity

audiometric having to do with audiometry

audiometric test battery a group of tests performed in a routine audiologic assessment including speech and language screening, otoscopy, immittance, pure-tone, otoacoustic emission, and speech perception testing; see also **audiologic evaluation**

audiometric test booth a sound-treated or sound-proof enclosure in which hearing tests are performed

audiometric zero the zero line as a function of frequency on an audiogram that represents the average thresholds for young normal ears; 0 dB HL/HTL

audiometrist a technician who works under the supervision of an audiologist; performs basic audiometric procedures for establishing hearing thresholds; may be credentialed in some states

audiometry assessment of peripheral or central auditory function by means of behavioral and electrophysiologic procedures; see also **audiology**

audiometry, air-conduction hearing tests that use pure-tone signals presented via earphones to establish thresholds

audiometry, automatic automatic hearing measurement through a computerized audiometer

audiometry, behavioral hearing tests that involve some form of participation or response from the patient to indicate that a stimulus was heard (e.g., raising a hand or pushing a button in response to a pure-tone signal)

audiometry, behavioral observation (BOA) the lowest developmental test procedure in which a controlled, calibrated sound stimulus is presented and an infant or child's unconditioned response behaviors are observed

audiometry, behavioral play play conditioning technique used for children ages 3 to 4 that utilizes some motivational activity (e.g., dropping a block in a bucket) to indicate that a sound was heard

audiometry, Békésy a technique of semiautomatic audiometry sweeping across a set frequency range where the listener controls the intensity of the signal to plot threshold or suprathreshold responses to continuous and interrupted tones; differentiates cochlear versus retrocochlear sites of lesion

audiometry, bone-conduction hearing tests that use pure-tone signals presented via a bone vibrator to establish thresholds

audiometry, brief-tone test used to determine a cochlear site of lesion in which tones of different durations are presented; in normals, threshold levels improve with longer durations up to a certain point

audiometry, conditioned play behavioral test of hearing that is effective for preschoolers above the age of 2½ years; the child's responses to sound are conditioned by incorporating them into a game activity

audiometry, electrodermal outdated test procedure that consisted of accompanying clearly audible signals with a small electric shock; anticipation of the shock resulted in a drop in skin resistance detected by surface electrodes; procedure was used with suspected malingerers, but is no longer used today

audiometry, evoked response (ERA) the use of electrophysiologic results from auditory stimuli to predict the viability of the hearing system

audiometry, galvanic skin response a change in the response of the skin to a conditioned stimulus; used in pseudohypacusis by measuring the skin response to sound after pairing the sound with a mild electric shock during conditioning; also known as **electrodermal audiometry**

audiometry, identification the process of applying simple measures to large numbers of individuals in order to identify those with a high probability of hearing disorders; intended to be a screening procedure rather than a diagnostic test; guidelines are available for hearing screening failures that identify people who are at risk for hearing loss

audiometry, immittance battery of tests used to assess middle ear function, including tympanometry, static admittance, and acoustic reflex thresholds and decay

audiometry, play the highest level of pediatric task in hearing testing; involves the active cooperation of the child as an auditory stimulus is paired with an operant task, such as dropping a block in a bucket

audiometry, pure-tone the procedure most commonly used for the measurement of hearing impairment; pure tones are presented via air conduction and bone conduction and the patient's sensitivity to discrete frequencies is measured; see also **air conduction (AC), bone conduction (BC)**

audiometry, speech measurement of speech perception skills including speech awareness and speech recognition; one component of an audiometric test battery; (e.g., speech recognition threshold and word identification testing)

audiometry, tangible reinforcement operant conditioning (TROCA) a pediatric behavioral audiometry technique that reinforces a response to auditory signals with food; the patient is conditioned to manipulate the reinforcer; used mainly with individuals who are mentally handicapped or developmentally delayed

audiometry, visual reinforcement (VRA) a pediatric behavioral audiometry procedure that reinforces localization responses to acoustic signals with a visual event (e.g., an animal playing an instrument)

audiometry, visual reinforcement operant conditioning (VROCA) a behavioral procedure used in pediatric audiometry that reinforces localization responses to acoustic signals with a visual event (e.g., an animal playing a musical instrument); it differs from visual reinforcement audiometry in that the child can manipulate the reinforcer

audioprosthology the study of prosthetic devices for hearing

audioprosthologist one who studies prosthetic devices for hearing; term used by some hearing aid dispensers to describe themselves; not a universally accepted term

Audioscan portable instrumentation for test-ing the electroacoustic characteristics of hearing aids and performing probe microphone measurements

audiovisual use of hearing and vision simultaneously

audiovisual feature test a closed-set speech feature perception test for young children in which they hear a phoneme or one-syllable word; child chooses from a representative set of pictures

audiowipes hygiene sterile cloths used to clean earmolds, hearing aids, and other audiometric surfaces to control infection

audition having to do with the sensation of hearing; see also **acusis, audibility**

auditory relating to the sense of hearing

auditory adaptation the temporary reduction in the audibility of a signal over time; associated with auditory nerve lesions; see also **adaptation; tone decay**

auditory agnosia total or partial loss of the ability to recognize familiar auditory signals including speech; results from damage to the auditory cortex

auditory area region on an audiogram enclosed by the curves defining the threshold of pain and the threshold of audibility as functions of frequency

auditory association area primary auditory cortex located in the temporal lobe; area that receives acoustic radiations from the medial geniculate body

auditory behavior index (ABI) classification of the type of response and level of adequate stimuli needed to elicit a behavioral response at various ages of normal development for infants and young children

auditory behaviors behaviors displayed by infants and children in response to acoustic stimulation; may be categorized as being attentive or reflexive in nature

auditory blending test a central auditory processing test in which the patient hears each phoneme of a word separated by short pauses and then must repeat the word as a whole

auditory brainstem implant (ABI) an implant similar to a cochlear implant that is placed on the cochlear nucleus for individuals with severed VIIIth nerves

auditory brainstem response (ABR) an objective test that measures the electrical potential produced in response to sound stimuli by the synchronous discharge of the first-through sixth-order neurons in the auditory nerve and brainstem; also known as **brainstem auditory evoked potential (BAEP)** and **brainstem auditory evoked response (BAER)**

auditory closure the ability to complete and make whole an incomplete form; uses inductive and deductive reasoning along with contextual cues and knowledge of language; communication strategy used by listeners who are hearing impaired

auditory comprehension understanding spoken language

auditory cortex primary auditory association area located in the temporal lobe; area that receives acoustic radiations from the medial geniculate body

auditory decoding deficit poor auditory closure abilities characterized by poor performance on tests of

monaural low-redundancy speech and speech-in-noise

auditory deprivation complete lack of, or partial reduction in, auditory stimulation

auditory development the development of audition and appropriate auditory behaviors

auditory discrimination the ability to distinguish one sound stimulus from another

auditory discrimination test specific measure of auditory discrimination skills for fine differences between phonemes used in English

auditory durations patterns test a central auditory processing test in which the patient must listen to triads of tones differing only in duration and then indicate which were short or long tones

auditory evoked potential (AEP) electrical activity evoked by sounds arising from auditory portions of the peripheral or central nervous system traveling from cranial nerve VIII to the cortex; recorded with electrodes; also known as **auditory evoked response (AER)**

auditory evoked response (AER) electrical activity evoked by sounds arising from auditory portions of the peripheral or central nervous system traveling from cranial nerve VIII to the cortex; recorded with electrodes; also known as **auditory evoked potential (AEP)**

auditory fatigue the temporary increase in the threshold of audibility resulting from a previous auditory stimulus; considered a mild temporary threshold shift lasting up to several minutes; see also **adaptation, auditory adaptation, temporary threshold shift (TTS)**

auditory feedback (1) aural perception of vocalizations made by oneself; (2) an audible response from an outside source (e.g., someone providing a verbal answer to another person's communication)

auditory figure-ground tasks in which an individual must discriminate an auditory signal, such as speech, from competing background noise

auditory flutter the wavering auditory sensation produced by periodically interrupting a continuous sound at a sufficiently slow rate

auditory fusion the phenomenon in which a series of (primary) sounds of short duration with successive arrival times at the ear(s) produce the sensation of a single (secondary) sound

auditory habilitation intervention for persons who have not developed listening, speech, and language skills; may include diagnosis, speech perception training, speech and language therapy, manual communication, and educational management; also known as **aural habilitation**; see also **auditory rehabilitation (AR)**

auditory integration therapy (AIT) a controversial audiological approach for the treatment of auditory hypersensitivity for children with learning disabilities, hearing disorders, and autism

auditory late response (ALR) electrical activity evoked by sounds, that originates from portions of the auditory cortex, is measured with electrodes placed on the scalp, and occurs within 100 to 300 ms after the sound is presented; also known as **long latency response**

auditory memory capacity to encode, process, and retrieve auditory signals

auditory middle latency response (AMLR) an auditory evoked potential occurring between 12 and 80 ms; provides information from the precortical region; see also **middle latency response**

auditory nerve cranial nerve VIII; consists of two sets of fibers: the anterior branch or cochlear nerve and the posterior branch or vestibular nerve; conducts neural signals from the inner ear to the brain; see also **acoustic nerve, auditory-vestibular nerve, VIIIth nerve**

auditory nerve compound action potential (1) gross neural potential; summed or averaged activity of action potentials of cranial nerve VIII in response to acoustic stimulation; (2) in auditory evoked potential measurements, it is the whole-nerve response of cranial nerve VIII; the main component of the electrocochleogram and wave I of the auditory brainstem response; also known as **action potential (AP)**

auditory nerve fibers neurons arising from cranial nerve VIII

auditory nervous system the peripheral (outer, middle, and inner ear structures including the auditory nerve) and central structures (including the cochlear nucleus, superior olivary complex, lateral lemniscus, inferior colliculus, medial geniculate body, and auditory cortex) involved in the process of hearing and perception

auditory neuropathy a pattern of abnormal findings for multiple audiometric measures (e.g., auditory brainstem response, pure-tone and speech audiometry, and/or acoustic reflexes, yet normal findings for otoacoustic emissions); various patterns may occur

auditory numbers test (ANT) an audiologic test using numbers for young children with severe-to-profound hearing loss

auditory pathway the route followed by auditory signals from the cochlea through the central auditory system to the auditory cortex for processing sound

auditory perception experience of a listener to any auditory event, includes such factors as memory, attention, and learning

auditory pit embryologic structure made of ectoderm; forms an indentation on either side of the neural groove; precursor to the inner ear; also known as **otic pit**

auditory placode thickening of ectoderm in the neural folds of the human embryo; precursor to the inner ear; also known as **otic placode**

auditory pointing test a central auditory processing test that assesses auditory memory and sequencing

auditory processing those processes that occur within the central auditory nervous system in response to acoustic stimuli; see also **central auditory processing (CAP)**

auditory processing disorder an impairment in the ability of the central auditory system to process and utilize auditory signals; heterogeneous disorder involving an observed deficit in one or more of the central auditory processes responsible for generating the auditory evoked potentials (i.e., electrocochleography, auditory brainstem response, auditory middle latency response, auditory late response, and auditory event-related response) and such behavioral phenomena as: sound localization and lateralization; auditory discrimination; auditory pattern recognition; temporal aspects of audition (including temporal resolution, temporal masking, temporal integration, and temporal ordering); auditory performance with competing acoustic signals; and auditory performance with degraded acoustic signals; also known as **central auditory processing disorder (CAPD)**

auditory radiations flow of information via auditory nerve fibers from the medial geniculate body to the auditory cortex; also known as **acoustic radiations**

auditory regression occurs when patients have forgotten sounds that they used to hear

auditory rehabilitation (AR) intervention aimed at minimizing and alleviating the communication difficulties associated with hearing loss that occurred after speech and language developed; may include diagnosis of hearing loss and communication handicap, amplification, counseling, communication strategies training, speech perception training, speech and language therapy, and educational management; also known as **aural rehabilitation**; see also **auditory habilitation**

auditory resolution the ability of the inner ear structures and their associated neural systems to generate patterns of neural activity that reflect spectral and temporal differences among sound patterns

auditory response cradle (ARC) an automatic, microprocessor-based newborn hearing screening system designed to examine several infant motor responses following programmed presentations of auditory stimuli; see also **crib-o-gram**

auditory selective attention test a central auditory processing test which assesses auditory figure-ground abilities that enable a patient to focus auditory attention on a signal in the presence of background noise

auditory sequencing the appropriate ordering of sounds and words perceptually

auditory sequential memory test an assessment of auditory recall via a digit span approach designed for children ages 5 to 8 years

auditory summating potential a sustained direct current shift in the endocochlear potential that occurs when the organ of Corti is stimulated by sound; a direct-current electrical potential of cochlear origin that can be measured using electrocochleography

auditory synthesis central auditory processing task in which a patient is required to listen to words one phoneme at a time and then say the word as a whole

auditory system a term used to describe the entire structure and function of the ears and the process of hearing

auditory toughening the auditory system's ability to modify its susceptibility to damage from noise depending on previous exposures

auditory trainer (AT) personal or group amplification system used frequently in classroom settings to enhance the signal-to-noise ratio for persons having hearing losses by effectively reducing the distance between the talkers' and listeners' ears; see also **assistive listening device (ALD)**

auditory training instruction designed to maximize an individual's use of residual hearing by means of formal and informal listening practice

auditory tube a canal that connects the middle ear with the nasal part of the pharynx (back of the throat); serves to equalize air pressure on two sides of the tympanic membrane; also known as **eustachian tube**

auditory vesicle embryologic structure formed by the closing of the auditory pit; lined with ectoderm; known as the early otocyst (developing inner ear); also known as **otic vesicle**

auditory visual enhancement tests lipreading tasks that measure a patient's abilities with and without the addition of auditory information

auditory-oral approach method of auditory habilitation that emphasizes auditory and speechreading cues; manual communication is not included; also known as **auditory, auditory-verbal,** or **aural-oral method**

auditory-verbal approach method of auditory habilitation that emphasizes auditory and speechreading cues; manual communication is not included; also known as **auditory, auditory-oral,** or **aural-oral method**

auditory-vestibular nerve cranial nerve VIII responsible for hearing and balance functions; see also **auditory nerve (AN)**

aural of or having to do with the ear

aural atresia congenital absence or complete closure of a body orifice; in hearing usually affects the ear canal (congenital absence of the external auditory meatus) causing a conductive hearing loss

aural discharge drainage from the ear; typically due to outer or middle ear pathology

aural domes circumaural earphones used to attenuate ambient noise during pure-tone testing; also known as audio cups

aural forceps device used in removing cerumen lodged in the ear canal

aural fullness sensation of fullness in the ear; associated with middle and inner ear pathologies

aural habilitation intervention for persons who have not developed listening, speech, and language skills; may include diagnosis, speech perception training, speech and language therapy, manual communication, and educational management; also known as **auditory habilitation**; see also **aural rehabilitation (AR)**

aural harmonic a harmonic generated in the ear as a result of nonlinearity and asymmetry in the auditory transducer; a whole-number multiple of the fundamental frequency of a complex wave; see also **harmonic, overtone**

aural irrigator device used to flush excess cerumen out of the ear canal; also used in caloric testing; see also **irrigator**

aural polyps benign neoplasms in or around the outer ear

aural rehabilitation (AR) intervention aimed at minimizing and alleviating the communication difficulties associated with hearing loss that occurred after speech and language developed; may include diagnosis of hearing loss and communication handicap, amplification, counseling, communication strategies training, speech perception training, speech and language therapy, and educational management; also known as **auditory rehabilitation (AR)**; see also **aural habilitation**

aural speculum a metal or plastic device with a nonreflective inner surface that is used to visualize the ear canal and tympanic membrane

aural suction unit a device with an aspirator and suction tip used for cerumen extraction

aural-oral method method of auditory habilitation that emphasizes auditory and speechreading cues; manual communication is not included; also known as **auditory** or **auditory- verbal method**

aures unitas (AU) both ears together (Latin term)

auricle/auriculae the external portion of the ear that consists of elastic cartilage with a complex shape and an extension about one third of the way down the ear canal; useful in localization of sounds; also known as **pinna/pinnae**

auricularis muscle muscle that inserts into the cartilage of the ear; innervated by the facial nerve; branches include anterior, posterior, superior, transverse, and oblique

auriculostomy deep canal hearing aid fitting performed in 1974 by placing the receiver into an earmold embedded as deeply as possible in the ear canal and isolating it from the microphone; see also **completely-in-the-canal (CIC) hearing aid**

auris dextra (AD) right ear (Latin term)

auris sinistra (AS) left ear (Latin term)

auropalpebral reflex (APR) eye blink reflex associated with stimulation or startle from loud sounds; also known as **cochleopalpebral reflex (CPR)**

auroscope a type of otoscope used specifically for pneumatic otoscopy

autism disorder associated with impaired social interactions, extreme withdrawal, and inability to communicate with others

autoimmune disease disorder characterized by an alteration in the immune system that produces antibodies that fight the body's own cells

autoimmune inner ear disease an autoimmune disease that not only affects the body's immune system, but also has an adverse effect on the inner ear, such as otosyphilis

automated auditory brainstem response audiometry (AABR) the use of auditory brainstem response measurement for newborn hearing screening programs; see also **ALGO**

automatic audiometry automatic hearing measurement through a computerized audiometer; see also **Békésy audiometry**

automatic brain operated noise suppressor option (ABONSO) acronym coined by Mead Killion to describe how the brain and hearing mechanism should operate for hearing in noise

automatic gain control (AGC) a feature in some hearing aids that reduces amplification at high input intensity levels; a nonlinear process in which the gain changes as a function of changing signal levels; see also **automatic volume control (AVC), compression**

automatic gain control-input (AGC-I) type of hearing aid compression circuit in which the volume control setting does not affect the level of the compression threshold; AGC circuit is placed before the volume control in the hearing aid

automatic gain control-output (AGC-O) type of hearing aid compression circuit in which the volume control setting affects the level of the compression threshold; AGC circuit is placed after the volume control in the hearing aid

automatic signal processing (ASP) an adaptive circuit that reduces background noise interference, primarily by reducing low-frequency amplification, thus making speech easier to hear and understand; also known as **adaptive signal processing (ASP)**

automatic speech recognition (ASR) sensory aid for discrete word recognition that allows for reasonably accurate recognition of speech for persons who are profoundly hearing impaired

automatic volume control (AVC) a type of automatic signal processing for hearing aids that limits output; see also **automatic gain control (AGC), compression**

autonomic nervous system (ANS) the part of the nervous system associated with independent or involuntary function

autophony condition produced by some middle-ear or eustachian tube abnormalities, such as patulous eustachian tube, in which the patient perceives his or her voice as louder than normal

autosomal dominant (1) expression of a gene when it is carried by only one of a pair of homologous chromosomes; (2) pertaining to an autosome that is any chromosome except a sex chromosome

autosomal recessive expression of a trait by a gene only when both members of a pair of homologous chromosomes are present

autosome any chromosome other than a sex chromosome

AVC automatic volume control; a type of automatic signal processing for hearing aids that limits output; also known as **automatic gain control (AGC)**

AVCN anterior ventral cochlear nucleus; divi-sion of the cochlear nucleus; the lower brainstem nucleus into which the auditory nerve terminates

Award for Continuing Education (ACE) honor presented to individuals who have completed a requisite number of continuing education units; awarded by the American-Speech-Language-Hearing Association

axon long slender extension of a neuron that conducts nerve impulses

azimuth the angular direction of the sound source relative to the listener; plane around the head used for specifying the angle of the direction of sound sources in degrees

B

B susceptance; a component of impedance that is the reciprocal of reactance; energy flow is associated with reactance

B-weighted scale filter network used by a sound level meter that attenuates frequency components below 300 Hz; approximates the 70 phon equal loudness contour; measurement is reported in **dBB**

babble random speechlike utterances, sometimes used as a form of masking (e.g., multitalker noise)

babbling early nonmeaningful vocalizations that are syllabic and repetitive in structure

Babinski reflex flexion of the foot and fanning of the toes in response to stimulation of the sole of the foot; normal reflex found in newborns and in children; abnormal reflex in adults having a lesion in the pyramidal tract

background noise ambient noise, often in competition with a speech signal; a major complaint of hearing aid users

backward masking the condition in which the masking sound appears after the masked sound and results in a threshold shift; the amount of the threshold shift is affected by the interstimulus interval; see also **forward masking, masking**

bacterial meningitis inflammation of the membranes covering the brain caused by a bacterial infection (e.g., *Streptococcus pneumoniae*); see also **meningitis**

bacterial otitis externa a bacterial infection of the external ear canal that often develops after water immersion; see also **external otitis, swimmer's ear**

BAEP brainstem auditory evoked potential; an objective test that measures the electrical potential produced in response to sound stimuli by the synchronous discharge of the first- through sixth-order neurons in the auditory nerve and brainstem; also known as **auditory brainstem response (ABR), brainstem auditory evoked response (BAER)**

BAER brainstem auditory evoked response; an objective test that measures the electrical potential produced in response to sound stimuli by the synchronous discharge of the first- through sixth-order neurons in the auditory nerve and brainstem; also known as **auditory brainstem**

response (ABR), brainstem auditory evoked potential (BAEP)

balance normal state of equilibrium; the function of the vestibular system

band in acoustics, a group of frequencies

band, octave range of frequencies divided by doublings of frequency (octaves)

band, side range of frequencies lying on either side of the center frequency of the band

band-pass filter a filter that passes energy in a specifiable band of frequencies between a lower cutoff frequency and an upper cutoff frequency; see also **filter**

band-reject filter a filter that rejects energy for frequencies between an upper and lower cutoff frequency; see also **filter**

banded electrodes a series of tapered pure platinum bands on a silastic carrier used in some cochlear implants

bandwidth the width of the band of frequencies that are passed by the filter; see also **filter**

Barany box an instrument that contains a simple clockwork mechanism that produces a loud white noise; also known as **noise box**

barotrauma traumatic inflammation of tissue, especially in the middle ear, caused by a sudden and large negative change in atmospheric pressure

barrel effect the perception of increased loudness when the outer ear is occluded with a hearing aid; often affects the users' perception of the

quality of their voices; see also **occlusion effect**

basal toward the bottom; refers to the base; the lowest level possible

basal cell carcinoma malignant epithelial cell tumor; can be found in the outer ear; see also **carcinoma**

basal ganglia subcortical nuclear masses derived from the telencephalon; consists of the caudate nucleus, putamen, globus pallidus, and amygdaloid nuclear complex

base of cochlea the lower portion of the cochlea; high-frequency sounds are represented in the basal region; see also **cochlea**

baseline documented level of response used for comparison with future measures; reflects reliability or stability of repeated measurement

baseline audiogram original audiogram used as a reference for comparison of future audiograms; used to monitor hearing and determine any change in hearing sensitivity

basement membrane delicate noncellular layer on the bottom of the epithelium of Reissner's membrane that separates cell layers of the scala vestibuli from those of the scala media

basilar artery artery arising from the base of the skull; provides blood supply to the inner ear and brainstem

basilar crest prominence emanating from the spiral ligament in the organ of Corti; lies near the basilar membrane

basilar membrane fibrous plate extending from the osseous spiral lamina to the spiral ligament on the outer wall of the cochlea; separates the scala media from the scala tympani and supports the organ of Corti; see also **cochlea, organ of Corti, osseous spiral lamina**

bass increase at low levels (BILL) nonlinear circuitry in a hearing aid that is activated by the overall level of background noise; it increases low-frequency amplification at low levels and decreases low-frequency amplification at high levels

battery (1) a cell that provides electrical power; a container holding materials that produce electricity by chemical action; (2) a set of diagnostic tests

battery door the hinged part of a hearing aid faceplate that houses the battery

battery pill device used in hearing aid analyzers to represent the constant load of the hearing aid when measuring battery drain

BBN broad-band noise; band of noise covering a wide range of frequencies

BC bone conduction; sound delivered to the cochleas by directly vibrating the bones of the skull of a listener; component of pure-tone audiometry

BEAM brain electrical activity mapping; topographic display (color, shading, or numeric) of auditory evoked response amplitudes recorded from multiple electrodes on the scalp; a form of **brain imaging**

beam forming microphone used with some cochlear implants and some

hearing aids to enhance the reception of signals to the front of the listener

beat frequency the rate at which periodic increases and decreases in sound amplitude occur; see also **beats**

beats periodic fluctuations that are heard when sounds of slightly different frequencies are superimposed; see also **beat frequency**

Beckwith-Wiedemann syndrome autosomal dominant disorder characterized by hypotonia, possible cognitive impairment, accelerated growth, creases in earlobes, enlarged liver, spleen, and kidneys; conductive hearing loss from chronic middle ear disease secondary to cleft palate

Beethoven's deafness chronic bone disease of one or many bones of the skull that results in disordered and active reconstruction of bone with alternating resorption of bone; can be associated with conductive and/or sensorineural hearing loss; also known as **Paget disease**

behavioral audiogram audiogram obtained using behavioral hearing tests that involve some form of participation/response from the patient to indicate that a stimulus was heard

behavioral audiometry hearing tests that involve some form of participation/response from the patient to indicate that a stimulus was heard (e.g., raising a hand or pushing a button in response to a pure-tone signal)

behavioral observation audiometry (BOA) the lowest developmental test procedure in which a controlled, calibrated sound stimulus is presented and an infant or child's unconditioned response behaviors are observed

behavioral play audiometry play conditioning technique used for children ages 3 to 4 years that utilizes some motivational activity (e.g., dropping a block in a bucket) to indicate that a sound was heard; see also **conditioned play audiometry, play audiometry**

behavioral response usually a verbal or motor response made by an individual in response to a stimulus (e.g., raising the hand when a tone is heard or turning the head to localize a sound in space)

behavioral techniques tests that elicit a behavior, measure the behavior, and infer function; can be used to evaluate the function of the auditory system

behind-the-ear (BTE) hearing aid hearing aid that sits completely behind the ear over the pinna and is typically coupled to the ear canal by an earmold

Békésy audiometer hearing measurement instrumentation that allows the patient control of the intensity level of the signal via a push-button attenuation control; used in the method of adjustment; see also **Békésy audiometry**

Békésy audiometry a technique of semiautomatic audiometry sweeping across a set frequency range where the listener controls the intensity of

the signal to plot threshold or suprathreshold responses to continuous and interrupted tones; differentiates cochlear versus retrocochlear sites of lesion; also known as **automatic audiometry**

Békésy traveling wave the wavelike action of the basilar membrane arising from stimulation of the perilymph of the scala vestibuli and scala tympani; the traveling wave moves from the base of the cochlea to the apex, and the point of maximum displacement of the basilar membrane indicates the frequency location where the stimulus is perceived; also known as **traveling wave**

bel unit of a logarithmic scale expressing relative intensity of a sound; a ratio of the power of a sound to that of a reference sound, usually 10^{-16} watts per cm^2, the approximate threshold of the human ear at 1000 Hz

belled bore the canal portion of an earmold or custom hearing aid shell that is flared at the end to enhance high-frequency amplification; a type of acoustic modification; see also **Libby horn**

Bell's palsy unilateral weakness or paralysis of the facial nerve due to trauma or disease, usually temporary; idiopathic facial paralysis

Bencze syndrome autosomal dominant disorder characterized by facial asymmetry, strabismus, amblyopia, submucous cleft palate; associated with conductive hearing loss from chronic middle ear disease secondary to cleft palate

benign indicating noncancerous or not malignant; often used in reference to growths or tumors

benign paroxysmal positional nystagmus (BPPN) nystagmus produced as a result of benign paroxysmal positional vertigo; characterized by a sudden, transient burst of rotatory nystagmus provoked by head motion or changes in body position (e.g., Dix Hallpike maneuver)

benign paroxysmal positional vertigo (BPPV) a specific vestibular disorder that causes vertigo, light-headedness, and rotatory nystagmus when provoked by head motion or changes in body position (e.g., Dix Hallpike maneuver); often seen in older persons

Berger prescriptive method one of the first prescriptive methods used in hearing aid fitting that prescribes the amount of real-ear gain needed for specific frequencies using threshold measures; essentially based on the half-gain rule with some modifications

Berman syndrome autosomal recessive disorder characterized by lysosomal storage disease, puffy face, strabismus, and variable cognitive impairment; associated with variable progressive sensorineural hearing loss ranging from moderate to severe

Bernoulli principle the effect dictating that given a constant volume flow of air or fluid at a point of constriction, there will be a decrease in air pressure perpendicular to the flow and an increase in velocity of the flow

beta rhythm electroencephalogram activity within the 13 to 30 Hz region; normally of low amplitude

Better Hearing Institute (BHI) a non-profit educational organization that provides national public information programs about hearing problems for individuals who are hearing impaired and their families; established in 1973

BHI Better Hearing Institute; a non-profit educational organization that provides national public information programs about hearing problems for individuals who are hearing impaired and their families; established in 1973

bi- prefix: two

BI-CROS bilateral contralateral routing of signals; an amplification arrangement consisting of a complete hearing aid on one ear with an additional microphone connected via a thin cable or FM transmission to the contralateral ear; used for individuals with normal or better hearing in one ear and no hearing in the other

BI-CROS hearing aid an amplification arrangement consisting of a complete hearing aid on one ear with an additional microphone connected via a thin cable or FM transmission to the contralateral ear; used for individuals with normal or better hearing in one ear and no hearing in the other; see also **CROS**

bifurcate two-forked; to split into two parts or channels

bilateral on both sides; having two symmetrical sides

bilateral conductive hearing loss hearing loss with a conductive component (outer and/or middle ear pathology) that is symmetrical in both ears

bilateral hearing loss hearing loss affecting both ears

bilateral sensorineural hearing loss hearing loss with a sensorineural component (inner ear and/or auditory nerve pathology) that is symmetrical in both ears

bilateral weakness finding in electronystagmography caloric testing suggesting hypoactivity of the vestibular system from both ears; often results from bilateral peripheral vestibular lesions

bilaterally symmetrical hearing loss hearing loss that is identical in type, degree, and configuration for both ears

bilirubin pigment found in the blood used to break down hemoglobin in red blood cells

BILL bass increase at low levels; nonlinear circuitry in a hearing aid that is activated by the overall level of background noise; it increases low-frequency amplification at low levels and decreases low-frequency amplification at high levels

Billeau ear loops stainless steel or plastic looped tools of varying size used to extract cerumen from the ear canal

bimodal the use of two different modalities; used to refer to a communication method that incorporates two different modalities simultaneously (e.g., using both auditory and visual information for speech perception)

binaural (1) having two ears; (2) using two loudspeakers or sources of sound reproduction or transmission to produce a three-dimensional or stereophonic auditory effect; (3) use of two hearing aids

binaural advantage using two ears to improve sound detection, localization, and understanding in noise; see also **binaural hearing**

binaural amplification wearing two hearing aids rather than one to utilize the binaural advantage

binaural beats periodic fluctuations that are heard when sounds of slightly different frequencies (<5 Hz) are presented to each ear simultaneously; results from interactions within the central auditory system

binaural diplacusis a tone of fixed frequency evokes different pitches in the left and right ears; see also **diplacusis**

binaural fusion the speech signal presented to the subject is split in such a way that neither portion contains sufficient information, but when presented simultaneously, one to each ear, the message is "fused" to give a representation of the whole; see also **binaural integration, binaural summation**

binaural fusion test a central auditory test in which the patient must repeat words that are presented with the high-frequency portion to one ear and the low-frequency portion to the other ear

binaural hearing the use of both ears simultaneously producing binaural advantages such as improved localization, speech perception in noise, acuity, etc.; see also **binaural advantage**

binaural integration the ability of a listener to process different information being presented to both ears simultaneously; see also **binaural fusion, binaural summation**

binaural interaction auditory processing involving the two ears and their neural connections; see also **binaural fusion, binaural summation**

binaural localization using both ears to determine the location of sounds in space

binaural masking level difference (BMLD) the difference in threshold of the signal when the signal and a masker have the same phase and level relationships at the two ears and when the interaural phase and/or level relationships of the signal and masker differ; see also **binaural release from masking, masking level difference (MLD)**

binaural release from masking a measure of the improvement in the detectability of a signal that can occur under dichotic binaural listening conditions; see also **binaural masking level difference (BMLD), masking level difference (MLD)**

binaural representation sound from each ear is represented in both the right and left hemispheres of the brain due to decussation along the central auditory nervous system

binaural separation the ability of a listener to process an auditory message coming into one ear while ignoring a separate message being presented to the opposite ear at the same time

binaural squelch the ability of the auditory system to reduce the effects of noise or reverberation more efficiently when input is received from two ears rather than one; the improvement in speech intelligibility in noise resulting from interaural phase and intensity differences

binaural summation the advantage in dB of binaural over monaural listening; the binaural threshold is approximately 3 dB better than the monaural threshold; see also **binaural fusion, binaural integration, minimal audible field, minimal audible pressure**

binaural temporal discrimination summation of sound power over durations less than 200 ms using both ears; see also **temporal integration**

Bing test a bone-conduction test in which one ear is occluded; in normal ears, low-frequency sounds will lateralize to the occluded ear; if middle ear dysfunction is present, this lateralization does not occur; see also **Weber test;** also known as **Bing test of occlusion (BING TOO)**

Bing test of occlusion (BING TOO) a test to determine if the occlusion effect will be a problem for a hearing aid user and if the existing fitting is reducing the occlusion effect; see also **Bing test**

biocompatible materials materials placed in the body that do not cause infection and are not rejected by the body

biofeedback training techniques, often relaxation procedures, that allow an individual to gain voluntary control over autonomic functions to produce a desired physiologic response

biologic calibration (1) performing a listening check on audiometric equipment to determine that it is functioning appropriately; (2) determining audiometric zero from the average hearing thresholds obtained from a normal-hearing population

biomechanics the study of mechanical laws and their application to human organisms

biphasic pulse square wave that has equal positive and negative amplitudes

bipolar refers to an electrode or electrode pair that measures electrical events (action potentials) at two distinct points

bipolar electrode electrode or electrode pair that measures electrical events (action potentials) at two distinct points; in electrophysiology, the resulting signals are usually supplied one to an inverting input, the other to a noninverting input of a differential amplifier

bipolar plus one (BP+1) the stimulation mode used in some cochlear implants in which there is one electrode in between the active and indifferent electrodes

bipolar plus three (BP+3) the stimulation mode used in some cochlear implants in which there are three electrodes between the active and indifferent electrodes

bipolar plus two (BP+2) the stimulation mode used in some cochlear implants in which there are two electrodes between the active and indifferent electrodes

bipolar stimulation (BP) the stimulation mode used in some cochlear implants and other signal processing strategies in which the active and indifferent electrodes that are stimulated are beside each other; two-electrode array

bisensory training training that emphasizes the integration of information between senses; for example, combining auditory and visual stimuli in auditory (re)habilitation training

bisyllabic nonsense syllables non-meaningful speech stimuli presented in a consonant-vowel-consonant-vowel context; see also **consonant-vowel-consonant-vowel (CVCV)**

bit the abbreviation for a binary digit; the fundamental unit of information in a digital system; a bit has two possible values, conventionally expressed as 0 or 1; 16 bits equal one byte

bithermal caloric stimulation test part of the electronystagmography test battery that assesses vestibular function when warm and cool water are injected into the external auditory canals to stimulate the horizontal semicircular canals

Bixler syndrome autosomal recessive disorder characterized by cleft lip and palate, microtia, short stature, cognitive impairment, heart anomalies, kidney anomalies, and anomalous ossicles; associated with conductive hearing loss

blood-brain barrier walls of capillaries in the brain that serve to separate the central nervous system and brain tissue from many substances in blood

BMLD binaural masking level difference; the difference in threshold of the signal when the signal and a masker have the same phase and level relationships at the two ears and when the interaural phase and/or level relationships of the signal and masker differ; see also **binaural release from masking (BMLD), masking level difference (MLD)**

BOA behavioral observation audiometry; the lowest developmental test procedure in which a controlled, calibrated sound stimulus is presented and an infant or child's unconditioned response behaviors are observed

body baffle effect the mass of the patient's body reduces the input of a hearing aid; see also **head shadow effect**

body hearing aid a hearing aid in which the microphone, amplifier, and fitting controls are in a housing carried on the body or in a pocket and the receiver is inserted in the ear and connected to the main unit by a cord

BOF syndrome branchio-oculo-facial syndrome; autosomal dominant disorder characterized by cleft lip and palate, lacrimal duct stenosis, eye anomalies, malformed auricles, premature grey hair, preauricular pits, cervically displaced thymus gland, thin skin on neck; associated with conductive hearing loss, usually mild to moderate

bone conduction (BC) sound delivered to the cochleas by directly vibrating the bones of the skull of a listener; a component of pure-tone audiometry

bone oscillator the piece of audiometric equipment, which looks like a small black box attached to a headband, used to present sounds (vibrations) to the skull in bone-conduction pure-tone or speech audiometry; used to obtain bone-conduction thresholds; also known as **bone-conduction oscillator**

bone vibrator the piece of audiometric equipment, which looks like a small black box attached to a headband, used to present sounds (vibrations) to the skull in bone-conduction pure-tone or speech audiometry; used to obtain bone-conduction thresholds; also known as **bone oscillator**

bone-anchored hearing aid a hearing aid with a direct contact, through a percutaneous coupling, between a screw-shaped implant placed in the bone of the mastoid process and the transducer; also known as **bone-conduction hearing aid**

bone-conducted click a short-duration pulse delivered via a bone-conduction oscillator; usually used in auditory brainstem response measurement

bone-conduction audiometry hearing tests that use pure-tone signals presented via a bone vibrator to establish thresholds

bone-conduction couplers a mechanical coupler for bone receivers that uses a vibration pickup to measure the vibration at a central point of the bone receiver face; also known as bone-conduction receivers

bone-conduction hearing aid a hearing aid in which the transducer is positioned over the mastoid process and vibrations are transmitted through the skin of the skull; also known as **bone-anchored hearing aid**

bone-conduction implant a hearing aid with a transcutaneous (Audiant) or percutaneous (BAHA) implanted transducer that is placed in the bone of the mastoid process

bone-conduction oscillator the piece of audiometric equipment, which looks like a small black box attached to a headband, used to present sounds (vibrations) to the skull in bone-conduction pure-tone or speech audiometry; used to obtain bone-conduction thresholds; also known as **bone oscillator**

bone-conduction speech audiometry hearing testing using speech stimuli presented via bone conduction

bone-conduction threshold absolute hearing threshold perceived from a bone-conducted pure-tone signal providing information about sensorineural function

bony labyrinth the osseous cavities of the inner ear; houses the membranous labyrinth containing the inner ear sense organs

boom microphone microphone used with some FM systems that is suspended out from the speaker's head

BOR syndrome branchio-oto-renal syndrome; autosomal dominant disorder characterized by ossicular anomalies, cochlear anomalies, vestibular anomalies, branchial clefts, preauricular pits, malformed auricles, lacrimal duct stenosis, renal anomalies; associated with conductive, sensorineural, or mixed hearing loss that may be progressive, ranges from mild to profound

border cells single row of supporting cells lying on the inward side of the inner hair cells in the organ of Corti

bore, belled the canal portion of an earmold or custom hearing aid shell that is flared at the end to enhance high-frequency amplification; a type of acoustic modification; see also **Libby horn**

bore, sound the portion of the earmold through which amplified sound is directed into the external auditory canal; modifications to the shape and length of this hole can affect the acoustic nature of the sounds going through the sound bore

Borud syndrome mitochondrial disorder characterized by myopathy, cardiomyopathy, encephalopathy, ataxia; associated with progressive sensorineural hearing loss

bottom-up processing information processing that is data driven; properties of the data are primary determinants of higher level representations

boundary noise assessment a legal assessment of noise that escapes over the boundary line of personal property into neighboring property

Boyles' law posits that there is an inverse relationship between volume and pressure; as volume decreases, pressure increases; this law has an important impact on fitting hearing aids on young children who have smaller ear canal volumes than adults; it also has an impact on deep-canal or completely-in-the-canal hearing aids that fit deep into the ear, thus decreasing volume and increasing pressure at the ear drum

BP bipolar; refers to an electrode or electrode pair that measures electrical events (action potentials) at two distinct points

BP+1 bipolar plus one; the stimulation mode used in some cochlear implants in which there is one electrode in between the active and indifferent electrodes

BP+2 bipolar plus two; the stimulation mode used in some cochlear implants in which there are two electrodes between the active and indifferent electrodes

BP+3 bipolar plus three; the stimulation mode used in some cochlear implants in which there are three electrodes between the active and indifferent electrodes

BPPN benign paroxysmal positional nystagmus; nystagmus produced as a result of benign paroxysmal positional vertigo; characterized by a sudden, transient burst of rotatory nystagmus provoked by head motion or changes in body position (e.g., Dix Hallpike maneuver)

BPPV benign paroxysmal positional vertigo; a specific vestibular disorder that causes vertigo, lightheadedness, and rotatory nystagmus when provoked by head motion or changes in body position (e.g., Dix Hallpike maneuver); often seen in older persons

brachium of inferior colliculus upper arm of the central auditory structure called the inferior colliculus; a fiber bundle passing from the inferior colliculus on either side of the brainstem along the lateral border of the superior colliculus to the thalamus; part of the major ascending auditory pathway

brachycephaly a disproportionate shortening of the head; a reduction of the anterior-posterior dimension of the head

brain abscess a cavity surrounded by inflamed tissue in the brain

brain attack a contemporary term for cerebral stroke; also used as a synonym for cerebrovascular accident (CVA); term usage believed to help potential victims appreciate the urgency for rapid medical care with the onset of CVA symptoms, as is recognized for heart attack symptoms; see also **cerebrovascular accident (CVA)**

brain electrical activity mapping (BEAM) topographic display (color, shading, or numeric) of auditory evoked response amplitude recorded from multiple electrodes on the scalp; a form of **brain imaging**

brain imaging procedures used to map the structure and metabolic and electrophysiological properties of the brain; includes magnetic resonance imaging, functional magnetic resonance imaging, computed tomography, positron emission topography, regional cerebral blood flow, and brain electrical activity mapping

brainstem lower portion of the brain comprising the pons, medulla, and midbrain; responsible for motor, sensory, and reflex functions

brainstem auditory evoked potential (BAEP) an objective test that measures the electrical potential produced in response to sound stimuli by the synchronous discharge of the first- through sixth-order neurons in the auditory nerve and brainstem; also known as **brainstem auditory evoked response (BAER)**

brainstem auditory evoked response (BAER) an objective test that measures the electrical potential produced in response to sound stimuli by the synchronous dis-

charge of the first- through sixth-order neurons in the auditory nerve and brainstem; also known as **brainstem auditory evoked potential (BAEP)**

brainstem evoked response (BSER) an objective test that measures the electrical potential produced in response to sound stimuli by the synchronous discharge of the first-through sixth-order neurons in the auditory nerve and brainstem; also known as **brainstem auditory evoked potential (BAEP), brainstem auditory evoked response (BAER)**

brainstem implant an implant similar to a cochlear implant that is placed on the cochlear nucleus for individuals with severed VIIIth nerves; also known as **auditory brainstem implant (ABI)**

brainstem lesion abnormality in the brainstem

branchial arches embryonic structures in the pharynx shaped like arches from which structures of the outer and middle ears develop

branchio-oculo-facial syndrome BOF syndrome; autosomal dominant disorder characterized by cleft lip and palate, lacrimal duct stenosis, eye anomalies, malformed auricles, premature grey hair, preauricular pits, cervically displaced thymus gland, thin skin on neck; associated with conductive loss, usually mild to moderate

branchio-oto-renal syndrome BOR syndrome; autosomal dominant disorder characterized by ossicular anomalies, cochlear anomalies vestibular anomalies, branchial clefts, preauricular pits, malformed auricles, lacrimal duct stenosis, renal anomalies; associated with conductive, sensorineural, or mixed hearing loss that may be progressive, ranges from mild to profound

brief-tone audiometry test used to determine a cochlear site of lesion in which tones of different durations are presented; in normals, threshold levels improve with longer durations up to a certain point

broad-band click short-duration, transient click stimulus producing a response affecting a wide range of frequencies

broad-band noise a band of noise covering a wide range of frequencies; also known as **wide-band noise**

Broca's area region in the dominant cerebralhemisphere responsible for motor planning for speech and components of expressive language; Brodmann's areas 44 and 45

Brodmann's areas regions of the cerebral hemisphere, identified by numeric characterization based on functional and anatomical organization; named for Korbinian Brodmann (1868–1918)

Bruhn method an outdated, traditional approach to lipreading therapy that emphasized analytic training techniques

BSER brainstem evoked response; an objective test that measures the electrical potential produced in response to sound stimuli by the synchronous discharge of the first-through sixth-order neurons in the auditory nerve and brainstem

BTE behind-the-ear; hearing aid that sits completely behind the ear over the pinna and is typically coupled to the ear canal by an earmold

buffer electronic device that permits temporary storage of incoming data to allow a printer to keep pace with a computer or to free the computer for other tasks during printing

bullous myringitis an inflammatory disorder of the middle ear resulting from fluid-filled vesicles on the tympanic membrane that cause severe ear pain; often a complication from otitis media

bumetanide loop diuretic used in the treatment of congestive heart failure and pulmonary edema; can be ototoxic

bus a connecting system for the components of a microcomputer system; the type of bus determines the compatibility of add-in boards for a system

button receiver a small circular sound transducer that is attached to a snap-ring earmold; used with body hearing aids and some FM systems; see also **body hearing instrument**

byte abbreviation for binary term; a unit of storage capable of holding a single character; equal to 8 bits on nearly all modern personal computers; large amounts of memory are indicated in terms of kilobytes (1024 bytes), megabytes (1,048,576 bytes), and gigabytes (1,073,741,824 bytes); see also **bit**

C

C-weighted scale filter network used by a sound level meter with the weighting switch on C; permits nearly a flat frequency response to input sound; measurement is reported in dBC; see also **dBC**

CA chronologic age; age of an individual calculated from the date of birth

calibration electronic or psychoacoustic determination that an electrical device or an acoustic transducer functions according to defined characteristics; also implies correction of the device if necessary

calibration tone a 1000-Hz tone presented at the beginning of recorded speech materials used to make appropriate adjustments to the VU meter of the audiometer; important for consistency in presentation level; also known as cal tone

California Consonant Test (CCT) consonant identification test in a closed-set format; test of phoneme recognition with four rhyming response alternatives

caloric irrigation process of injecting warm or cool water into the external auditory canal during caloric testing as part of the electronystagmography test battery

caloric nystagmus type of nystagmus induced by stimulation of the horizontal semicircular canal with warm or cool water

caloric stimulation irrigation of warm or cool water into the external auditory canal during caloric testing as part of the electronystagmography test battery; see also **caloric testing**

caloric testing a test of function of the horizontal semicircular canals that are stimulated by warm and cool air or water; a subtest of the electronystagmography test battery; used to determine if there is a unilateral vestibular weakness

canal earmold type of earmold that fits primarily into the external auditory canal leaving the concha area of the pinna open

canal hearing aids hearing aids that fill the entire ear canal, but do not extend as deeply in the canal as completely-in-the-canal hearing aids, nor do they fill the concha portion of the external ear; see also **in-the-canal hearing aids**

canal-lock earmold a canal earmold with a built-in extension that lies along the bottom of the concha to keep the earmold in place

cancellation phenomenon that occurs in acoustics in which the amplitude of an auditory signal is reduced to zero due to interference with another signal that is equal in amplitude and frequency but 180° out of phase

CANS central auditory nervous system; the auditory brainstem, subcortical pathways, auditory cortex, and corpus callosum; responsible for processing auditory stimuli; see also **central auditory processes**

canthus the angle of the eye; medial and lateral margins of the eyelid

CAOHC Council for Accreditation in Occupational Hearing Conservation; organization that sponsors training workshops and provides appropriate certification for individuals responsible for the development and maintenance of hearing conservation programs

CAP (1) compound action potential; simultaneously occurring action potentials from thousands of nerve fibers; (2) central auditory processes or processing; auditory system mechanisms and processes responsible for sound localization and lateralization; auditory discrimination; auditory pattern recognition; temporal aspects of audition including temporal resolution, temporal masking, temporal integration, and temporal ordering; auditory performance with competing acoustic signals; and auditory performance with degraded acoustic signals; these auditory system mechanisms and processes generate electric brain waves or auditory evoked potentials (i.e., electrocochleography, auditory brainstem response, auditory middle latency response, auditory late response, and auditory event-related response) in response to acoustic stimuli

capacitance the ability of a circuit or condensor to maintain a flow of electric current determined by the amount of electric charge a condensor can receive and store; commonly expressed in farads

capacitive reactance the opposition to changes in voltage through storage

capacitor electronic component that functions to acquire, store, and discharge electrical energy in a predictable and predetermined manner; the impedance of a capacitor decreases as the frequency of alternating current decreases; a capacitor passes high frequencies and blocks low frequencies

CAPD central auditory processing disorder; an impairment in the ability of the central auditory system to process and utilize auditory signals; heterogeneous disorder involving an observed deficit in one or more of the central auditory processes responsible for generating the auditory evoked potentials (i.e., electrocochleography, auditory brainstem response, auditory middle latency response, auditory late response, and auditory event-related response) and such behavioral phenomena as: sound localization and lateralization; auditory discrimination; auditory pattern recognition; temporal aspects of audition (including temporal resolution, temporal masking, temporal integration, and temporal ordering); auditory performance with competing acoustic signals; and auditory performance with degraded acoustic signals; also known as **auditory processing disorder**

captioning, closed (CC) printed text or printed dialog on the screen that corresponds to the auditory speech signal from a television program or movie; requires specific circuitry to be operational; see also **open captioning**

captioning, open printed text or printed dialog on the screen that corresponds to the auditory speech signal from a television program or movie without the need for specific circuitry to be operational

captioning, real-time provides a typed dialog of a person's speech in real-time on a computer screen; can be used with a notebook computer or can be displayed on a large screen; see also **closed captioning, open captioning**

carbon hearing instrument a hearing aid used in the early 1900s that consisted of a sensitive carbon microphone, a magnetic receiver, and a battery

carbon microphone early microphone that converted acoustic energy into electrical energy using carbon granules

carboplatin antineoplastic drug used in the treatment of cancer and tumors that is potentially ototoxic; second generation analog of cisplatin developed to be a less toxic alternative than cisplatin

carcinoma a malignant tumor of epithelial cells that can metastasize to distant sites in the body; see also **basal cell carcinoma, squamous cell carcinoma**

cardoid a heart-shaped curve that describes the direction of sound reception of a microphone; used in psychoacoustics and amplification; see also **polar response curve**

Carhart notch a decrease in bone-conduction hearing in the 2000 Hz region of patients with otosclerosis; usually not present after stapedectomy

carotid artery main artery providing blood supply to the head and neck

carrier (1) a phenotypically normal person who is heterozygous for a recessive condition; (2) a person or animal that harbors a specific infectious agent in the absence of discernible disease and serves as a potential source of infection; (3) a very high-frequency signal that is used to modulate other auditory signals as in amplitude modulation or frequency modulation

carrier phrase a phrase such as "say the word _____" that precedes a stimulus word during word recognition measurement in speech audiometry; its purpose is to prepare the patient for the test word and allow clinicians to monitor their presentation level during monitored-live-voice presentation of the stimuli

carryover generalization of treatment effects to everyday activities

case history information gained from the patient pertaining to identification data, medical history, education, prenatal information, family history, etc.

CAST computer-aided speechreading training; component in a comprehensive auditory rehabilitation program using a computer platform with a videocassette playback to train speechreading skills

CAT scan a computer-generated picture of a section of the brain compiled from sectional radiographs obtained from the same plane; outdated term; see also **computed tomography**

categorical perception the ability to identify a signal as speech and categorize its elements by comparing them with previously stored categories and analyzing the signal in terms of appropriate categories representing content and meaning

catenary principle belief that the buckling action of the tympanic membrane during vibration provides a slight increase in pressure adding to the transformer action of the middle ear; see also **middle ear transformers**

cathode negative electrode of an electrode pair; negative portion of a battery; see also **anode**

caudal toward the tail; inferior in position (e.g., in the central nervous system, the brainstem is caudal to the cerebrum)

caudate nucleus a major deep brain cell body of gray matter that is part of the basal ganglia

cauliflower ear disorder of the external ear caused by repeated trauma to the pinna; results in thickening of the cartilage and skin which diminishes the visibility of the traditional landmarks of the pinna

cavum concha inferior portion of the concha; a landmark of the pinna; see also **concha**

cc cubic centimeter; unit of measurement for volume; 1 cc = 1 ml

CC closed captioning; printed text or printed dialog on the screen that corresponds to the auditory speech signal from a television program or movie

CCB clinical certification board; working group that is part of the American Speech-Language-Hearing Association responsible for defining and enforcing guidelines for obtaining clinical certification from the organization

CCC certificate of clinical competence; American Speech-Language-Hearing Association certification that requires a graduate level degree, completion of a clinical practicum, and a passing score on the National

Examination in Speech-Language Pathology and Audiology (NESPA)

CCM contralateral competing message; a form of the Synthetic Sentence Identification test for assessment of central auditory function; stimuli are presented with a competing message presented simultaneously to the contralateral ear

CCT California Consonant Test; consonant identification test in a closed-set format; test of phoneme recognition with four rhyming response alternatives

CD (1) compact disc; high-fidelity digital recording of analog signals presented on a disc that uses a laser-read mechanism; (2) communication disorder; an impairment in in an individual's ability to communicate (e.g., disordered use of speech, language, or hearing)

CDP computerized dynamic posturography; a type of vestibular assessment that focuses on the function of the balance system in maintaining postural stability in a variety of simulated conditions; computer-induced platform movements evaluate motor responses that include strength, symmetry, and latency of muscle response; also known as **posturography**

CDT continuous discourse tracking; aural rehabilitation technique in which the listener attempts to repeat text verbatim that is presented by a speaker; performance is summarized as the number of words repeated per minute; also referred to as connected discourse tracking

ceiling effect phenomenon occurring during data analysis in which scores are so high that it is difficult to determine the distribution of performance among those scoring at the maximum

cell membrane boundary of all cells in the body that controls permeability for cell entry and exit

center frequency (CF) the arithmetic center of a constant bandwidth filter, or the geometric center (midpoint on a logarithmic scale) of a constant percentage filter

central auditory assessment use of a battery of tests designed to assess the central auditory processing skills of an individual; see also **central auditory processing, central auditory processing disorder (CAPD)**

central auditory dysfunction an impairment in the ability of the central auditory system to process and utilize auditory signals; heterogeneous disorder involving an observed deficit in one or more of the central auditory processes responsible for generating the auditory evoked potentials (i.e., electrocochleography, auditory brainstem response, auditory middle latency response, auditory late response, and auditory event-related response) and such behavioral phenomena as: sound localization and lateralization; auditory discrimination; auditory pattern recognition; temporal aspects of audition (including temporal resolution, temporal masking, temporal integration, and temporal ordering); auditory performance with competing acoustic signals; and auditory performance with degraded acoustic signals; also known as **auditory processing disorder**

central auditory nervous system (CANS) the auditory brainstem, subcortical pathways, auditory cortex, and corpus callosum; structures responsible for processing auditory stimuli

central auditory nuclei central nervous system structures making up the afferent central auditory pathway; include the cochlear nuclei, superior olivary complex, inferior colliculus, and medial geniculate body

central auditory processes auditory system mechanisms and processes responsible for sound localization and lateralization; auditory discrimination; auditory pattern recognition; temporal aspects of audition including temporal resolution, temporal masking, temporal integration, and temporal ordering; auditory performance with competing acoustic signals; and auditory performance with degraded acoustic signals; these auditory system mechanisms and processes generate electric brain waves or auditory evoked potentials (i.e., electrocochleography, auditory brainstem response, auditory middle latency response, auditory late response, and auditory event-related response) in response to acoustic stimuli

central auditory processing the ability to achieve sound localization

and lateralization; auditory discrimination; auditory pattern recognition; temporal aspects of audition including temporal resolution, temporal masking, temporal integration, and temporal ordering; auditory performance with competing acoustic signals; and auditory performance with degraded acoustic signals; these auditory system mechanisms and processes generate electric brain waves or auditory evoked potentials (i.e., electrocochleography, auditory brainstem response, auditory middle latency response, auditory late response, and auditory event-related response) in response to acoustic stimuli

central auditory processing disorder (CAPD) an impairment in the ability of the central auditory system to process and utilize auditory signals; heterogeneous disorder involving an observed deficit in one or more of the central auditory processes responsible for generating the auditory evoked potentials (i.e., electrocochleography, auditory brainstem response, auditory middle latency response, auditory late response, and auditory event-related response) and such behavioral phenomena as: sound localization and lateralization; auditory discrimination; auditory pattern recognition; temporal aspects of audition (including temporal resolution, temporal masking, temporal integration, and temporal ordering); auditory performance with competing acoustic signals;

and auditory performance with degraded acoustic signals; also known as **auditory processing disorder**

central deafness profound impairment of hearing that occurs when there is damage in the auditory pathways or the auditory centers of the brain; results in auditory processing difficulty; often occurs when peripheral hearing is normal or near normal; see also **central hearing loss**

central hearing loss the impairment of hearing that occurs when there is damage in the auditory pathways or the auditory centers of the brain; results in auditory processing difficulty; often occurs when peripheral hearing is normal or near normal; also known as **central deafness**

Central Institute for the Deaf (CID) program for deaf children that emphasizes the aural-oral approach to auditory habilitation in St. Louis, Missouri; affiliated with Washington University and contains undergraduate and graduate programs in audiology, speech-language pathology, and deaf education

central masking masking that occurs in the higher auditory pathways of the brain when a masked sound is presented to one ear and a masking sound to the other

central nervous system (CNS) the spinal cord, brainstem, cerebellum, and cerebrum; the axis or central core of the nervous system; cranial nerves and other nerves are part of the peripheral nervous system

central perforation perforation or hole in the central area of the tympanic membrane; as opposed to a **marginal perforation**

central presbycusis age-related changes in hearing sensitivity resulting from degeneration of central auditory function

central processing unit (CPU) term for the component of a personal computer containing the hardware

CEOAE click evoked otoacoustic emission; otoacoustic emission measured in the external auditory canal in response to a click stimulus; useful technique for determining cochlear function in infants; also known as **transient evoked otoacoustic emission (TEOAE)**; see also **otoacoustic emission (OAE)**

ceramic microphone type of piezoelectric microphone in which electric current is produced by applied mechanical emphasis

cerebellopontine angle (CPA) the angle formed or bordered by the cerebellum and the lateral surface of the pons; located in the posterior fossa; cranial nerve VIII passes through the cerebellopontine angle; a common site for auditory nerve tumors

cerebellum portion of the brain located behind the brainstem; consists of two lateral hemispheres united by a middle portion, the vermis; responsible for coordinating voluntary muscle activity

cerebral cortex gray matter on the surface of the cerebral hemispheres;

responsible for high-level processing, general movement, and behavioral reactions

cerebral dominance the concept that certain higher level brain functions, such as language, music, art, or logical thought, are localized more in one hemisphere of the brain than the other; for speech, the left cerebral hemisphere is typically dominant

cerebrospinal fluid (CSF) the watery-appearing liquid in which the brain is bathed and that fills the ventricles in the brain and the column in the spinal cord

cerebrovascular accident (CVA) a stroke; brain damage resulting from interruption of blood supply to the brain; see also **brain attack**

cerebrum portion of the brain that is the highest and largest, mainly the cerebral hemispheres and basal ganglia; responsible for integrative functioning as well as sensory and motor functions; see also **cortex**

certificate of clinical competence (CCC) American Speech-Language-Hearing Association certification that requires a graduate level degree, completion of a clinical practicum, and a passing score on the National Examination in Speech-Language Pathology and Audiology (NESPA)

cerumen a waxy secretion of the ceruminous and sebaceous glands within the external auditory meatus commonly known as ear wax; lubricates and cleanses the external auditory canal

cerumen impaction accumulation of cerumen in the ear canal that is caused by lack of keratinocytic separation; usually completely closes off the ear canal resulting in a conductive hearing loss

cerumen management the extraction of cerumen usually through manual extraction, suctioning, or irrigation

cerumen softening the use of ear wax solvents to soften hard and firmly attached cerumen; see also **cerumenolytic**

cerumen spoon a blunt ear curette or wire curette used to remove chunks of cerumen

cerumenolytic any ear wax solvent; commercially available products and other agents used to soften cerumen (e.g., mineral oil); see also **cerumen softening**

ceruminoma benign or malignant tumor of the ceruminous glands

ceruminous glands glands found in the lateral one third of the external auditory canal; secrete cerumen together with the sebaceous and apocrine glands

cervical tinnitus a clinical type of tinnitus related to movement of the head and neck

CF (1) center frequency; the arithmetic center of a constant bandwidth filter, or the geometric center (midpoint on a logarithmic scale) of a constant percentage filter; (2) characteristic frequency; the frequency at which the threshold of a given single neuron is lowest (i.e., the frequency at which it is most sensitive); (3) clinical fellowship; supervised clinical experience that must be completed after graduate work to obtain certification from ASHA; can range from 9 to a maximum of 36 months; (4) crossover frequency; the frequency or frequencies representing the cutoff frequencies of the filters that divide the frequency range into separate bands; used in filters and some hearing aids

CFA continuous flow adapter; type of earmold that contains a single snap-in/snap-out elbow with a constant internal diameter; provides a relatively smooth frequency response and emphasizes high frequencies during amplification

change/no change test test that measures detection of an acoustic change in the suprasegmental or segmental features of speech; includes nine subtests; considered an alternative to word-recognition tasks

channel (1) a single set of inputs into an evoked response system or a stimulus generator; (2) the number of separate stimulation sites in the cochlea that can be selectively stimulated in a cochlear implant; does not always correspond to the number of electrodes; (3) band of selected frequencies through which some hearing aids present signals

chaos (1) a qualitative description of a dynamic system that seems unpredictable, but actually has a "hidden" order; (2) a mathematic theory that involves fractal geometry and nonlinear dynamics

characteristic frequency (CF) the frequency at which the threshold of a given single neuron is lowest (i.e., the frequency at which it is most sensitive)

characteristic impedance the ratio between sound pressure and particle velocity

Charcot-Marie-Tooth disease progressive neural muscular atrophy; weakness of distal muscles of arms and feet; can be associated with hearing loss

CHARGE syndrome a collection of newborn defects; letters of the acronym refer to the following disorders: c = coloboma of the eye; h = heart anomaly; a = atresia (stenosis) of choanae (in nose); r = retardation of growth and/or development; g = genital hypoplasia; e = ear abnormalities and/or deafness; possible sensorineural hearing loss and/or mixed hearing loss

Children's Auditory Test speech perception test for children consisting of monosyllabic words, spondees, trochees, and polysyllables; scored by the number of syllables correctly categorized and by the number of words correctly identified

Children's Implant Profile (CHIP) a protocol for evaluating candidacy for a cochlear implant that reviews factors believed to be related to implant benefit

Children's Vowel Perception Test picture vowel recognition test for young children; includes five sets of pictures, each with four items that differ by only the medial vowel

chloral hydrate common medication used for sedation during auditory brainstem response measurement in children

cholesteatoma benign mass in the middle ear composed of cholesterol and epithelial cells usually resulting from chronic otitis media; contains enzymes that can destroy adjacent structures; requires surgical removal

cholesterol granuloma a pathology created by cholesterol crystals deposited in the submucosa with a surrounding foreign body giant cell reaction

chopper response neural responses characterized by a periodic, chopped temporal pattern that is present throughout stimulation

chopper-s response a fast sustained chopper response variant characterized by short onset latencies, brief interspike intervals, and high discharge rates; see also **chopper response**

chopper-w response a wide and slow chopper variant characterized by long onset latencies, high thresholds, long interspike intervals, and low discharge rates; see also **chopper response**

chorda tympani nerve branch of cranial nerve VII (facial) passing through the middle ear and conveying taste information from the anterior two thirds of one side of the tongue

chromosomal disorder anomaly based on structure and/or number of chromosomes

chromosomes long strands of deoxyribonucleic acid (DNA) and protein that carry the genetic material (genes) that guides the formation of offspring; in a double strand of DNA, humans have 46 chromosomes or 23 pairs; 22 pairs are homologous pairs of autosomes and there is 1 pair of sex chromosomes

chronic slow developing and lasting a very long time; a disease process can be considered chronic

chronic external otitis slow developing and long lasting external otitis (inflammation of the outer ear); see also **external otitis**

chronic otitis media slow developing and long lasting inflammation or infection of the middle ear; see also **otitis media, otitis media with effusion**

chronologic age (CA) age of an individual calculated from the date of birth

CI cochlear implant; a device that delivers electrical stimulation to cranial nerve VIII (auditory nerve) via an electrode array surgically implanted in the cochlea; consists of a microphone, signal processor, and electrode system; used in cases of profound and total deafness

CIC completely-in-the-canal; extremely small hearing aid that fits deeply in the ear canal; usually appropriate for mild-to-moderate hearing losses

CIC coupler specially designed coupler for connecting completely-in-the-canal hearing aids to electroacoustic analysis equipment for evaluation

CICI Cochlear Implant Club International; a non-profit organization dedicated to supporting cochlear implant users and their families that provides information and support for social, educational, and political purposes; established in 1978

CID Central Institute for the Deaf; program for deaf children that emphasizes the aural-oral approach to auditory habilitation in St. Louis, Missouri; affiliated with Washington University and contains undergraduate and graduate programs in audiology, speech-language pathology, and deaf education

CID Auditory Test W-1 early test of speech perception measuring threshold of intelligibility; developed at the Central Institute for the Deaf (CID)

CID Auditory Test W-2 open-set test for rapid estimation of the intelligibility threshold by sweeping intensity; developed at the Central Institute for the Deaf (CID)

CID Auditory Test W-22 monosyllabic word-recognition test with mul-

tiple randomized lists; developed at the Central Institute for the Deaf (CID)

CID Everyday Sentences speech perception assessment test that allows direct comparison with a wealth of data for hearing-impaired adults and children and provides a measure of one's ability to understand sentences in an open-set context; developed at the Central Institute for the Deaf (CID)

CID Lipreading Enhancement Test Battery test that measures the degree to which lipreading improves when audition is added; stimulus materials are hierarchical in terms of linguistic content and task demands; developed at the Central Institute for the Deaf (CID)

CID Monster Test test designed to assess the perception of prosodic information in children with profound hearing loss; consists of four words presented in three different prosodic forms (monosyllables, trochees, and spondees); developed at the Central Institute for the Deaf (CID)

CID Phonetic Inventory assessment tool that can be used with children of any age that focuses on the ability to produce phonemes; results can be a useful part of program planning; developed at the Central Institute for the Deaf (CID)

CID Speech Perception Battery a battery of tests that evaluates the auditory-only speech perception performance of children with profound hearing loss (based on a 7-point scale); includes a test of lipreading enhancement; developed at the Central Institute for the Deaf (CID)

circuit the path of an electric current flow, including the wiring, connections, and often the energy source and electronic components

circuit, integrated (IC) a group of small transistors built into one circuit designed to provide power to a hearing aid

circuit noise undesirable sound created by the functioning of the circuitry in a hearing aid

circumaural encircles the ear (e.g., circumaural cushion on earphones and/or earmuffs)

CIS continuous interleaved sampling; strategy used in the Clarion cochlear implant that sends the speech signal to the electrodes through a series of very rapid pulses

cisplatin an antineoplastic agent shown to be effective against various cancers; may be ototoxic; results in cochlear damage in the high frequencies with progression to the lower-frequency region; early detection of ototoxicity can be observed if thresholds above 8000 Hz are monitored regularly

Clarion cochlear implant type of multichannel cochlear implant that processes the full spectrum of information; has up to eight channels; capable of implementing simultaneously compressed analog strategies

class A amplifier power output amplifier that consumes the peak requirement battery current at all times; typically used in linear amplification devices; simple and inexpensive; useful for individuals requiring mild gain hearing aids

class B amplifier power output amplifier referred to as push-pull; consumes battery current in proportion to the output required; has 10 times more battery life than class A amplifiers; see also **push-pull circuitry**

class D amplifier hearing aid amplifier design that produces a dramatic improvement in undistorted high-frequency output with reduced battery drain; provides more headroom than class A and class B amplifiers

classroom accommodation modifying the child's learning environment to help him or her cope with hearing loss; modifications include preferential seating, peer assistance, and alerting and teaching techniques; see also **accommodation**

classroom acoustics the noise and reverberation (echo) characteristics of a classroom as determined by sound sources inside and outside the classroom, classroom size, shape, surface material, furniture, persons, and other physical characteristics

classroom amplification assistive listening devices used to benefit individuals with hearing impairment in the classroom (e.g., FM systems, sound field FM systems, infrared systems, induction loops); see also **assistive listening device (ALD)**

Claudius cells cells that lie on the outward (lateral) side of the cells of Hensen in the organ of Corti; cochlear support cells

cleft lip failure of both sides of the lips to fuse together during development; congenital defect

cleft palate failure of both sides of the palate to fuse together during development; congenital defect; often associated with otitis media

click an abrupt onset and brief duration broad-band sound produced by delivering an electrical pulse to a transducer; broad spectrum stimulates many nerve fibers

click, broad-band an abrupt onset and brief duration click stimulus producing a response affecting a broad range of frequencies

click, condensation an abrupt onset and brief duration broad-band sound produced by the positive-polarity click delivered to an earphone

click, rarefaction an abrupt onset and brief duration broad-band sound produced by the negative-polarity click delivered to an earphone

click evoked otoacoustic emission (CEOAE) otoacoustic emission measured in the external auditory canal in response to a click stimulus; useful technique for determining cochlear function in infants; also known as **transient evoked otoacoustic emission (TEOAE)**; see also **otoacoustic emission (OAE)**

Client Oriented Scale of Improvement (COSI) method for measuring the efficacy of treatment (e.g., hearing aid satisfaction and improvement) by having patients define and rank order areas of perceived communication difficulty with and without amplification

clinical audiometer an electronic instrument that delivers calibrated pure-tone, speech, and noise stimuli for the clinical assessment of hearing sensitivity; has broad capabilities to perform routine tests as well as advanced techniques such as masking, special testing, and dual-channel testing

clinical certification board (CCB) working group that is part of the American Speech-Language-Hearing Association responsible for defining and enforcing guidelines for obtaining clinical certification from the organization

clinical fellowship (CF) supervised clinical experience that must be completed after graduate work to obtain certification from the American Speech-Language-Hearing Association; can range from 9 to a maximum of 36 months

closed captioning (CC) printed text or printed dialog on the screen that corresponds to the auditory speech signal from a television program or movie

closed set presentation of all possible choices to the individual before giving a test item; having a finite number of choices

closed-loop irrigation process of injecting warm or cool water into the external auditory canal during caloric testing in which the water enters an expandable, silastic balloon in the ear canal

Closed-Response Nonsense Syllable Test (CR-NST) test of phoneme recognition using meaningless syllables presented in a closed-set format (e.g., test uses seven subtests of seven to nine syllables per test)

closure the ability to complete and make whole an incomplete form; uses inductive and deductive reasoning along with contextual cues and knowledge of language; communication strategy used by listeners who are hearing impaired; also known as **auditory closure**

CM cochlear microphonic; an alternating current electrical potential from the hair cells of the cochlea that resembles the input signal; recorded during electrocochleography

CMR common mode rejection; when an electrical signal that is detected by two electrodes is the same (common) and is rejected or subtracted from itself by the differential amplifier; used in auditory evoked potential measurement to minimize electrical noise and enhance the response

CMRR common mode rejection ratio; the ratio (often in dB) between the amplitude of the output of a differential amplifier, when a signal is fed to only one input, with the other input shorted to ground, and the amplifier output when the same signal is supplied to both inputs of a differential amplifier

CMV cytomegalovirus; viral infection caused by the herpes family of viruses; also known as cytomegalic inclusion disease; most common viral cause of mental retardation and congenital progressive hearing impairment

CN (1) cochlear nucleus; initial brainstem nucleus of the auditory neural pathway found within the pons and subdivided into anteroventral, posteroventral, and dorsal cochlear nuclei; primary origin of sources of the lateral lemniscus, or central auditory pathway; (2) cranial nerve; 12 pairs of nerves originating at the base of the brain that carry messages for such functions as hearing, vision, swallowing, phonation, tongue movement, smell, eye movement, pupil contraction, equilibrium, mastication, facial expression, glandular secretion, taste, head movement, and shoulder movement; starting with the most anterior, cranial nerves are enumerated by Roman numerals; (CN I) olfactory, (CN II) optic, (CN III) oculomotor, (CN IV) trochlear, (CN V) trigeminal, (CN VI) abducens, (CN VII) facial, (CN VIII) acoustic (cochleovestibular), (CN IX) glossopharyngeal, (CN X) vagus, (CN XI) accessory, (CN XII) hypoglossal

CNC consonant-nucleus-consonant; word recognition material consisting of monosyllabic words with three phonemes; the initial and final phonemes are consonants and the middle phoneme is a vowel

CNS central nervous system; the spinal cord, brainstem, cerebellum, and cerebrum; the axis or central core of the nervous system; cranial nerves and other nerves are part of the peripheral nervous system

CNT could not test

CNV contingent negative variation; a low-frequency negative-voltage evoked response in the 300 to 500 ms region associated with anticipation of a stimulus condition

coarticulation the overlapping effect of one sound upon another

cochlea medial most portion of the inner ear that is continuous with the bony vestibule; consists of a base with $2\frac{5}{8}$ turns ending at the apex; the membranous portion of the cochlea which houses the organ of Corti is known as the **cochlear duct**

cochlear pertaining to the sensory portion of the inner ear (i.e., cochlea)

cochlear amplifier refers to the nonlinearities observed in basilar membrane motion; an active process requiring energy that is located between the auditory nerve fibers and the basilar membrane; contributes to the sharp tuning of the hair cells and the auditory nerve fibers

cochlear aqueduct part of the membranous labyrinth of the cochlea containing perilymph that is a small opening between the scala vestibuli and the subarachnoid space of the cranial cavity

cochlear artery artery supplying blood to the majority of the cochlea

cochlear concussion temporal bone fracture that results in at least a high-frequency hearing loss, usually with a dip in the pure-tone audiogram at 4000 Hz

cochlear conductive presbycusis a type of presbycusis (hearing loss due to aging) that does not affect the organ of Corti, spiral ganglion, or stria vascularis; manifested by a loss of sensitivity caused by mechanical changes in the basilar membrane, spiral ligament, and/or other structures

cochlear distortion product distortion product that is believed to be generated by the intrinsic nonlinear mechanical properties inherent in the cochlear organ of Corti; see also **distortion product otoacoustic emission (DPOAE), otoacoustic emission (OAE)**

cochlear duct the portion of the membranous labyrinth contained within the cochlea; endolymph-filled duct following the spiral shape of the cochlea; cavity of the cochlear duct is called the **scala media**

cochlear echo an output of sound from the inner ear produced in response to a sound stimulus; an otoacoustic emission; see also **otoacoustic emission (OAE)**

cochlear endolymphatic shunt an operation that creates a permanent communication between the perilymphatic space and the hydropic endolymphatic compartment by creating a small fistula in the osseous spiral lamina

cochlear fluids three different fluids coursing through the membranous labyrinth of the cochlea: endolymph, perilymph, and cortilymph; see also **cortilymph, endolymph, perilymph**

cochlear hearing loss hearing loss due to some sensory pathology in the cochlea of the inner ear; often associated with loudness recruitment; distinguished from retrocochlear hearing loss; see also **sensorineural hearing loss (SNHL)**

cochlear hydrops cochlear dysfunction resulting in a fluctuating sensorineural hearing loss with no vestibular signs or symptoms; see also **Ménière's disease**

cochlear implant (CI) a device that delivers electrical stimulation to cranial nerve VIII (auditory nerve) via an electrode array surgically implanted in the cochlea; consists of a microphone, signal processor, and electrode system; used in cases of profound and total deafness

Cochlear Implant Club International (CICI) a non-profit organization dedicated to supporting cochlear implant users and their families that provides information and support for social, educational, and political purposes; established in 1978

cochlear implant mapping the process of setting or adjusting the speech processor for an individual's cochlear implant device; the dynamic range of each electrode and electrode pair is determined by establishing threshold and loudness discomfort levels for electrical stimuli; also known as **mapping**

cochlear labyrinth intricate passageways within the cochlea including the spiral organ (cochlear duct) and perilymphatic channels (scalae tympani and vestibuli)

cochlear lesion lesion or pathology in the cochlear structures resulting in a sensorineural hearing loss

cochlear microphonic (CM) an alternating current electrical potential from the hair cells of the cochlea that resembles the input signal; recorded during electrocochleography

cochlear nerve cranial nerve VIII; consists of two sets of fibers: the anterior branch or cochlear nerve and the posterior branch or vestibular nerve; conducts neural signals from the inner ear to the brain; preferred terminology is auditory nerve; see also **auditory nerve, auditory-vestibular nerve, VIIIth nerve**

cochlear nerve action potential (1) gross neural potential; summed or averaged activity of action potentials of cranial nerve VIII in response to acoustic stimulation; (2) in auditory evoked potential measurements, it is the whole- nerve response of cranial nerve VIII; the main component of the electrocochleogram and wave I of the auditory brainstem response; also known **auditory nerve action potential, action potential (AP)**

cochlear neuritis inflammation of cranial nerve VIII resulting in a significant retrocochlear disorder; etiology is often viral

cochlear nuclei collection of neuronal cell bodies in the lower brainstem (pons) that synapse with fibers from cranial nerve VIII leading from the cochlea; consists of dorsal cochlear nucleus, anterior ventral cochlear nucleus, posterior ventral cochlear nucleus

cochlear nucleus (CN) initial brainstem nucleus of the auditory neural pathway found within the pons and subdivided into anteroventral, posteroventral, and dorsal cochlear nuclei; primary origin of sources of the lateral lemniscus, or central auditory pathway

cochlear nucleus implant an implant that places electrodes over the dorsal cochlear nucleus to stimulate neural tissue rather than the auditory nerve; see also **auditory brainstem implant (ABI)**

cochlear otosclerosis bony growth or softening involving the endosteal layer of the otic capsule adjoining the cochlea around the footplate of the stapes; see also **otosclerosis**

cochlear partition term used to describe collectively the partitions of the scala media, the most significant of which are the basilar membrane, the tectorial membrane, and the organ of Corti; see also **cochlear duct**

cochlear potentials bioelectric potentials generated in the cochlea

cochlear reserve the auditory response that is considered to reflect largely the condition of the cochlea; refers to the functioning structures of the cochlea

cochlear vasculature refers to the rich blood supply to the cochlea; blood is supplied by an artery running spirally around the modiolus with arterioles radiating out over the scala vestibuli and spiral lamina

cochleopalpebral reflex (CPR) eye blink reflex associated with stimulation or startle from loud sounds; also known as **auropalpebral reflex (APR)**

cochleostomy removal of the cochlea during preparation for some cochlear implant surgery

cochleotoxic the poisonous effect of toxic substances to the structures of the cochlea, particularly hair cells in the organ of Corti; see also **ototoxicity, vestibulotoxicity**

cochleovestibular nerve cranial nerve VIII; consists of two sets of fibers: the anterior branch or cochlear nerve and the posterior branch or vestibular nerve; conducts neural signals from the inner ear to the brain; see also **auditory nerve, auditory-vestibular nerve, VIIIth nerve**

Cockayne syndrome an autosomal recessive disorder characterized by dwarfism, mental retardation, retinal atrophy, and blindness; infant often appears normal at birth and by the second year of life starts to lag behind in motor and mental development; associated with severe, progressive sensorineural hearing loss

code of ethics (1) guidelines for ethical practice for audiologists and speech-language pathologists developed by the American Speech-Language-Hearing Association; (2) guidelines for ethical practice for audiologists developed by the American Academy of Audiology

coincidence effect the passing of a certain band of sound waves through a partition almost without attenuation when the projected wavelength of a sound in air is the same as the wavelength of the bending waves of the partition

cold running speech rapidly delivered, monotonous speech with a relatively consistent intensity level

collapsed ear canals condition that results from pressure of the supra-aural cushion on the pinna resulting in some degree of occlusion of the canal; condition gives rise to artefactually depressed air-conduction thresholds

coloboma tumor of the iris, retina, or optic nerve

coloboma lobuli congenital opening in the earlobes

columella the ossicular structure found in the middle ear of birds that is formed somewhat like a column or piston; comparable to the ossicular chain in humans

combination tone produced when two tones act simultaneously on a nonlinear transducer; may have a frequency equal to the difference between the two tones or any of their harmonics (difference tones) or it may have a frequency equal to the sum of two tones or any of their harmonics (summation tones)

comfort level maximum level for different stimuli that does not produce an uncomfortable loudness sensation; used to determine the maximum level for a series of pulses that does not produce an uncomfortable loudness sensation for a hearing aid or cochlear implant user

comfortable loudness level intensity level that is judged to be comfortable to listen to a sound; also known as **most comfortable level (MCL)**; see also **comfort level**

commissure a group of axons of neurons passing from one side of the brain to a similar structure on the opposite side of the brain

commissure of Probst one of at least five decussations or crossed-fiber groups connecting the right and left sides of the central auditory system; connects the lateral lemniscus to the inferior colliculus

commissurotomy surgical sectioning of the posterior portion of the corpus callosum

common electrode the relationship of one electrode to a second electrode; usually refers to the noninverting electrode

common ground stimulation stimulation mode that allows for the use of all 22 electrodes in a cochlear implant; when one electrode is chosen as the active electrode, all of the remaining electrodes are connected together and become the indifferent electrode

common mode rejection (CMR) when an electrical signal that is detected by two electrodes is the same (common) and is rejected or subtracted from itself by the differential amplifier; used in auditory evoked potential measurement to minimize electrical noise and enhance the response

common mode rejection ratio (CMRR) the ratio (often in dB) between the amplitude of the output of a differential amplifier, when a signal is fed to only one input, with the other input shorted to ground, and the amplifier output when the same signal is supplied to both inputs of a differential amplifier

Common Objects Token Test test designed to pinpoint children with the potential to identify open-set materials correctly; uses a closed-set task of increasing complexity

Common Phrases Test test designed to measure a child's speech perception of short, highly predictable, and familiar phrases; assesses the role of context in speech perception

communication the process by which a message is transferred from one person to another; can be accomplished via numerous methods including the use of verbal and nonverbal speech, sign language, manual communication, total communication, writing, hand gestures, and augmentative communication boards

communication breakdown instance in the course of a conversation when one participant does not recognize the message presented by another

communication disorder (CD) an impairment in an individual's ability to communicate (e.g., disordered use of speech, language, or hearing)

communication handicap psychosocial disadvantages that result from a communication disorder (e.g., hearing loss, speech, or language impairment) including the limitations that occur in performing the activities of everyday life

communication strategy a course of action taken to enhance communication; methods of coping with difficult listening situations including planning ahead, manipulating the environment, and using various repair techniques

communicative competence the functional and pragmatic use of language form and style to express effective messages that are listening oriented, coherent, fluent, and composed of adult grammar

compact disc (CD) high-fidelity digital recording of analog signals presented on a disc that uses a laser-read mechanism

comparative-prescriptive fittings procedure used in hearing aid fittings in which specific electroacoustic requirements, or hearing aid models, are recommended based on comparative tests; specifies a set of optimum electroacoustic characteristics that are to be integrated into the patient's hearing aids

compensated static acoustic immittance static acoustic immittance that has been compensated or corrected for the acoustic immittance of the external auditory meatus

compensated tympanometry a measurement of acoustic immittance that has been compensated or corrected for the acoustic immittance of the external auditory meatus (or other specified values of acoustic immittance)

compensation rehabilitative approach directed toward reducing the negative impact of a disorder or disease not amenable to complete recovery through treatment; see also **communication strategy**

Competing Message Test method used to measure speech understanding in the presence of a background competing message or noise

Competing Sentences Test test used to assess auditory processing and central auditory nervous system functioning; different sentences are presented simultaneously to each ear at different dB HLs; patient attempts to repeat each sentence correctly in the target ear

complete recruitment a high-intensity tone is perceived as being equally loud in both ears although the thresholds are sustained differently; possible result of the alternate binaural loudness balancing test; see also **alternate binaural loudness balancing (ABLB), loudness recruitment, recruitment**

completely-in-the-canal (CIC) hearing aid extremely small hearing aid that fits deeply in the ear canal; usually appropriate for mild-to-moderate hearing losses

complex aperiodic tone a sound wave containing simple sinusoidal components of different frequencies that is without periodicity

complex periodic tone a sound wave containing simple sinusoidal components of different frequencies whose waveform repeats itself regularly as a function of time

complex tone (1) a sound wave containing simple sinusoidal components of different frequencies; (2) a sound sensation characterized by more than one pitch

complex waveform a sound wave containing simple sinusoidal components of different frequencies displayed as amplitude as a function of time

compliance elasticity of the tympanic membrane measured during tympanometry; the point of maximum compliance reflects the point where the eardrum is most mobile and where ear canal pressure is equal to middle ear pressure

compound action potential (CAP) simultaneously occurring action potentials from thousands of nerve fibers; see also **action potential (AP), compound whole-nerve action potential**

compound threshold shift (CTS) threshold shift as a result of noise exposure that contains the combination of a temporary (TTS) and permanent (PTS) component

compound whole-nerve action potential refers to the summed or averaged activity of action potentials of cranial nerve VIII in response to acoustic stimulation; see also **compound action potential (CAP)**

comprehension a sophisticated level of auditory skill development, characterized by an ability to understand connected speech easily; highest step to be obtained in auditory training

compressed analog processing signal processing strategy used in cochlear implants in which signals are divided into frequency bands and delivered to the appropriate frequency-specific electrode pairs

compressed speech speech that has had segments removed and then compressed and yet maintains intact frequency composition

compressed speech test behavioral test used in the assessment of the central auditory nervous system using monosyllabic words presented in time compression monaurally resulting in a percent correct score

compression (1) a type of automatic gain control that produces reduced output levels for given changes in input levels; used in nonlinear amplification devices; (2) the portion of a signal that has an increase in the density of air molecules corresponding to the positive component of a sine wave

compression, syllabic type of hearing aid compression system that is characterized by short time constants (attack and release times) and a low compression threshold; results in compression of virtually all signals presented to the listener; see also **wide-dynamic range compression (WDRC)**

compression, wide-dynamic range (WDRC) a type of compression circuitry that can provide much greater amplification for low-intensity signals than for medium-intensity signals while providing less or no gain for high-intensity signals; useful for individuals with a very narrow dynamic range; has a low compression threshold; see also **syllabic compression**

compression amplification a hearing aid or amplification device that reduces the intensity range among audio signals while increasing the overall intensity of all signals; (e.g., automatic gain control, output limiting, wide-dynamic range compression)

compression circuits hearing aid circuitry capable of providing different forms of compression amplification

compression kneepoint minimum intensity level to activate compression; also known as **compression threshold**

compression range (CR) range of input levels over which the compression function of a hearing aid operates

compression ratio (CR) ratio of the change in output level of a hearing aid that results from a given change in the input level in a compression amplifier; e.g., for every 10 dB of input, the output increases by 5 dB; CR = 10/5 = 2:1

compression threshold (CT) the lowest input level at which the compression operates; the level that activates compression; also known as **compression kneepoint**

computed tomography (CT) specialized x-ray scan that produces thin (usually 10-mm thick) cross-sectional reconstructions of the body using computer back-projection techniques; highly sophisticated, computer-intense process for measuring and analyzing multiplane (multicut) X-rays; also known as **CAT scan** (obsolete usage); see also **computerized axial tomography, positron emission tomography (PET)**

computer averaging a technique of averaging successive samples of encephalographic activity time-locked to a stimulus to reduce unrelated signals and thus enhance the measurement of the desired response by improving the signal-to-noise ratio; also known as **signal averaging**

computer-aided speechreading training (CAST) component in a comprehensive auditory rehabilitation program using a computer platform with a videocassette playback to train speechreading skills

computerized axial tomography/ CAT scan a computer-generated picture of a section of the brain compiled from sectional radiographs obtained from the same plane; see also **computed tomography (CT)**

computerized dynamic posturography (CDP) a type of vestibular assessment that focuses on the function of the balance system in maintaining postural stability in a variety of simulated conditions; computer-induced platform movements evaluate motor responses that include strength, symmetry, and latency of muscle response; see also **sensory organization test**

concha landmark of the auricle; bowl in the center of the outer ear leading to the external auditory meatus

concha-related Helmholtz resonance acoustic characteristic of the concha resulting in a natural resonance between 4000 and 5000 Hz; sound energy in this frequency region is maintained with completely-in-the-canal hearing aids, but lost with in-the-ear and in-the-canal hearing aids

concurrent validity criterion-related validity index employed to predict real-life performance

condensation (1) the portion of a signal that has an increase in the density of air molecules corresponding to the positive component of a sine wave; (2) polarity; positive-voltage electrical signal producing an outward movement of the transducer diaphragm with associated sound waves

condensation stimulus polarity positive-voltage electrical signal producing an outward movement of the transducer diaphragm with associated sound waves

condenser microphone a microphone with a diaphragm separated from a back plate by a small volume of air and a preamplifier; type of input transducer used in hearing aids

conditioned orientation reflex (COR) a method for establishing auditory thresholds in young children; requires conditioning the child to make a response to a sound (e.g., head turn) that is reinforced; see also **visual reinforcement audiometry (VRA)**

conditioned play audiometry behavioral test of hearing that is effective for preschoolers above the age of 2 ½ years; the child's responses to sound are conditioned by incorporating them into a game activity; see also **behavioral play audiometry, play audiometry**

conditioned response a behavior that occurs as a result of training (conditioning); elicited by a conditioned stimulus

conditioned stimulus a stimulus that is used to train an individual to perform a particular behavioral response

conductance (G) reciprocal of resistance; refers to the ease of flow of energy

conductive hearing loss type of hearing impairment resulting from an interruption of sound transmission through an abnormal outer and/or middle ear

conductive mechanism the part of the auditory system that includes the outer and middle ears and is responsible for conduction of sound to the inner ear

conductor a substance that transfers or conveys a form of energy, such as electricity

condyle rounded prominence at an extreme end of a bone; the process of the mandible that inserts into the temporomandibular joint

cone of light triangular-shaped light reflex seen when a light is shone down the external auditory canal toward the tympanic membrane with an otoscope; also known as **light reflex**

confidentiality process of keeping personal information about an individual's medical, psychological, and audiological health care private; such information is only available to others when the individual authorizes such activity in writing

configuration term used to describe the shape or pattern of an audiogram; how hearing loss varies as a function of test frequency; the three main configurations are sloping, rising, and flat

confusion matrix a visual representation of the stimulus-response paradigm in which the stimuli are listed down the side of the matrix and the responses are represented across the top in the same order as the stimuli; may also be called a symmetric matrix; useful tool for analyzing phonemic perceptual errors

congenital present at birth

congenital deafness profound hearing loss (deafness) that occurs prior to the development of speech and language, usually before or at birth; also known as **prelingual hearing loss**

congenital hearing impairment a hearing impairment that occurs prior to the development of speech and language, usually before or at birth; also known as **prelingual hearing loss**

congenital sensorineural hearing loss a hearing impairment affecting the inner ear and/or auditory nerve that occurs prior to the development of speech and language, usually before or at birth

conjugate eye movements paired activity of the eyes such that both eyes move in the same direction at the same time

Connected Speech Test (CST) test of intelligibility of everyday speech; uses an open-set format of 48 passages of conversationally produced connected speech; scored using key words

consanguinity relationship by descent from a common ancestor

conservation, hearing prevention or reduction of hearing loss through a program of identifying and minimizing risk, monitoring hearing sensitivity, education, and providing protection from noise exposure

conservation, speech active intervention as part of auditory rehabilitation to preserve the speech production skills of an individual who is hard-of-hearing

consonance the phenomenon in which tones presented together produce a blended or pleasant sensation; see also **dissonance**

consonant a speech sound formed by restricting, channeling, or directing air flow with the tongue, teeth, and/or lips

Consonant Confusion Test a closed-set speech perception test that compares words that have similar consonants

Consonant-Nucleus-Consonant (CNC) Test word-recognition material consisting of monosyllabic words with three phonemes; the initial and final phonemes are consonants and the middle phoneme is a vowel

consonant-vowel (CV) a nonsense syllable or a real word comprised of a consonant followed by a vowel (e.g., ba, da, ga, to, do, me)

consonant-vowel ratio relationship between the intensity of a consonant and its adjacent vowel(s)

consonant-vowel-consonant (CVC) a nonsense syllable or real word comprised of a consonant followed by a vowel followed by a consonant (e.g., kik, pip, sis, bat, hit)

consonant-vowel-consonant-vowel (CVCV) a bisyllabic nonsense syllable comprised of a consonant followed by a vowel followed by another consonant-vowel combination (e.g., /sufɛ/); as used in the Edgerton-Danhauer Nonsense Syllable Test

construct validity statistical term meaning the extent to which a test measures what it is supposed to measure, usually a trait or a skill; the extent to which a test measurement corresponds to theoretical concepts (as when a measure expected to vary over time does so)

content validity statistical term referring to the extent to which a test adequately samples what it is supposed to measure (the domain studied); e.g., measurement for sentence perception would include sentence or phrase stimuli

context linguistic and/or environmental support available for identifying a target word, phrase, or sentence

contextual cues clues available in the communication environment that enhance the understanding of speech; taking advantage of such linguistic or situational information allows one to perform closure (i.e. fill in the gaps of missing information)

contingent negative variation (CNV) a low-frequency negative-voltage evoked response in the 300 to 500 ms region associated with anticipation of a stimulus condition

continuous discourse tracking (CDT) aural rehabilitation technique in which the listener attempts to repeat text verbatim that is presented by a speaker; performance is summarized as the number of words repeated per minute; also referred to as connected discourse tracking

continuous flow adapter type of earmold that contains a single snap-in/snap-out elbow with a constant internal diameter; provides a relatively smooth frequency response and emphasizes high frequencies during amplification

continuous interleaved sampling (CIS) strategy used in the Clarion cochlear implant that sends the speech signal to the electrodes through a series of very rapid pulses

continuous spectrum a plot of a sound wave displaying amplitude as a function of frequency; the components of the signal are continuously distributed over a frequency region; see also **line spectrum**

contraindication any factor negating a particular treatment

contralateral originating on the opposite side

contralateral acoustic reflex acoustic reflex activating signals are presented in the ear opposite that containing the probe; assesses the integrity of the contralateral acoustic reflex arc and provides diagnostic information regarding possible site of lesion; also known as **crossed acoustic reflex**

contralateral competing message (CCM) a form of the Synthetic Sentence Identification test for assessment of central auditory function; stimuli are presented with a competing message presented simultaneously to the contralateral ear

contralateral ear effect dominance of performance by one ear over the other in central auditory assessment; often seen as a contralateral ear effect where the ear opposite the site of lesion has the poorer performance; also known as **ear effect**

contralateral masking type of masking in which a masking noise is presented to the ear opposite the test ear

contralateral routing of signals (CROS) a hearing aid arrangement originally developed for patients with unilateral hearing losses; a microphone is located at the poorer ear and the signal is routed to the better ear and delivered through an "open" earmold

contralateral suppression the reduction in otoacoustic emission amplitude when contralateral acoustic stimulation is generated in the opposite ear; see also **efferent suppression**

convergence coming together toward a common point; coordinated inward movement of both of the eyes toward the nose; opposite of divergence

conversion deafness psychogenic hearing disorder caused by emotional trauma; severe anxiety becomes the physical appearance of deafness; hearing loss of no physiologic origin; also known as conversion hysteria or **hysterical deafness**; see also **functional hearing loss, inorganic hearing loss**

cookie bite an outdated term for an audiogram configuration characterized by decreased hearing sensitivity in the mid-frequency region only; was often seen in individuals affected by prenatal rubella

cookie bite audiogram an audiometric configuration characterized by decreased hearing sensitivity in the mid-frequency region only; was often seen in individuals affected by prenatal rubella

COR conditioned orientation reflex; a method for establishing auditory thresholds in young children; requires conditioning a child to make a response to sound (e.g., head turn) that is reinforced; see also **visual reinforcement audiometry (VRA)**

CORFIG coupler response for flat insertion gain; a set of correction factors used to predict hearing aid insertion gain from coupler performance

Cornelia de Lange syndrome characterized by short stature, cognitive impairment, digital anomalies, coarse facies, microcephaly, irritability, seizures, hypertonia, lack of facial expression, cleft palate, anomalous auricles, short neck, renal anomalies, intestinal anomalies, cardiac malformations, and micrognathia; associated with conductive or sensorineural hearing loss from mild to profound in approximately 50% of the cases; also known as **de Lange syndrome**

corneoretinal potential an electrical potential of the eyes resulting from the positive electrical charge from the cornea and the negative electrical charge from the retina; the electrical potential is about 1 mV; the eye acts as a dipole (molecule having two equal and opposite charges); used in the measurement of eye movements during electronystagmography testing

corner audiogram an audiogram configuration that displays a profound hearing loss with thresholds measurable only in the low frequencies; also known as left-corner audiogram

cornua horn

corona crown

coronal section a cross section dividing, by actually cutting or through imaging methods, the body into a vertical plane perpendicular to the median plane (front and back halves); see also **frontal section**

corpus callosum major collection of fibers connecting the two cerebral hemispheres

correct rejection the event that occurs in a detection situation during a specified observation interval when a "noise-alone" response (output) follows a "noise-alone" stimulus (input)

cortex gray matter on the surface of the cerebral hemispheres; responsi-

ble for high-level processing, general movement, and behavioral reactions; outer layer of a body organ or structure; different regions of the cortex are differentiated for specialized functions

cortical deafness damage from bilateral lesions of the temporal lobe primary receptive area; peripheral pure-tone hearing may be normal

cortical evoked response audiometry electrical activity evoked by sounds, that originates from portions of the auditory cortex, is measured with electrodes placed on the scalp, and occurs within 100 to 300 ms after the sound is presented; also known as **long latency response**

cortical lesion lesion or pathology in the cortex or brain

cortilymph fluid within the tunnel of Corti located between the pillars or rods of Corti

COSI Client Oriented Scale of Improvement; method for measuring the efficacy of treatment (e.g., hearing aid satisfaction and improvement) by having patients define and rank order areas of perceived communication difficulty with and without amplification

cost-benefit analysis (CBA) an economic evaluation of medical care costs that compares monetary benefit between a variety of health interventions

cost-effective analysis (CEA) economic analysis for determining the best use of funds available for medical care; often conducted on the basis of cost per unit achieved

cough reflex cough reflex is observed in some patients whenever something is placed into the ear canal due to stimulation of the vagus cranial nerve (e.g., during earmold impression taking or cerumen management)

Council for Accreditation in Occupational Hearing Conservation (CAOHC) organization that sponsors training workshops and provides appropriate certification for individuals responsible for the development and maintenance of hearing conservation programs

counseling process used by audiologists to provide personal-adjustment support and informational counseling; process used to help patients and their families accept their hearing losses and subsequent consequences and make decisions regarding treatment

coupler device connecting a receiver and a measuring microphone; contains an air-filled chamber with a given shape that serves to load the receiver; various coupler sizes exist for measuring hearing aid performance or performing calibration procedures

coupler, CIC specially designed coupler for connecting completely-in-the-canal hearing aids to electroacoustic analysis equipment for evaluation

coupler, HA-1 standard direct access 2-cc coupler for connecting in-the-ear and in-the-canal hearing aids to electroacoustic analysis equipment for analysis; uses putty to seal the shell of the hearing aid to the coupler

coupler, HA-2 standard 2-cc coupler for connecting hearing aids that are not integrated into an ear piece (e.g., behind-the-ear and body hearing aids) to electroacoustic analysis equipment for analysis; earhook of hearing aid fits into tubing for direct connection; includes a standard earmold simulator

coupler, HA-3 standard 2-cc coupler for connecting hearing aids that do not have nubs (e.g., insert receivers, earphones, and modular in-the-ear hearing aids) to electroacoustic analysis equipment for analysis

coupler, HA-4 standard 2-cc coupler for connecting hearing aids to electroacoustic analysis equipment for analysis that is a modification of the HA-2 coupler; used to couple eyeglass hearing aids and some behind-the-ear hearing aids using special tubing

coupler, 1.5-cc Zwislocki coupler used in Knowles Electronic Manikin for Acoustic Research designed to be analogous to the human ear canal

coupler, 6-cc a device for acoustic loading of earphones during calibration of audio equipment; designed to represent the volume of the human pinna and ear canal; measures the sound pressure level of the stimulus at the earphone under test; device meeting ANSI S3.6-

1989 specifications for coupling an earphone to a sound level meter for audiometer calibration

coupler, 2-cc a precisely bored tube in a metal block that represents the volume of air occupying the human ear canal for the use of checking hearing aid conformance to manufacturers' specifications

coupler, Zwislocki a 1.5-cc device for coupling a hearing aid for measurements of hearing aid performance developed in 1970; more closely resembles the real ear than the commonly used 2-cc coupler

coupler gain the amount of acoustic gain measured in a 2-cc coupler; see also **acoustic gain**

coupler response for flat insertion gain (CORFIG) a set of correction factors used to predict hearing aid insertion gain from coupler performance

CPA cerebellopontine angle; the angle formed or bordered by the cerebellum and the lateral surface of the pons; located in the posterior fossa; cranial nerve VIII passes through the cerebellopontine angle; a common site for auditory nerve tumors

CPR cochleopalpebral reflex; eye blink reflex associated with stimulation or startle from loud sounds; also known as **auropalpebral reflex (APR)**

cps cycles per second; unit of measurement for frequency; frequency is determined as the number of cycles per second; also represented by **Hz (Hertz)**

CPT codes current procedural terminology codes; a specialized set of numeric codes assigned to particular diagnostic and rehabilitative procedures; used for billing in medical and audiology practices

CPU central processing unit; term for the component of a personal computer containing the hardware

CR (1) compression range; range of input levels over which the compression function of a hearing aid operates; (2) compression ratio; ratio of the change in output level of a hearing aid that results from a given change in the input level in a compression amplifier; e.g., for every 10 dB of input, the output increases by 5 dB; $CR = 10/5 = 2{:}1$

CR-NST Closed-Response Nonsense Syllable Test; test of phoneme recognition using meaningless syllables presented in a closed-set format (e.g., test uses seven subtests of seven to nine syllables per test)

Craig lipreading inventory test of audiovisual perception; contains words and sentences in a four-choice closed-set context; utilizes pictures

cranial related to the head

cranial nerve I olfactory nerve; cranial nerve I responsible for the sense of taste

cranial nerve II optic nerve; cranial nerve II responsible for afferent innervation from the eyes

cranial nerve III oculomotor nerve; cranial nerve III responsible for movements of the eyes

cranial nerve IV trochlear nerve; cranial nerve IV responsible for efferent innervation for eye movement

cranial nerve V trigeminal nerve; cranial nerve V responsible for chewing, face sensitivity, and muscle innervation; innervates the tensor tympani middle ear muscle and muscles used to open and close the eustachian tube

cranial nerve VI abducens nerve; cranial nerve VI responsible for control of eye movements

cranial nerve VII facial nerve; cranial nerve VII innervates facial muscles; one branch of the facial nerve, known as the **chorda tympani nerve**, courses through the middle ear and provides taste sensation for the anterior two thirds of the tongue on each side

cranial nerve VIII auditory nerve; cochleovestibular nerve responsible for the sense of hearing and balance; has two branches: vestibular and cochlear

cranial nerve IX glossopharyngeal nerve; cranial nerve IX responsible for the sense of taste and secretion from certain glands

cranial nerve X vagus nerve; cranial nerve X named for its wandering course that extends through the neck, thorax, and abdomen; provides neural innervation to the external ear and the speech mechanism, including the larynx, tongue, and palate

cranial nerve XI accessory nerve; cranial nerve XI responsible for speech, swallowing, and head and shoulder movements

cranial nerve XII hypoglossal nerve; cranial nerve XII responsible for swallowing and moving the tongue

cranial nerves (CN) 12 pairs of nerves originating at the base of the brain that carry messages for such functions as hearing, vision, swallowing, phonation, tongue movement, smell, eye movement, pupil contraction, equilibrium, mastication, facial expression, glandular secretion, taste, head movement, and shoulder movement; starting with the most anterior, cranial nerves are enumerated by Roman numerals; (CN I) olfactory, (CN II) optic, (CN III) oculomotor, (CN IV) trochlear, (CN V) trigeminal, (CN VI) abducens, (CN VII) facial, (CN VIII) acoustic (cochleovestibular), (CN IX) glossopharyngeal, (CN X) vagus, (CN XI) accessory, (CN XII) hypoglossal

craniodiaphyseal dysplasia autosomal recessive disorder characterized by severe thickening of the bone of the face and skull, hypertelorism, eventual optic atrophy (possible blindness), progressive cognitive deterioration, early death is common; associated with mixed hearing loss secondary to osseous growth in the tympanum and eventual compression of the auditory nerve

craniofacial involving the head and face

craniofrontonasal dysplasia syndrome X-linked dominant disorder characterized by hypertelorism, orbital dystopia, cleft lip and palate, longitudinal splitting of fingernails, agenesis of corpus callosum, strabismus, craniofacial asymmetry, sloping shoulders, occasional cognitive impairment; associated with conductive hearing loss caused by middle ear effusion secondary to cleft palate

craniometaphyseal dysplasia autosomal dominant and autosomal recessive disorder characterized by bony overgrowth of face and skull, hypertelorism, nystagmus; associated with moderate to severe mixed hearing loss

crest ridge; bone prominence

crest factor difference in decibels between the peak sound pressure level (SPL) and the root mean square SPL

crib-o-gram an automated infant hearing screening device that utilizes a specially designed bassinet for detection of infant movement following presentation of an auditory stimulus through a small loudspeaker; see also **auditory response cradle (ARC)**

CRISCROS hearing aid binaural CROS hearing aid arrangement for bilateral severe sensorineural hearing loss in which the microphone on each ear transmits the signal to the opposite side (ear) allowing for considerable increase in gain without feedback; see also **contralateral routing of signals (CROS)**

crista ampularis the primary sense organ of the ampulla in the semicircular canals that responds to angular acceleration of the head; contains vestibular hair cells and stereocilia

criterion-related validity test effectiveness of an individual's behavior or abilities in specific situations

critical band (1) a region of noise surrounding a pure tone; when the SPL of the narrow band is the same as the SPL of the tone, the tone is barely perceptible; as the critical bandwidth is exceeded, the signal is perceived as being louder; (2) when sounds fall within one critical bandwidth, their total loudness is a function of the total loudness level; when sounds fall outside one critical bandwidth, their total loudness approaches the sum of their individual loudnesses; see also **critical ratio, loudness summation**

critical period the early years in a child's life during which the language and vocal patterns of the individual are acquired most easily

critical ratio based on indirectly derived measures of bandwidth; the ratio of the intensity of the tone to the intensity level per cycle of the noise or the dB difference between the masked threshold and level-per-cycle of noise; critical ratios underestimate critical bands by about 2.5 times; see also **critical band**

CROS contralateral routing of signals; a hearing aid arrangement originally developed for patients with unilateral hearing losses; a microphone is located at the poorer ear and the signal is routed to the better ear and delivered through an "open" earmold

CROS hearing aid a hearing aid arrangement originally developed for patients with unilateral hearing losses; a microphone is located at the poorer ear and the signal is routed to the better ear and delivered through an "open" earmold; allows for better localization of sounds

CROS-plus hearing aid the typical CROS amplification arrangement for the good ear combined with a second hearing aid for direct amplification to the poorer ear; the hearing aid on the poorer ear is a power in-the-ear hearing aid; see also **contralateral routing of signals (CROS)**

cross hearing sound stimulus presented to one (test) ear travels around or across the head (via bone conduction) to stimulate the other (non-test) ear; also known as **crossover**

cross-check principle concept of using a test battery approach to lessen the limitations of conventional behavioral audiometry; the principle states that the results of any single audiometric test cannot be considered valid without independent verification from another test; provides accurate information with which hearing loss can be identified and quantified

cross-modality matching a psychophysical method used primarily to scale sensations; the subject adjusts a stimulus along some dimen-sion until that stimulus appears equal to another stimulus received by a different sense modality

crossed acoustic reflex acoustic reflex activating signals are presented in the ear opposite that containing the probe; assesses the integrity of the contralateral acoustic reflex arc and provides diagnostic information regarding possible site of lesion; also known as **contralateral acoustic reflex**

crossover frequency (CF) the frequency or frequencies representing the cutoff frequencies of the filters that divide the frequency range into separate bands; used in filters and some hearing aids

Crouzon syndrome a condition associated with conductive hearing loss characterized by an abnormally shaped head, skull abnormalities, marked exophthalmus (bulging eyes), a beaklike nose, and a short upper lip

crown the topmost portion of a structure or organ, as the top of the head

crura the two pillars of the stapes connecting the head to the footplate; Latin for legs; plural

crus singular for crura; refers to one leg or arm

CSF cerebrospinal fluid; the watery-appearing liquid in which the brain is bathed and that fills the ventricles in the brain and the column in the spinal cord

CST (1) Competing Sentences Test; test used to assess auditory processing and central auditory nervous system functioning; different sentences are presented simultaneously to each ear at different dB HLs; patient attempts to repeat each sentence correctly in the target ear; (2) Connected Speech Test; test of intelligibility of everyday speech; uses an open-set format of 48 passages of conversationally produced connected speech; scored using key words

CT (1) compression threshold; the lowest input level at which the compression operates; the level that activates compression; the kneepoint; (2) computed tomography; specialized x-ray scan that produces thin (usually 10-mm thick) cross-sectional reconstructions of the body using computer back-projection techniques; highly sophisticated, computer-intense process for measuring and analyzing multiplane (multicut) X rays

CT scan specialized X-ray scan that produces thin (usually 10-mm thick) cross-sectional reconstructions of the body using computer back-projection techniques; highly sophisticated, computer-intense process for measuring and analyzing multiplane (multicut) X-rays; also known as **CAT scan** (obsolete usage); see also **computerized axial tomography**, **positron emission tomography (PET)**

CTS compound threshold shift; threshold shift as a result of noise exposure that contains the combination of a temporary (TTS) and permanent (PTS) component

cubic centimeter (cc) unit of measurement for volume; 1 cc = 1 ml

cubic distortion product (1) a reflection of the nonlinearity of the basilar membrane of the cochlea at high stimulus intensity levels; expressed by the formula $2f1 - f2$; (2) a major response parameter in measurement of distortion product otoacoustic emissions; see also **distortion product otoacoustic emission (DPOAE), otoacoustic emission (OAE)**

cue any signal that enhances the successful communication of a message; can be verbal or nonverbal (e.g., gestures, signs)

cued speech a communication system that combines auditory information and visual cues (hand and finger movements about the face) for sounds that cannot be easily identified by speechreading; a system for making all the sounds of speech visible; utilizes eight hand shapes, placed in four different locations around the face, to remove any ambiguity about what is seen and heard by a person with a hearing loss

cupula (1) a structure shaped like a cup or dome; (2) gelatinous structure in the crista ampularis in which the stereocilia and kinocilium of the vestibular hair cells are embedded

current the flow of electrons through a conductor; measured in amperes

current, alternating (AC) an electric current that periodically flows in one direction and then the other

current, direct (DC) electric current that only flows in one direction in a conductor or circuit

current procedural terminology (CPT) codes a specialized set of numeric codes assigned to particular diagnostic and rehabilitative procedures; used for billing in medical and audiology practices

currette instrument used in cerumen management

custom earmold earmold that is made from an ear impression to fit the individual ear specifically

custom earplugs earplugs made from ear impressions to fit difficult ear canals or to provide a comfortable fit

custom hearing aid hearing aids such as in-the-ear, in-the-canal, and completely-in-the-canal that are made for specific individuals from an ear impression

cuticular plate membrane at the superior region of each hair cell; stereocilia protude through this thickened membrane

cutoff frequency upper and lower frequencies for which the amplitude of the response is 3 dB less than the amplitude at the maximum frequency

CV consonant-vowel; a nonsense syllable or real word comprised of a consonant followed by a vowel (e.g., ba, da, ga, to, do, me)

CVA cerebrovascular accident; a stroke; brain damage resulting from interruption of blood supply to the brain; contemporary term is **brain attack**

CVC consonant-vowel-consonant; a nonsense syllable or real word comprised of a consonant followed by a vowel followed by a consonant (e.g., kik, pip, sis, bat, hit)

CVCV consonant-vowel-consonant-vowel; a bisyllabic nonsense syllable comprised of a consonant followed by a vowel followed by another consonant-vowel combination (e.g., /sufɛ/); as used in the Edgerton-Danhauer Nonsense Syllable Test

cycle one complete set of the recurrent values of a periodic quantity

cycles per second (cps) unit of measurement for frequency; frequency is determined as the number of cycles per second; also represented by **Hz (Hertz)**

cymba concha superior portion of the concha; see also **concha**

cyst benign growth of the skin containing epithelial tissue and/or fluid

cyt-, cyto- pertaining to a cell

cytocochleogram a display of the percentage of cochlear hair cell loss along the basilar membrane

cytomegalovirus (CMV) viral infection caused by the herpes family of viruses; also known as cytomegalic inclusion disease; most common viral cause of mental retardation and congenital progressive hearing impairment

Cz refers to the electrode location at the coronal (C) midline (z) according to the International 10–20 Electrode System; also referred to as the **vertex**

D

DAC digital-to-analog converter; an electronic device that converts a series of numeric values that are processed by a computer into a continuously varying electrical signal

DAF delayed auditory feedback; (1) a procedure that alters the time in which a listener's speech is presented to his or her ears, affecting the rate and fluency of speech production; (2) a technique that induces dysfluency in persons who can hear the signal; useful technique to identify malingerers; (3) a technique used to induce fluency in some stutterers

DAI direct audio input; a circuit in some hearing aids that directly connects them to some assistive listening devices and also to radios and televisions

damage risk criteria (DRC) the maximum safe allowable noise levels for different bandwidths as determined by the Occupational Safety and Health Administration; the level of sound to which a population may be exposed for a specified time with a specified risk of hearing loss

damper materials or filters placed in hearing aid tone hooks, earmolds, and receiver tubing and in hearing aid vents to reduce output and smooth peaks; available in varying ohm resistance; also known as acoustic damper

damping (1) any means of dissipating vibration energy within a vibrating system; (2) the action of frictional or dissipative forces on a dynamic system causing the system to lose energy and reduce the amplitude of movement; (3) removal of echoes by the use of sound-absorbing materials; also known as acoustic damping

damping ratio ratio of actual damping to critical damping at a resonant frequency

daPa decaPascal; unit of measurement used in immittance testing; 1daPa = 10 Pascals

Darwin's tubercle variation in the helix of the pinna; thickened, sometimes pointy, portion near the posterior tip of the pinna

DASL Developmental Approach to Successful Listening; test used with children to assess training needs and determine placement in an auditory training program by indicating which levels of developmental skills have been obtained

DAT digital audiotape; type of magnetic tape recording that uses digital signals that have been converted from analog inputs

dB decibel; unit of sound intensity; one-tenth of a bel; a logarithm of the sound pressure of a sound to a reference sound pressure (0.0002 dyne/cm^2) or the logarithm of the sound power to a reference sound power (10^{-16} watts/cm^2)

dB HL decibels hearing level; a decibel scale referenced to accepted standards for normal hearing (0 dB is average normal hearing for each audiometric test frequency)

dB HTL decibels hearing threshold level; a decibel scale referenced to a patient's threshold of sensitivity

dB nHL decibels normalized hearing level; a decibel scale used in auditory brainstem response measurement referenced to the average behavioral threshold for a click stimulus of a small group of normal-hearing subjects

dB peSPL refers to peak equivalent sound pressure level; equal to the amplitude of a 1000-Hz tone as if it were equivalent to the peak of a transient signal such as a click; used to determine the intensity level of a click

dB SL decibels sensation level; sound intensity described in reference to an individual patient's behavioral threshold for an audiometric frequency or some other measure of hearing threshold

dB SPL decibels sound pressure level; a decibel scale referenced to a physical standard for pressure intensity (e.g., 0.0002 dyne/cm^2 or 20 μPa)

dBA measurement in dB from a sound level meter with the weighting switch on A; filters out low-frequency components of the sound to compensate for less sensitive human hearing for low frequencies; approximates the 40 phon equal loudness contour

dBB measurement in dB from a sound level meter that attenuates frequency components below 300 Hz and approximates the 70 phon equal loudness contour

dBC measurement in dB from a sound level meter with the weighting switch on C; permits nearly a flat frequency response to input sound

DC direct current; electric current that only flows in one direction in a conductor or circuit

DCA digitally controlled analog; a hearing aid that has analog components but is controlled digitally; commonly referred to as programmable

DCN dorsal cochlear nucleus; dorsal (posterior) division of the cochlear nuclei; exhibits the greatest diversity in response relative to the other cochlear nuclei; dominated by inhibition; involved in processing spatial or spectral information needed in the detection of threshold level signals embedded in a narrow spectral band or in complex feature detection during speech

de Lange syndrome characterized by short stature, cognitive impairment, digital anomalies, coarse facies, microcephaly, irritability, seizures, hypertonia, lack of facial expression, cleft palate, anomalous auricles, short neck, renal anomalies, intestinal anomalies, cardiac malformations, and micrognathia; associated with conductive or sensorineural hearing loss from mild to profound in approximately 50% of the cases; also known as **Cornelia de Lange syndrome**

dead ear an audiologic/otologic slang term for a profound hearing impairment (i.e., an ear that does not respond to or has little response to sound)

deaf hearing sensitivity poorer than 90 dB bilaterally; minimal or no hearing; inability to hear well enough to understand speech, even with amplification; see also **deafness**

Deaf community persons who do not view deafness as a handicap but as a cultural identity; see also **Deaf culture**

Deaf culture a subculture in society that shares a common language (American Sign Language), beliefs, customs, arts, history, and folklore; comprised primarily of individuals who have prelingual deafness; see also **Deaf community**

deaf English nonstandard features of the English language used by deaf persons; also referred to as deaf speech

deaf mute slang, politically incorrect term used for someone who is deaf and does not speak

deafisms deviant structures of grammar that approximate standard English produced by the deaf

deafness hearing loss so profound that acquisition of oral language is not possible without amplification and intense special educational methods; traditional amplification may provide little benefit; types of deafness include **central, congenital, conversion, cortical, familial, postlingual, prelingual,** and **sensorineural**; see also **deaf**

deafness, central the impairment of hearing that occurs when there is damage in the auditory pathways or the auditory centers of the brain; results in auditory processing difficulty; often occurs when peripheral hearing is normal or near normal

deafness, congenital profound deafness that occurs prior to the development of speech and language, usually before or at birth; also known as **prelingual hearing loss**

deafness, conversion psychogenic hearing disorder caused by emotional trauma; severe anxiety becomes the physical appearance of deafness; hearing loss of no physiologic origin; see also **pseudohypacusis**

deafness, cortical damage from bilateral lesions of the temporal lobe primary receptive area; peripheral pure-tone hearing may be normal; see also **central deafness**

deafness, familial profound deafness in members of the same family

deafness, hysterical psychogenic hearing disorder caused by emotional trauma; severe anxiety becomes the physical appearance of deafness; hearing loss of no physiologic origin; see also **pseudohypacusis**

deafness, postlingual profound hearing loss (deafness) that occurs after the normal development of speech and language (usually age 5 years or older)

deafness, prelingual the loss of hearing before the development of speech and language; may include congenitally deaf and those deafened before the age of 2 years

Deafness Research Foundation (DRF) scientific society that funds research in the areas of hearing, hearing loss, and deafness

decaPascal (daPa) unit of measurement used in immittance testing; 1 daPa = 10 Pascals

decay time the amount of time it takes a gated signal to reach its minimum; usually defined from about two-thirds maximum; see also **fall time**

decibel (dB) unit of sound intensity; one-tenth of a bel; a logarithm of the sound pressure of a sound to a reference sound pressure (0.0002 dyne/cm^2) or the logarithm of the sound power to a reference sound power (10^{-16} watts/cm^2)

decompression (1) gradual decrease in atmospheric pressure to allow the body time to adapt to normal atmospheric pressure after being exposed to high levels of pressure; (2) surgical procedure for removal of pressure caused by gas or other structures

deconvolution reducing a complex waveform with multiple frequencies into individual frequencies as in spectral analysis; see also **Fourier analysis**

decruitment loudness growth is abnormally decreased resulting in the opposite effect of recruitment; possible result of the alternate binaural loudness balancing test; see also **alternate binaural loudness balancing (ABLB), recruitment**

decussation a crossing of fibers from one side of the central nervous system to the other; the corpus callosum is a major decussation

deductive reasoning reasoning from the general to the specific

deep far from the surface

deep canal hearing aid term that includes both completely-in-the-canal and peritympanic hearing aid fittings; the hearing aid terminates beyond the second bend of the external auditory canal; see also **completely-in-the-canal (CIC) hearing aid**

DEEPtrode ECochG electrocochleography measurement using DEEPtrodes where the normative value is <45%; see also **electrocochleography**

deferoxamine drug used for iron-overloaded patients who require multiple blood transfusions due to severe anemia; potentially ototoxic

degenerative disease any disease in which there is deterioration of structure and function

degraded speech speech that has been altered to reduce its acoustic redundancy; see also **extrinsic redundancy, intrinsic redundancy**

Deiter's cells several rows of supporting cells that extend from the basilar membrane and support the outer hair cells in the organ of Corti; large cup-shaped cells that lie beneath each outer hair cell; see also **phalangeal process**

delayed auditory feedback (DAF) (1) a procedure that alters the time in which a listener's speech is presented to his or her ears, affecting the rate and fluency of speech production; (2) a technique that induces dysfluency in persons who can hear the signal; useful technique to identify malingerers; (3) a technique used to induce fluency in some stutterers

delayed latency in evoked potential testing, an abnormal prolongation of the time between the stimulus onset and peak of the wave; has diagnostic significance regarding possible auditory pathology

demyelination a disease process that attacks the myelin sheath surrounding nerve fibers

dendrite a branched protoplasmic process of a neuron that conducts impulses to the cell body; dendrites form contacts with other neurons

dendritic branching dendrites branch out in various directions, thus increasing the surface area available for synapses with the axons of other nerve cells; see also **dendrite**

density that attribute of auditory sensation used to describe the volume of a sound; perception may be ordered on a scale running from dense to diffuse; the density of a tone increases with increased intensity and also with increased frequency

Denver Scale of Communication Function self-assessment inventory designed to allow patients to rate the psychological, social, vocational, and emotional handicaps imposed by their hearing loss

depolarization a change in electrical potential from a large negative value to a less negative value caused by sodium flow into a cell and ionic changes with stimulation; see also **sodium-potassium pump**

derived response a waveform that is the result of some statistical/mathematical manipulation of other waveforms; usually is a difference waveform (i.e., the difference between two waveforms); see also **mismatched negativity**

descending method procedure for establishing audiometric thresholds by decreasing the intensity of the signal from audibility to inaudibility

desired sensation level (DSL) approach approach to selecting characteristics of hearing aids in which desired sensation levels for the amplified speech spectrum are determined at each frequency for all degrees of sensorineural hearing loss; a hearing aid fitting method geared primarily for children; see also **desired sensation level (DSL-I/O)**

desired sensation level (DSL-I/O) modification of the desired sensation level approach to hearing aid fitting for nonlinear amplification; target values for soft, average, and loud speech are adjusted to consider the effects of nonlinear amplification; see also **desired sensation level (DSL)**

detection the ability to hear that sound is present

detection threshold the lowest intensity level at which a person can detect the presence of a speech or nonspeech signal; it approximates the best hearing level in the 250 to 8000 Hz audiometric frequency region; also known as **speech awareness threshold (SAT), speech detection threshold (SDT)**

developmental age a manifestation of a child's maturational growth based on the acquisition of specific developmental milestones in areas such as speech, language, motor, and social skills

Developmental Approach to Successful Listening (DASL) placement test test used with children to assess training needs and determine placement in an auditory training program by indicating which levels of developmental skills have been obtained

developmental delay lagging behind in development relative to age-matched peers

DFD Distinctive Feature Difference Test; picture identification task that assesses word-recognition ability using distinctive feature scoring

DI directivity index; a loudspeaker characteristic defined by its sound intensity increase in dB along the major axis in which the speaker is pointed as compared to omnidirectional radiation of the speaker from the same origin; DI = 10 log Q

diabetes mellitus a complex metabolic disorder resulting from a lack of insulin; may affect the central nervous system and can be associated with progressive sensorineural hearing loss; also referred to as diabetes

diabetic (1) pertaining to diabetes; (2) a person who has diabetes mellitus; see also **diabetes mellitus**

diagnosis identification of a disorder by evaluation of symptoms, case history information, physical findings, and test results

diagnostic audiology differentiates among peripheral and retrocochlear hearing losses and central auditory processing problems to classify peripheral hearing loss into types and to obtain specific information to guide the implementation of appropriate management techniques; see also **differential diagnosis, site of lesion test battery**

Diagnostic Rhyme Test (DRT) a two-alternative forced-choice, minimal pairs, monosyllabic word-recognition test that determines an individual's perception of various distinctive features of speech

diagonal vent type of vent that runs up to the sound bore and branches into it (i.e., intersects the sound bore); results in a decrease in high-frequency gain of as much as 10 dB more than a parallel vent; the effect increases as vent diameter increases

dichotic simultaneous presentation of a different sound to each ear; mostly used as a design for tests of central auditory nervous system function

Dichotic Binaural Fusion Test test of central auditory function in which the listener must repeat words when the high-frequency portion of a stimulus is presented to one ear and the low-frequency portion is presented to the other ear

Dichotic Consonant-Vowel Test test of central auditory function in which different consonant-vowel nonsense stimuli are presented simultaneously to both ears

Dichotic Digits Test a measure of central auditory function that utilizes dichotically presented numbers

Dichotic Listening Tasks tasks that present different signals to each ear

simultaneously designed to determine which ear has greater difficulty processing auditory signals when a competing message is presented to the opposite ear

Dichotic Low-Redundancy Speech Test measure of central auditory function utilizing speech signals that are degraded by modifying or distorting the frequency, temporal, or spectral characteristics of the signal; different degraded signals are presented to both ears simultaneously

dichotic monosyllabic digits a measure of central auditory function that utilizes dichotically presented numbers

dichotic nonsense syllables test of central auditory function in which different nonsense stimuli are presented simultaneously to both ears

Dichotic Rhyme Test (DRT) central auditory test utilizing rhyming monosyllabic words presented simultaneously to both ears

Dichotic Sentence Identification (DSI) an audiologic measure utilizing dichotically presented synthetic sentences to assess central auditory processing disorders

difference limen (DL) the minimal increment in a stimulus needed to produce a just-noticeable difference in sensation; the relative difference limen is the ratio of the difference limen to the value of the stimulus to which it is added; also known as **dif-**

ferential threshold, just-noticeable difference (jnd); see also **Weber fraction**

difference limen for frequency (DLF) the just-noticeable difference in the frequency of a signal; the smallest detectable difference between two frequencies

difference limen for intensity (DLI) the just-noticeable difference in the intensity of a signal; the SISI procedure is based on a patient's ability to detect small changes in the intensity of a pure tone

difference limen for time (DLT) the just-noticeable difference in the duration of a signal; the smallest detectable difference between two signal durations

difference tone a combination tone with a frequency equal to the difference between the frequencies of two primary tones or of their harmonics

difference waveform the mathematical difference between two waveforms such as observed in the mismatched negativity or in binaural interaction waveforms

differential amplifier an electrical device with two inputs that subtracts the voltage of one input from the other and then increases the amplitude (strength) of this voltage difference; used in the process of common mode rejection; see also **common mode rejection (CMR)**

differential diagnosis analyzing the results of various tests to determine the particular site of lesion for a disorder, (e.g., process used to identify if the test results suggest a cochlear lesion or a retrocochlear lesion); see also **site of lesion test battery**

differential loudness summation technique used to predict the amount and slope of an individual's hearing loss by comparing reflex thresholds to pure-tone stimuli with reflex thresholds to noise; see also **sensitivity prediction of the acoustic reflex (SPAR)**

differential threshold the minimal increment in a stimulus needed to produce a just-noticeable difference in sensation; the relative difference limen is the ratio of the difference limen to the value of the stimulus to which it is added; see also **Weber fraction**

diffraction the bending or changing of the direction of a wave that results from striking an edge or entering a narrow opening or a new medium

digital (1) the measurement of a signal in terms of a series of zeros and ones, not in terms of continuously varying numbers; (2) pertaining to a digit (e.g., finger or toe); (3) slang term used for a digital hearing aid

digital audiotape (DAT) type of magnetic tape recording that uses digital signals that have been converted from analog inputs

digital circuits circuits that are characterized by signal measurement into discrete numbers rather than a continuous sample; see also **digital signal processing (DSP)**

digital hearing aid hearing aid utilizing digital technology to process the signal; see also **digital, digital signal processing (DSP) hearing aid**

digital signal processing (DSP) conversion of continuous time analog signals into sampled discrete time data points (numbers); allows for the use of multiple algorithms for processing signals; see also **digital**

digital signal processing (DSP) hearing aid hearing aid that utilizes digital signal processing; the signal is converted from an analog to a digital signal, it is manipulated according to a processing algorithm, and then the signal is converted back into an analog signal; also known as **digital hearing aid**

digital-to-analog converter (DAC) an electronic device that converts a series of numeric values that are processed by a computer into a continuously varying electrical signal; see also **analog-to-digital converter (ADC)**

digitally controlled analog (DCA) hearing aid a hearing aid that has analog components but is controlled digitally; commonly referred to as programmable

digitally programmable hearing instrument digitally controlled analog hearing aid; a hearing aid that has analog components but is con-

trolled digitally; commonly referred to as programmable

digitized speech storage of a person's actual words and sentences in the form of "digitized" sounds which are recorded by a peripheral device that converts sound input from a stereo system, an instrument, or a microphone into a form that a computer can process, store, and play back as speech synthesis

dihydrostreptomycin antibiotic drug that can be ototoxic

diotic (1) the condition in which the sound stimulus presented at each ear is identical; (2) presenting the same sound to both ears simultaneously (*di* = two, *otic* = ears)

DIP Discrimination by the Identification of Pictures; a pediatric picture identification speech audiometry task for very young children

diplacusis hearing a pure-tone signal as having a different pitch in the two ears; hearing a pure-tone signal in one ear as a chord or noise; see also **binaural diplacusis**

dipole a neuron with a positive and negative pole; an electrical source (as in the brain) with an axis that has a positive voltage charge at one end and a negative voltage charge at the other end

direct audio input (DAI) a circuit in some hearing aids that directly connects them to some assistive listening devices and also to radios and televisions

direct current (DC) electric current that only flows in one direction in a conductor or circuit

direction-changing positional nystagmus abnormal nystagmus that changes the direction of the nystagmus beat with the head held in a stable position; sign of a central lesion

direction-fixed positional nystagmus type of abnormal nystagmus that continues to beat in the same direction despite changes in head position; sign of a peripheral vestibular lesion

directional hearing the ability to determine the location of sounds within (lateralization) and outside (localization) the head

directional hearing aids amplification devices that employ directional microphones to improve reception of signals at the front relative to those from the rear

directional microphone (DMic) a microphone that is more sensitive to sound coming from one direction than from another direction; also known as **unidirectional microphone**

directional preponderance comparison of the amplitude of right-beating nystagmus (right warm (RW) + left cool (LC)) to the amplitude of left-beating nystagmus (right cool (RC) + left warm (LW)) in caloric stimulation during electronystagmographic vestibular assessment

directivity factor (Q) a loudspeaker characteristic that can be calculated from its directivity index; log Q = DI/10; see also **directivity index (DI)**

directivity index (DI) a loudspeaker characteristic defined by its sound intensity increase in dB along the major axis in which the speaker is pointed as compared to omnidirectional radiation of the speaker from the same origin; DI = 10 log Q; see also **directivity factor (Q)**

disability the consequences of an impairment on the functional performance and activity of an individual (e.g., difficulty hearing in noisy places as a result of a hearing impairment)

disarticulation (1) the separation of a joint; (2) a break in the ossicular chain; also known as ossicular disarticulation or **ossicular discontinuity**

discharge rate the rate of energy release from a neuron; how quickly a neuron can fire (respond to stimulation)

discomfort level level at which sound is perceived to be uncomfortable; a level of loudness that a patient would not want to listen to for an extended period of time; see also **loudness discomfort level (LDL)**

discrete Fourier transform a version of the Fourier transform applicable to a finite number of discrete samples; see also **fast Fourier transform**

discrete-frequency signals individual distinct frequencies; not part of a complex tone

discrimination the ability to hear that one sound is the same or different from another

Discrimination After Training Test test that assesses recognition of words on the basis of nonphonetic or prosodic cues; performance reflects perception of temporal and amplitude changes in speech

Discrimination by the Identification of Pictures (DIP) Test a pediatric picture identification speech audiometry task for very young children

discrimination score outdated term referring to the percentage of monosyllabic words correctly repeated when presented at an intensity well above the speech recognition threshold; more appropriate term is **word-recognition score (WRS)**

disequilibrium loss of balance; inability to maintain an upright posture

disorder abnormality in general functioning of a structure or system

dispenser the Food and Drug Administration term for any person who sells hearing aids; includes ear, nose, and throat physicians, audiologists, and hearing aid specialists

displacement (1) a change in position; specified by calculating the distance from a reference or starting position to a new or ending position; (2) in amplitude, refers to the distance that an acoustic sound wave is deflected from the zero crossing point; (3) in cochlear physiology, refers to the deflection of the basilar membrane to provide information regarding the frequency of a signal

dispraxia a disorder caused by damage to the brain and characterized by an inability to execute a motor response, especially a speech act

dissonance the phenomenon in which tones presented together produce a harsh or unpleasant sensation; see also **consonance**

distal away (distant) from the center or medial portion of a structure (e.g., the cochlea is at the distal end of the auditory nerve); opposite of proximal

distinctive feature property that distinguishes a given unit (e.g., phoneme) from others

Distinctive Feature Difference (DFD) Test picture identification task that assesses word-recognition ability using distinctive feature scoring

distortion an undesirable change in wave-form; perversion of a sound or waveform resulting in false reproduction; see also **acoustic distortion**

distortion, amplitude erroneous reproduction of sound waves in which the output is not linear with respect to the input; often occurs when the system is saturated

distortion, harmonic additional spurious frequencies (nonlinearities) in the output signal that were not present in the input signal but that are related to the fundamental frequency; in a hearing aid expressed as a percentage of the total signal at the point of measurement; measured at 500, 800, and 1600 Hz

distortion, intermodulation additional frequencies produced when two frequencies are presented to the ear simultaneously; the output contains the 2 frequencies of the input, plus arithmetic additions or subtractions of the input frequencies

distortion product (DP) otoacoustic emission recorded in the external ear canal that represents the cubic distortion product (2f1–f2) following simultaneous presentation of combinations of two pure tones (f1 and f2); see also **cubic distortion product**

distortion product otoacoustic emission (DPOAE) otoacoustic emission recorded in the external ear canal that represents the cubic distortion product (2f1–f2) following simultaneous presentation of combinations of two pure tones (f1 and f2); see also **cubic distortion product**

distortional bone conduction one of the three mechanisms of bone-conduction hearing; vibrations of the skull are transmitted directly to the inner ear which produce biomechanical events that result in activation of the cochlear hair cells

Distraction Test behavioral test of hearing for infants of about 7 months of age; auditory stimuli are presented at ear level and out of the child's visual field; a response is reported when the infant's head turns toward the sound source

diuretics loop diuretics commonly used in patients with heart failure and peripheral edema; may cause reversible high-frequency hearing loss; may be irreversible if used along with aminoglycosides

Dix-Hallpike maneuver brisk movement of the patient's head by the examiner into hanging right or hanging left positions; used in electronystagmography testing to determine the presence of nystagmus after a positioning movement; also known as **Hallpike maneuver**

dizziness general term referring to an inability to maintain normal balance; can be described as lightheadedness, sensation of spinning, vertigo, etc.

dizziness handicap inventory a questionnaire designed to measure the physical, functional, and psychological impact of balance and dizziness symptoms

DL difference limen; the minimal increment in a stimulus needed to produce a just-noticeable difference in sensation; the relative difference limen is the ratio of the difference limen to the value of the stimulus to which it is added; also known as **just-noticeable difference (jnd)**; see also **Weber fraction**

DLF difference limen for frequency; the just-noticeable difference in the frequency of a signal; the smallest detectable difference between two frequencies

DLI difference limen for intensity; the just-noticeable difference in the intensity of a signal; the SISI procedure is based on a patient's ability to detect small changes in the intensity of a pure tone

DLT difference limen for time; the just-noticeable difference in the duration of a signal; the smallest detectable difference between two signal durations

DMic directional microphone; a microphone that is more sensitive to sound coming from one direction than from another direction; also known as **unidirectional microphone**

DNE did not evaluate

DNT did not test

doctor of audiology (AuD) an earned postbaccalaureate professional degree primarily designed to prepare audiologists to be competent to perform the wide array of diagnostic, remedial, and other services associated with the current practice of audiology

Doerfler-Stewart Test a test useful in confirming malingering (functional or inorganic hearing loss) that assesses speech recognition in quiet versus noise

doppler effect phenomenon in which the pitch of a sound seems to decrease as the sound source moves away from the individual

dorsal posterior; pertaining to the back

dorsal cochlear nucleus (DCN) dorsal (posterior) division of the cochlear nuclei; exhibits the greatest diversity in response relative to the other cochlear nuclei; dominated by inhibition; involved in processing spatial or spectral information needed in the detection of threshold level signals embedded in a narrow spectral band or in complex feature detection during speech; see also **cochlear nuclei**

dosimeter a type of sound level meter (can be portable) that can read sound levels directly or store a sequence of sound levels, categorize them in various ways, and transfer those data to a printer; often used to obtain an individual's personal total (dose) of noise exposure over a specified period of time

dosimetry the process of obtaining an individual's personal total (dose) of noise exposure over a specified period of time; uses a dosimeter that can read sound levels directly or store a sequence of sound levels over a designated time period

Down syndrome a chromosomal, congenital condition that results from the presence of an extra chromosome on chromosome 21; characterized by flat occiput, upslanting eyes, strabismus, small ears, large protruding tongue, short neck, micropenis, inguinal hernias, brachydactyly, short 5th finger, hyperextensible joints, obesity, cognitive impairment, small teeth, maxillary hypoplasia, heart anomalies, immune deficiency, blood disorders, occasional cleft lip and palate, airway obstruction, and hypertrophic lymphoid tissue; hearing is usually normal although conductive hearing loss secondary to chronic otitis media is common; also referred to as **trisomy 21**

down-beating nystagmus a type of vertical nystagmus in which the fast phase beats downward; can be pathological

downward spread of masking the masking of low-frequency components in a signal as a result of a spread of energy from intense high-frequency components

DP distortion product; otoacoustic emission recorded in the external ear canal that represents the cubic distortion product (2f1–f2) following simultaneous presentation of combinations of two pure tones (f1 and f2)

DPgram a graph of distortion product otoacoustic emission amplitude in the ear canal (in dB SPL) as a function of the frequencies of the stimulus tones (in Hz)

DPOAE distortion product otoacoustic emission; otoacoustic emission recorded in the external ear canal that represents the cubic distortion product (2f1–f2) following simultaneous presentation of combinations of two pure tones (f1 and f2)

DR dynamic range; the difference in dB between hearing threshold and discomfort level; the auditory area that is used when fitting amplification devices

DRC damage risk criteria; the maximum safe allowable noise levels for different bandwidths as determined by the Occupational Safety and Health Administration; the level of sound to which a population may be exposed for a specified time with a specified risk of hearing loss

dri-aid kit an accessory that can be used with hearing aids to remove any moisture build-up in the devices; useful for those who perspire frequently

drop attack a very abrupt and violent attack of vertigo; usually causes the patient to fall; possible symptom of Ménière's disease; see also **Lermoyez's syndrome**

DRT Diagnostic Rhyme Test; a two-alternative forced-choice, minimal pairs, monosyllabic word-recognition test that determines an individual's perception of various distinctive features of speech

DSI Dichotic Sentence Identification; an audiologic measure utilizing dichotically presented synthetic sentences to assess central auditory processing disorders

DSL desired sensation level; approach to selecting characteristics of hearing aids in which desired sensation levels for the amplified speech spectrum are determined at each frequency for all degrees of sensorineural hearing loss; a hearing aid fitting method geared primarily for children

DSL (I/O) desired sensation level (input/output); modification of the desired sensation level approach to hearing aid fitting for nonlinear amplification; target values for soft, average, and loud speech are adjusted to consider the effects of nonlinear amplification

DSP digital signal processing; conversion of continuous time analog signals into sampled discrete time data points (numbers); allows for the use of multiple algorithms for processing signals

ductus reuniens a tube containing endolymph that connects the saccule of the vestibular apparatus with the scala media of the cochlea

duration the length of time (usually in ms) from the beginning to the end of a stimulus

Duration Patterns Test test of temporal ordering in which the frequency of the tones is held at a constant 1000 Hz and duration is the factor to be discriminated

dynamic platform posturography a type of vestibular assessment that focuses on the function of the balance system in maintaining postural stability in a variety of simulated conditions; computer-induced platform movements evaluate motor responses that include strength, symmetry, and latency of muscle response; see also **sensory organization test**

dynamic range (DR) the difference in dB between hearing threshold and discomfort level; the auditory area that is used when fitting amplification devices

dynamic range compression a type of compression circuitry that can provide much greater amplification for low-intensity signals than for medium-intensity signals while providing less or no gain for high-intensity signals; useful for individuals with a very narrow dynamic range; has a low compression threshold; see also **syllabic compression**

dyne unit of force required to move 1 gram 1 centimeter per second

dyne/cm² the unit of sound pressure; a dyne is defined as the force that will produce a change of velocity of 1 centimeter per second in a gram mass in 1 second

dysacusis suprathreshold hearing impairment in which loud sounds can cause pain or discomfort

dysarthria any of several motor speech disorders that originate in the central or peripheral nervous system; any disturbance of articulation due to paralysis, incoordination, and the like

dysmetria an inaccuracy in horizontal saccadic movement of the eyes; may be considered undershoot or overshoot

dysmorphology the study of congenital anomalies for the purposes of diagnosis, delineation, and classification

dysphagia abnormality of swallowing

dysphasia a disorder caused by damage to the brain and characterized by an impairment of language production and/or comprehension

dysphonia a voice disorder of phonation characterized by a loss of voice; also known as **aphonia**

dysplasia an abnormality in the development of tissue or organs

E

E-wave expectancy wave; a wave seen as part of the contingent negative variation that results in the "readiness" of the individual to make a response

EAA Educational Audiology Association; professional organization comprised mainly of educational audiologists

EAC external auditory canal; the canal of the outer ear leading from the concha to the tympanic membrane

EAM external auditory meatus; the external auditory canal; the canal that conducts sound vibrations from the auricle to the tympanic membrane

ear anatomical structure responsible for hearing and balance; consists of an outer ear, middle ear, inner ear (including cochlear and vestibular systems)

ear, cauliflower disorder of the external ear caused by repeated trauma to the pinna; results in thickening of the cartilage and skin which diminishes the visibility of the traditional landmarks of the pinna

ear, external the portion of the ear that is normally visible; major components include the pinna, concha, tragus, and external auditory canal

ear, glue serous otitis media or otitis media with effusion; fluid is very thick and viscous with the consistency of glue

ear, inner the medialmost peripheral structure of the ear housing the sense organ for hearing (cochlea) and the sense organs for balance (vestibule and semicircular canals)

ear, middle an air-filled tympanic cavity within the mastoid portion of the temporal bone that contains the three auditory ossicles; communicates with the eustachian tube and the mastoid air cells

ear, nontest (NTE) the ear not intended to be tested during an audiometric procedure; the ear receiving the masking noise during clinical masking

ear, nose, and throat (ENT) physician medical professional whose specialty is the diagnosis and treatment of diseases of the ear, nose, and throat; also known as **otolaryngologist, otologist, otorhinolaryngologist**

ear, outer peripheral part of the auditory mechanism that includes the pinna, the concha, and the external auditory canal

ear, swimmer's informal term for external otitis resulting from infection transmitted in the water of a swimming pool; see also **external otitis, otitis externa**

ear, test (TE) the ear to be evaluated in audiometric procedures

Ear and Hearing scientific journal of the American Auditory Society

ear canal the canal of the outer ear leading from the concha to the tympanic membrane; see also **external auditory canal (EAC)**

ear canal abrasion laceration or cut of the external auditory canal due to foreign bodies, hearing aids, etc.

ear canal acoustics the unaided frequency response as measured in a human ear canal; represents the combined acoustic effects of the pinna, concha, and external ear canal resonances; see also **ear canal resonance**

ear canal dynamics (1) vibrant and active link to the human sense of hearing that the ear canal possesses; (2) refers to changes in the ear canal shape as a result of jaw movement; see also **ear canal acoustics, ear canal resonance, external ear effects (EEE)**

ear canal resonance natural acoustic amplification in the external auditory canal of about 10 dB seen in the 2000-to-7000 Hz frequency region; amount of resonance and its frequency peak vary individually; see also **external ear effects (EEE)**

ear canal volume (ECV) measurement used in immittance audiometry to determine the volume of the ear canal; also used in calculation of static admittance; see also **admittance, static admittance**

ear candles hollow cones, about 7 to 10 inches long, made of beeswax and cloth; used to remove excessive cerumen; see also **cerumen management**

ear cup anomaly of the auricle involving a downward folding and deficiency of the superior aspect of the helix; often associated with maldevelopment of the concha

ear impression mold made from a patient's external auditory canal and concha for the purposes of fabricating ear plugs, earmolds, and hearing aids

ear infection inflammation of the ear; can affect all portions of the ear (e.g., outer, middle, and inner ears)

ear simulator a device that takes into account the equivalent volumes or loading of the receiver of the hearing instrument with the same average frequency-dependent impedance of the human ear in the hearing frequency range

ear trumpet historic amplification device once used to increase amplification of sound funneled into the ear

ear wax a waxy secretion of the ceruminous and sebaceous glands within the external auditory meatus; lubricates and cleanses the external auditory canal; also referred to as **cerumen**

ear wax removal the extraction of cerumen usually through manual extraction, suctioning, or irrigation; see also **cerumen management**

ear wax solvents any cerumen solvent; commercially available products and other agents used to soften cerumen (e.g., mineral oil); see also **cerumen softening**

earache a pain in the ear characterized as sharp, burning, or dull

eardrum the membranous separation between the outer and middle ears; responsible for initiating the mechanical impedance-matching process of the middle ear; has three layers: cutaneous, fibrous, mucous; also known as **tympanic membrane (TM)**

earhook the curved apparatus of a behind-the-ear hearing aid and some other types of listening devices that connects the device case to the earmold and hooks over the pinna

early intervention concerns the management of a child with a hearing loss before the primary school years, especially before 2 years of age to insure normal speech and language development

early latency response an objective test that measures the electrical potential produced in response to sound stimuli by the synchronous discharge of the first- through sixth-order neurons in the auditory nerve

and brainstem; includes electrococochleography and auditory brainstem responses that occur within the first 10 to 12 ms after stimulus onset

Early Speech Perception (ESP) Test test of closed-set perception of single words through auditory-only cues; used with young children who are profoundly hearing impaired and have limited vocabulary and language skills

earmold fitting that couples a hearing aid to the ear; major types or variations of earmolds include canal, open, standard, shell, skeleton, and vented versus nonvented

earmold, canal type of earmold that fits primarily into the external auditory canal leaving the concha area of the pinna open

earmold, canal-lock a canal earmold with a built-in extension that lies along the bottom of the concha to keep the earmold in place

earmold, custom earmold that is made from an ear impression to fit the individual ear specifically

earmold, nonoccluding an open earmold that markedly reduces low-frequency amplification by allowing low-frequency energy to enter the ear without being amplified; useful device for a high-frequency steeply sloping hearing loss; also useful in ears that require substantial ventilation because it does not close off the ear canal

earmold, open an earmold fitting consisting of only a piece of tubing inserted into the ear canal to deliver sound from a hearing aid; sometimes referred to as a tube fit

earmold, shell type of earmold that completely fills the concha; can be made of silicone or lucite materials

earmold, skeleton type of earmold that fits around the outer portion of the concha but does not completely fill it

earmold acoustics the influence of an earmold's configuration and structure, such as bore length and venting, on the acoustic properties of the sound delivered to the tympanic membrane by a listening device; see also **external ear effects (EEE)**

earmold bore a hole in an earmold through which an amplified auditory signal travels

earmold impression cast made of the concha and ear canal to custom-fit hearing protection and hearing aids; also known as **ear impression**

earmold vent a canal drilled in the earmold for the purpose of aeration or alteration of the audio signal; see also **vent, venting**

earmuffs a kind of ear protection, made of earcups that seal around the ear for the purpose of sound attenuation; see also **hearing protection device (HPD)**

earphone a device for presenting a sound stimulus to the ear that consists of an acoustic transducer for converting an electrical signal into an acoustic signal and a cushion that couples the transducer to the ear; see also **insert earphone, supra-aural earphones**

earplugs a kind of ear protection, consisting of a material that is inserted into the ear canal for the purpose of sound attenuation; various types of materials are inserted into the external auditory canal to seal it off from ambient noise (e.g., semi-aural protectors); see also **hearing protection device (HPD)**

ec- prefix: out of

echo wave that has been reflected or otherwise returned with sufficient magnitude and delay to be detected as a wave distinct from that directly transmitted; see also **otoacoustic emission (OAE)**

ECochG electrocochleography; early evoked responses originating from the cochlea and auditory nerve; includes the summating potential, the cochlear microphonic, and the N1 or action potential component; occurs within the first 1.5 to 2 ms after stimulation

ecto- prefix: on the outer side; toward the surface

ectodermal abnormalities anomalies occurring in the ectodermal layer during embryological development; often associated with syndromes as well as hearing loss

ECV ear canal volume; measurement used in immittance audiometry to determine the volume of the ear canal; also used in calculation of static admittance

ED-NST Edgerton-Danhauer Nonsense Syllable Test; a 25-item list of meaningless consonant-vowel-consonant-vowel items presented in open-set to assess listeners' phoneme identification

edema inflammation of a tissue structure or area due to an abnormal accumulation of fluid

Edgerton-Danhauer Nonsense Syllable Test (ED-NST) a 25-item list of meaningless consonant-vowel-consonant-vowel items presented in open-set to assess listeners' phoneme identification

educational audiologist an audiologist responsible for the diagnosis and management of children (usually in the schools) who have some degree of hearing impairment

educational audiology subspecialty of audiology for audiologists who are responsible for the diagnosis and management of children who have hearing loss

Educational Audiology Association (EAA) professional organization comprised mainly of educational audiologists

Edwards syndrome autosomal recessive disorder characterized by short stature, obesity, nystagmus, blindness, cognitive impairment, and diabetes mellitus; associated with progressive sensorineural hearing loss; also known as **trisomy 18**

EEE external ear effects; the unaided frequency response as measured in a human ear canal; represents the combined acoustic effects of the pinna, concha, and external ear canal resonances

EEG (1) electroencephalogram; graphical representation of the electrical activity of the brain using electroencephalography; (2) electroencephalography; process of recording background electrical activity during evoked response measurement

effective masking (EM) the least amount of narrowband noise that is theoretically required to eliminate cross hearing; the hearing threshold level to which an ear will be shifted by a given amount of noise (i.e., refers to amount of threshold shift provided by a given level of noise); refers to the level of the test signal that a masker will just-mask; does not refer to the intensity level of the masker itself; see also **masking**

efferent transmission of neural information from the central nervous system out to a sensory receptor

efferent auditory system pathway from the auditory cortex to the cochlea that parallels the afferent system; includes both excitatory and inhibitory activity and has significant implications for function such as detection of a signal in a background of noise

efferent fibers motor fibers that carry impulses from the central nervous system to muscles and organs;

in the cochlea, efferent fibers are called **inner spiral** and **tunnel radial**

efferent nuclei nuclei in the efferent system that send tonotopically ordered fibers to the cochlea; include the medial geniculate body, inferior colliculus, and superior olivary complex; the majority of efferent fibers cross from the superior olivary complex to the contralateral cochlea bypassing the cochlear nucleus; see also **efferent olivocochlear system**

efferent olivocochlear system contains cell bodies and axons originating from specialized nuclei within and surrounding the brainstem superior olivary region; these descending centrifugal fiber bundles provide direct, bilateral input to the cochlea via the anatomically segregated medial and lateral efferent divisions; see also **efferent nuclei**

efferent suppression the reduction in otoacoustic emission amplitude when contralateral acoustic stimulation is generated; believed to be a result of the function of the efferent auditory system; also known as **contralateral suppression**

efficacy effectiveness, efficiency, and effects of treatments; documenting treatment efficacy requires demonstrating that a particular treatment produces the desired outcomes or behavior change in an efficient manner (e.g., cost-effective) as a result of the treatment

effusion exudation of body fluid from the middle ear membranous walls as a result of inflammation; see also **otitis media with effusion (OME)**

VIIIth cranial nerve the auditory-vestibular nerve; consists of two sets of fibers: the anterior branch or cochlear nerve and the posterior branch or vestibular nerve; conducts neural signals from the inner ear to the brain; see also **acoustic nerve, auditory nerve, auditory-vestibular nerve**

VIIIth nerve tumor tumor originating from nerve fibers of cranial nerve VIII; usually occurs on the vestibular branch of the nerve; see also **acoustic nerve tumor, auditory nerve tumor**

EIN equivalent input noise; electroacoustic quantity that expresses the level of internally generated random noise that occurs at each amplifier stage in a hearing aid; measured with the volume control at reference test position by calculating the average coupler sound pressure levels (SPLs) using a 60-dB SPL input and then removing the 60-dB SPL input signal and recording the SPL in the coupler caused by the inherent noise

elasticity the quality of a material that causes it to return to its original position after being distended

ELC equal loudness contours; curves plotted as a function of frequency showing the sound pressure level required to produce a given loudness level for a typical listener; referenced to a 1000-Hz tone at 40 dB SPL

electret microphone a type of condenser microphone with a diaphragm made of a dielectric material that exhibits permanent polarity, as in a magnet

electric response audiometry (ERA) an older, general term for auditory evoked responses; see also **auditory evoked responses (AER)**

electrical field an area surrounding a generator from which the spread of electrical activity occurs

electrical potential (1) a difference in electrical charge measured between two electrodes; (2) in evoked potential measurement, the source of electrical potentials is stimulus-evoked activity in sensory portions of the peripheral or central nervous system; (3) each cell in the body pumps ions across cell membranes to keep an electrical potential difference across the membrane: ions travel in and out of a cell through channels in the membrane; passive channels allow free movement; chemically gated channels are selective

electro-oculography (EOG) the recording of eye movement with the use of electrodes placed at both the outer edges and inner edges of the eye for horizontal eye movement, and above and beneath the eye for vertical eye movement; recording is DC coupled so that movement of the eye causes changes in the electrical field, which results in electrical activity; used as the basis for **electronystagmography (ENG)**

electroacoustic conversion of an acoustic signal to an electrical signal or an electrical signal to an acoustic signal

electroacoustic analysis measurements that determine whether a hearing aid and other listening devices are functioning according to the manufacturer's specifications

electroacoustic measures for amplification measurements that determine whether a hearing aid and other listening devices are functioning according to the manufacturer's specifications; also known as **electroacoustic analysis**

electrocochleogram a plot of the results obtained during electrocochleography displaying the magnitudes of the summating potential, cochlear microphonic, and action potential as a function of time

electrocochleography(ECochG) early evoked responses originating from the cochlea and auditory nerve; includes the summating potential, the cochlear microphonic, and the N1 or action potential component; occurs within 1.5 to 2 ms after stimulation

electrode a metal device (cup, needle, plate) that makes contact with the body; conducts bioelectrical activity from the body via a wire lead to recording equipment in all sensory 0evoked responses; may be used to deliver electrical stimulation to the body in somatosensory evoked response measurement

electrode, active usually refers to the noninverting electrode in auditory evoked potential measurements

electrode, bipolar electrode or electrode pair that measures electrical events (action potentials) at two distinct points; in electrophysiology, the resulting signals are usually supplied one to an inverting input, the other to a noninverting input of a differential amplifier

electrode, common the relationship of one electrode to a second electrode; usually refers to the noninverting electrode

electrode, ground the electrode in an electrophysiologic set-up that attaches the patient to the ground

electrode, inverting usually the second electrode in an electrode pair in evoked response measurement; also referred to as inactive or reference electrode; also known as **indifferent electrode**

electrode, monopolar the electrode of a pair that is detecting the response while the second electrode is inactive

electrode, noninverting a primary or active electrode usually leading to the positive voltage input of a differential amplifier; the vertex electrode in auditory evoked response measurements

electrode, surface an electrode placed on the skin's surface for audiometric testing

electrode, transtympanic a needle electrode that is inserted through the tympanic membrane and rests on the promontory at the medial end of the middle ear; used for electrophysiology measurements

electrode array (1) arrangement of electrodes for cochlear implants; (2) placement locations for electrodes in electrophysiologic assessments; also known as **electrode montage**

electrode impedance check process followed to check the interelectrode impedance for evoked potential testing; should be less than 5000 ohms to ensure proper contact with the skin; see also **impedance**

electrode montage (1) arrangement of electrodes for cochlear implants; (2) placement locations for electrodes in electrophysiologic assessments; also known as **electrode array**

electrodermal audiometry outdated test procedure that consisted of accompanying clearly audible signals with a small electric shock; anticipation of the shock resulted in a drop in skin resistance detected by surface electrodes; procedure was used with suspected malingerers, but is no longer used today

electroencephalogram (EEG) graphic representation of the electrical activity of the brain using electroencephalography

electroencephalograph an electronic device used to measure the ongoing electrical activity arising from the brain in electroencephalography

electroencephalography (EEG) process of recording background electrical activity during evoked response measurement

electromagnetic field a magnetic field induced around a wire when an electrical current passes through it; type of signal used in induction loop systems and telephones (telecoils)

electromagnetic induction the use of a copper wire to set up an electromagnetic field to transmit a signal; type of induction used in induction loop systems and telephones (telecoils)

electromyography (EMG) electrophysiologic recording of muscle activity, usually with hook electrodes embedded in muscle

electroneuronography (ENoG) electrophysiologic recording of facial nerve or muscle activity

electronystagmograph electronic instrumentation designed to record eye movements during electronystagmography

electronystagmography (ENG) a test of vestibular (balance) functioning in which nystagmus (eyeball movements) is recorded electrophysiologically during stimulation of the vestibular system; based on electrooculography; has a battery of tests divided into three groups: ocular motor, positional, and caloric tests

electrophonic effect the ability of an alternating current, of suitable frequency and intensity, to arouse a sensation of hearing when passed through a person's head

electrophysiology the study of electrical phenomena associated with cellular physiology (e.g., auditory evoked responses)

electrostatic field an electric field produced by electric charges that are stationary or at rest

electrostatic noise electrostatic fields capacitively coupled into cables from electrical charges caused by motor armature sparks, neon of fluorescent light gas discharge, and other sources

electrotactile device device that uses electrical signals to stimulate the sense of touch or vibration

EM effective masking; the least amount of narrowband noise that is theoretically required to eliminate cross hearing; the hearing threshold level to which an ear will be shifted by a given amount of noise (i.e., refers to amount of threshold shift provided by a given level of noise); refers to the level of the test signal that a masker will just-mask; does not refer to the intensity level of the masker itself; see also **masking**

eminence projection or prominence, especially of a bone

EMG electromyography; electrophysiologic recording of muscle activity, usually with hook electrodes embedded in muscle

en-, em- prefix: in

encephalitis an inflammatory condition of the brain that is often caused by a virus

encephalopathy a general term meaning any brain disease

endemic a condition or a disease found in a given community that prevails continually in a region, thereby distinguished from epidemic; see also **epidemic**

endo- prefix: toward the interior; within

endocochlear potential a type of cochlear potential that reflects the constant positive potential difference between the scala media and the peripheral scalae vestibuli and tympani; see also **endolymphatic potential, resting potential**

endogenous (1) growing from within the organism; arising from causes internal to the organism rather than imposed from the environment; (2) refers to evoked potentials generated by an internal response to an external event and is usually due to perception or cognition; the nature of the response changes according to the internalization of the event, not the dimensions of the external event; see also **exogenous**

endogenous hearing impairment a hearing impairment caused by genetic factors that have various probabilities of being passed on to children or to grandchildren

endolymph a pale, clear fluid within the scala media of the cochlea thought to be secreted by the stria vascularis; Latin word for clear fluid; see also **cortilymph, perilymph**

endolymphatic duct duct arising from the saccule of the vestibule, terminating blindly in the petrous portion of the temporal bone; ends in the endolymphatic sac that lies in the subarachnoid space

endolymphatic hydrops excessive accumulation of endolymph in the scala media; may cause fluctuating sensorineural hearing loss and vertigo; also known as **labyrinthine hydrops;** see also **cochlear hydrops, Ménière's disease**

endolymphatic potential cochlear electrical potential within the endolymph and its cells; endolymph in the scala media relative to the perilymph in the scala vestibuli and scala tympani is positive: +70 to 90 mV (± 20 mV); see also **endocochlear potential**

endolymphatic sac a sac at the end of the endolymphatic duct; part of the membranous labyrinth of the inner ear that contains endolymph; lies in the subarachnoid space; often becomes compressed in Ménière's disease due to an increase in endolymph

endolymphatic shunt treatment for Ménière's disease that redirects the flow of endolymph to release the pressure in the scala media; see also **Ménière's disease**

endoscopy visualization of internal organs and body cavities using an illuminated optic instrument (endoscope)

endosteal hyperostosis sclerosing bone dysplasia that results in auditory impairment

ENG electronystagmography; a test of vestibular (balance) functioning in which nystagmus (eyeball movements) is recorded electrophysiologically during stimulation of the vestibular system; based on electrooculography; has a battery of tests divided into three groups: ocular motor, positional, and caloric tests

ENoG electroneuronography; electrophysiologic recording of facial nerve or muscle activity

ENT ear, nose, and throat physician; medical professional whose specialty is the diagnosis and treatment of diseases of the ear, nose, and throat; also referred to as **otologist, otolaryngologist, or otorhinolaryngologist**

ento- prefix: toward the interior; within

envelope in acoustics, the shape of the overall waveform of an acoustic stimulus that follows the rise, plateau, and fall portions of the stimulus; also known as **waveform envelope**

environmental microphone microphone on an FM system that allows the user to hear sounds in the environment in addition to the FM signal; useful in the classroom if the child needs to hear the teacher (FM signal) as well as the other students in the classroom

Environmental Sounds Test (EST) objective measure of environmental sound recognition; often used as part of an auditory training program for individuals with minimal auditory capabilities

EOAE evoked otoacoustic emission; otoacoustic emission measured in the external auditory canal in response to some evoking stimulus (either a click or two tones presented simultaneously); includes **distortion product (DPOAE), click evoked otoacoustic emissions (CEOAE), transient otoacoustic emissions (TEOAE), and stimulus frequency otoacoustic emissions (SFOAE)**

EOG electro-oculography; the recording of eye movement with the use of electrodes placed at both the outer edges and inner edges of the eye for horizontal eye movement and above and beneath the eye for vertical eye movement; recording is DC coupled so that movement of the eye causes changes in the electrical field, which results in electrical activity; the basis for **electronystagmography (ENG)**

EP evoked potential; a series of electrical charges occurring in the peripheral and central nervous system following stimulation of an end organ or peripheral nerve

ep-, epi- prefix: on or above

epidemic a condition or disease that attacks many people in a community simultaneously but is not continually present, thereby distinguished from endemic; see also **endemic**

epidemiology the study of the incidence, distribution, and control of disease in a population and the significant factors controling its presence or absence

epidermal cyst an accumulation of fluid under the skin; often occurs in the external ear

epitympanic above the tympanic membrane (eardrum)

epitympanic recess the superior region of the middle ear space above the superior margin of the tympanic membrane; houses the head of the malleus and the body of the incus; also known as **attic**; see also **epitympanum**

epitympanum upper part of the middle ear space or attic; see also **antrum**; also known as **epitympanic recess**

epoch a time period, such as the analysis time in evoked response measurement

Epstein syndrome autosomal dominant disorder characterized by progressive renal failure, thrombocytopenia; associated with progressive sensorineural hearing loss with onset in childhood (usually after age 5), usually resulting in moderate to severe hearing loss

equal energy rule of noise exposure in calculating temporary threshold shift with noise exposure, for each doubling of a sound's duration, the sound power must be decreased by 3 dB to maintain equal threshold shift; also known as the **3-dB rule**

equal loudness contours (ELC) curves plotted as a function of frequency showing the sound pressure level required to produce a given loudness level for a typical listener; referenced to a 1000-Hz pure tone at 40 dB SPL; also known as **Fletcher-Munson curves**

equalizer (1) a device that excites a signal to enhance it in some way; (2) a device that can make adjustments across frequency that equalize output

equilibration the process by which the activity in a nerve subjected to repetitive stimulation achieves a steady state; the initial burst of activity in a nerve, as measured by the action potential, is greater than the final level of activity reached after prolonged stimulation

equilibrium a condition of balance; see also **balance**

equipotentiality having equal electrical charge

equivalent input noise (EIN) level electroacoustic quantity that expresses the level of internally generated random noise that occurs at each amplifier stage in a hearing aid; measured with the volume control at reference test position by calculating the average coupler sound pressure levels (SPLs) using a 60-dB SPL input and then removing the 60-dB SPL input signal and recording the SPL in the coupler caused by the inherent noise

equivalent level (Leq) a time-weighted energy average that represents the total sound energy experienced over a given period of time as if the sound was unvarying; also known as **equivalent sound level (Leq)**

equivalent sound level (Leq) a time-weighted energy average that represents the total sound energy experienced over a given period of time as if the sound was unvarying; also known as **equivalent level (Leq)**

equivalent volume a method of approximating the compliance component of aural immittance based on the volume of air with the physical property equivalent to the middle ear system

ER-3A insert earphones type of earphone that is inserted into the ear canal; uses disposable adult- and pediatric-sized recovery foam plugs for appropriate fit; have greater interaural attenuation than supra-aural earphones; also known as **insert earphones**

ERA electric response audiometry; an older, general term for auditory evoked responses; also known as **evoked response audiometry (ERA)**

erg unit of measurement for work

ERP event-related potential; term used to describe certain evoked responses, such as the 40-Hz response or the P300 response, that are elicited with stimuli other than a simple sequence of brief duration clicks or tones; usually elicited by an endogenous stimulus representing high-level processing (e.g., cognition)

erythema redness due to inflammation

erythroblastosis fetalis a grave hemolytic disease of the newborn that usually results from development of antibodies to the Rh factor of the blood in an Rh-negative mother carrying an Rh-positive fetus

erythromycin antibiotic agent used to treat many bacterial infections; can be ototoxic

Escobar syndrome autosomal recessive disorder characterized by small stature, downslanting drooping eyes, hypertelorism, micrognathia, cleft palate, lack of facial expression, webbing of neck; associated with possible conductive hearing impairment caused by middle ear effusion secondary to cleft palate

esotropia/exotropia abnormal eye alignment conditions

ESP Early Speech Perception Test; test of closed-set perception of single words through auditory-only cues; used with young children who are profoundly hearing impaired and have limited vocabulary and language skills

ESPrit™ speech processor in the Nucleus-24 cochlear implant system worn at ear level

EST Environmental Sounds Test; objective measure of environmental sound recognition; often used as part of an auditory training program for individuals with minimal auditory capabilities

ET eustachian tube; a canal that connects the middle ear with the nasal part of the pharynx (back of the throat); serves to equalize air pressure on two sides of the tympanic membrane

ethacrynic acid a loop diuretic used as treatment for edema as a result of cardiac or renal disease; can be ototoxic

etio- prefix: pertaining to cause or origin

etiology the study of all possible causes of a disease

etymotic gain another term for insertion gain; the difference in SPL produced by the hearing aid at a point in the ear canal and the SPL at the same point in the ear canal without the hearing aid; the difference between the two recordings (unaided versus aided frequency responses) is the insertion gain

eustachian tube (ET) a canal that connects the middle ear with the nasal part of the pharynx (back of the throat); serves to equalize air pressure on two sides of the tympanic membrane; also known as **auditory tube**

eustachian tube dysfunction situation where the eustachian tube does not function properly to equalize the air pressure of the middle and outer ears; can be the result of intrinsic (e.g., inflammatory disorders) or extrinsic (e.g., swollen tonsils and adenoids) eustachian tube disorders; common etiology for middle ear infections

event-related potential (ERP) term used to describe certain evoked responses, such as the 40-Hz response or the P300 response, that are elicited with stimuli other than a simple sequence of brief duration clicks or tones; usually elicited by an endogenous stimulus representing high-level processing (e.g., cognition)

evoked elicited, stimulated, or activated

evoked otoacoustic emission (EOAE) otoacoustic emission measured in the external auditory canal in response to some evoking stimulus (either a click or two tones presented simultaneously); includes **distortion product (DPOAE), click evoked otoacoustic emissions (CEOAE), transient otoacoustic emissions (TOAE), stimulus frequency otoacoustic emissions (SFOAE)**

evoked potential (EP) a series of electrical charges occurring in the peripheral and central nervous system following stimulation of an end organ or peripheral nerve

evoked potential audiometry the use of electrophysiologic results from auditory stimuli to predict the viability of the hearing system; also known as **evoked response audiometry (ERA)**

evoked response change in the electrical activity of the central nervous system in response to some stimulus; can refer to auditory, visual, and somatosensory stimuli

evoked response audiometry (ERA) the use of electrophysiologic results from auditory stimuli to predict the viability of the hearing system; also known as **evoked potential audiometry**

exceedence level sound measurement that describes the maximum acoustic condition allowable under certain circumstances; Lx, where L is the level in dB and x is the percent of time that level is exceeded (e.g., 95_{10} means that the sound level exceeds 95 dB 10% of the time)

excitation an external force or motion applied to a system that causes the system to respond in some way

excitation pattern the pattern of neural activity evoked by a given sound as a function of the characteristic frequency of the neurons being excited; term used to describe the effective level of excitation (in decibels) at each characteristic frequency

exogenous (1) something that develops or originates outside the organism; (2) refers to an evoked potential generated by an external stimulus; the nature of the response changes according to the dimensions of the external event; see also **endogenous**

exogenous hearing impairment a hearing impairment caused by environmental factors such as a virus, medications, or lack of oxygen and, therefore, cannot be passed on to offspring

exostosis a bony growth that arises from the surface of the bone; usually found in the osseous portion of the ear canal and results from prolonged exposures to cold water

expanded speech recorded speech altered by duplicating small segments of the signal so that the speech sounds as if it were produced with a slow speaking rate; no additional spectral information is introduced

expander a signal processor that for a given input amplitude range produces a larger output range than without the processing; see also **tubing expander**

expansion in the intensity domain, it refers to increasing the range of variation in the output sound pressure level (SPL) in relation to the input SPL; expansion, like compression, is produced in a system when the input signal exceeds a predetermined threshold level but is the opposite of compression; see also **compression**

expectancy wave a wave seen as part of the contingent negative variation that results in the "readiness" of the individual to make a response; also called the **E-wave**

explantation removal of electrode(s) from within the cochlea for the purpose of reinsertion of new electrode(s) for cochlear implant use

expressivity the extent to which a genetic trait demonstrates its effect; a trait with variable expression, or expressivity, may appear from mild-to-severe or in different forms among individuals

external on the exterior or outside of the body or a structure

external auditory canal (EAC) the canal of the outer ear leading from the concha to the tympanic membrane; also known as **ear canal, outer ear canal**

external auditory canal (EAC) atresia congenital absence or complete closure of the external auditory canal

external auditory meatus (EAM) the external auditory canal; the canal that conducts sound vibrations from the auricle to the tympanic membrane; also known as **external auditory canal (EAC)**

external auditory meatus (EAM) atresia congenital absence or complete closure of the external auditory meatus

external ear the portion of the ear that is normally visible; major components include the pinna, concha, tragus, and external auditory canal

external ear acoustics represents the combined acoustic effects of the pinna, concha, and external ear canal resonances; the unaided frequency response as measured in a human ear canal

external ear effects (EEE) the unaided frequency response as measured in a human ear canal; represents the combined acoustic effects of the pinna, concha, and external ear canal resonances; also known as **ear canal resonance**

external otitis an affliction of the external ear canal usually the result of a bacterial infection; also known as swimmer's ear; often develops after water immersion; characterized by edema, erythema, desquamation, and pus; also known as **otitis externa**; see also **bacterial external otitis**

external validity generalizability of results; results can lead to unbiased inferences about the target population and not just the study subjects

extra- prefix: outside of; without

extra-axial originating from or located outside of the brainstem (e.g., a tumor arising from within the cerebellopontine angle is extra-axial)

extra-tympanic lateral to (outside of) the tympanic membrane; can refer to electrodes located in the external ear canal

extracochlear implant electrical stimulation of cranial nerve VIII by a device transmitting the stimulation external to the scala tympani or without invasion of the cochlea

extracochlear stimulation activation of cranial nerve VIII via electrical impulses transmitted external to the scala tympani

extraocular nerve nerves that innervate the muscles of the eye

extrinsic from the outside

extrinsic redundancy superfluous information present in speech signals that assists in successful speech understanding even if some speech information is distorted or missing

exudate a fluid substance discharged from cells or blood vessels that is infected

eyeglass hearing aid style of hearing aid in which the hearing aid is housed in the temple piece of a pair of eyeglasses; also known as **spectacle hearing aid**

f frequency; the number of cycles occurring per unit of time, or which would occur per unit of time if all subsequent cycles were identical with the cycle under consideration; reciprocal of the period

F force; the product of mass and acceleration; force (F) = mass x acceleration (F = ma)

F_0, f_0 fundamental frequency; the lowest component frequency of a periodic wave or quantity

F1 formant 1; first formant; the first frequency band above the fundamental frequency that demonstrates high energy in the speech signal; represents resonances in the vocal tract

F2 formant 2; second formant; the second frequency band above the fundamental frequency that demonstrates high energy in the speech signal; represents resonances in the vocal tract

F3 formant 3; third formant; the third frequency band above the fundamental frequency that demonstrates high energy in the speech signal; represents resonances in the vocal tract

F4 formant 4; fourth formant; the fourth frequency band above the fundamental frequency that demonstrates high energy in the speech signal; represents resonances in the vocal tract

FAAA Fellow of the American Academy of Audiology; designation of membership in the American Academy of Audiology

Fabry syndrome X-linked recessive disorder characterized by multiple dark nodules on skin clustering in several areas, renal failure, severe burning pain in extremities, headaches, seizures, vascular abnormalities in brain; associated with high-frequency sensorineural hearing loss and diminished vestibular response

face validity how well test items represent what they claim to test

faceplate portion of an in-the-ear hearing aid that faces outward, away from the internal components of the instrument; usually contains the battery door, microphone, and volume control

facial nerve cranial nerve VII that innervates facial muscles; branch of the facial nerve, the chorda tympani, courses through the middle ear and innervates the anterior two thirds of the tongue for taste sensation

facial nerve canal a bony channel within the medial wall of the middle ear through which the facial nerve passes; also known as **fallopian canal**

facial nerve dysfunction reduction or complete loss of facial muscle control as a result of damage to the facial nerve

facial nerve monitoring close attention to electromyography results during surgeries that potentially could cause damage to the facial nerve; see also **electromyography, intraoperative monitoring**

facial nerve palsy/paralysis/paresis damage to the facial nerve that causes loss of facial motor control

facial nerve stimulation electrical stimulation of the facial nerve by an implant that produces synkinetic facial movements

facial nerve weakness weakness of facial muscles caused by facial nerve dysfunction or damage to the facial nerve during surgery

facioscapulohumeral muscular dystrophy autosomal dominant disorder characterized by weakness of facial and shoulder muscles, upper arm weakness, progressive course spreading to other muscle groups, cognitive impairment in about a third of the cases, retinal vascular anomalies; associated with bilateral sensorineural hearing loss, highly variable, from mild to profound, cochlear pathology

failure of fixation suppression (FFS) an inability to suppress nystagmus during caloric testing when visually fixating on an object; finding in electronystagmographic vestibular assessment

fall time the time (usually in milliseconds) from the maximum amplitude of a stimulus, or the end of the plateau, to some measure of baseline (zero voltage)

fallopian canal a bony channel within the medial wall of the middle ear through which the facial nerve passes; also known as fallopian aqueduct, **facial nerve canal**

false alarm the event that occurs in a signal detection situation, during a specified observation interval, when a "signal-plus-noise" response (output) follows a "noise-alone" stimulus (input); the patient indicates that the stimulus was present when it was actually absent

false negative (FN) in audiology, the outcome from a test indicating that the individual has normal hearing when in fact there is some degree of hearing loss

false positive (FP) in audiology, the outcome from a test indicating that the individual has some degree of hearing loss when in fact there is normal hearing

false-negative response an erroneous response in audiology; no response from a patient even though a signal was presented

false-positive response an erroneous response; in audiology, a positive response from a patient in the absence of a signal presentation

familial deafness profound deafness in members of the same family

fanconi pancytopenia syndrome autosomal recessive disorder characterized by short stature, microcephaly, cognitive impairment in a quarter of cases, small or absent thumbs bilaterally, hip dislocation, renal anomalies, small genitals in males, hematologic disorders (pancytopenia), nystagmus, strabismus; associated with conductive hearing loss in approximately 10% of cases caused by ossicular anomalies or external canal stenosis

far-field recording a response recorded with electrodes relatively distant from the generator of the response; see also **near-field**

FAS fetal alcohol syndrome; characterized by cognitive impairment, low birth weight, microcephaly, short palpebral fissures, heart anomalies, short nose, cleft palate, cleft lip, digital anomalies, and joint abnormalities; caused by maternal consumption of alcohol during pregnancy; associated with chronic otitis media and resulting conductive hearing loss

fast Fourier transform (FFT) a computerized technique, named after the French physicist and mathematician, for separating a complex waveform consisting of multiple frequencies into its individual frequency components; see also **discrete Fourier transform**

fast phase component of a nystagmus beat that is represented by the vertical movement in the tracing; represents the saccadic movement of the eye that occurs when it repositions the visual target on the fovea of the retina

fatigue (1) diminution of the response from the sensory and neural receptors of the ear after prolonged exposure to intense stimulation; also known as **temporary threshold shift (TTS)**; poststimulatory effect, occurs after exposure to stimulation; (2) auditory adaptation, a reduction in the audibility of a sound during extended stimulation; perstimulatory effect, occurs during exposure to stimulation

FDA Food and Drug Administration; U.S. government regulatory agency that stipulates and enforces standards regarding the sale and use of drugs, food, and cosmetics; purpose is to inhibit the sale and use of dangerous substances

FDC frequency dependent compression; a single-channel, automatic gain control (AGC) circuit having some form of low-frequency gain reduced via a tone control located prior to the AGC sensor

FDRC full-dynamic range compression; feature of a hearing aid or amplification device that compresses amplified output levels into a narrower range than the range of input levels; the compression occurs over an input range from about 40 to 90 dB SPL; see also **wide-dynamic range compression (WDRC)**

Feasibility Scale for Predicting Hearing Aid Use a self-assessment scale containing many prognostic factors in determining adult hearing aid use

feature detectors neurons that respond to specific characteristics of a stimulus

feature extraction providing selected information with emphasis on elements of a signal that relate specifically to speech by stimulating only certain electrodes of a cochlear implant

Fechtner syndrome autosomal dominant disorder characterized by late onset renal dysfunction, large platelets, and cataracts; associated with high-frequency sensorineural hearing loss that is late in onset and has variable severity

feedback (1) a process by which a system or device regulates or limits itself by feeding back part of its output; (2) sound from the receiver of an amplification system leaks back to the microphone and is re-amplified producing unwanted oscillations (e.g., whistling of hearing aids); see also **acoustic feedback**

feedback control a device that regulates feedback in a hearing aid

feedback loop self-monitoring of sensations associated with the pressure changes and location sensations of speech organs

feedback suppression reduction of acoustic feedback for hearing aid users by installing an adaptive filter into a hearing aid

feigned deafness term for pseudo-hypacusis or functional hearing loss; hearing loss with no physiologic origin; also known as **functional hearing loss, pseudohypacusis**

Fellow of the American Academy of Audiology (FAAA) designation of membership in the American Academy of Audiology

fenestra an opening or window

fenestration (1) an opening or window; (2) in otology, an outdated operation for treating hearing loss from otosclerosis; refers to the creation of a new window (fenestra) in the lateral semicircular canal in order to bypass a fixated ossicular chain; used to be a common treatment for otosclerosis

FET field effect transistor; element of an impedance converter that converts electrical impedance so that there is a relatively low-resistance output at the external microphone terminals; used in hearing aid microphones

fetal alcohol syndrome (FAS) characterized by cognitive impairment, low birth weight, microcephaly, short palpebral fissures, heart anomalies, short nose, cleft palate, cleft lip, digital anomalies, and joint abnormalities; caused by maternal consumption of alcohol during pregnancy; associated with chronic otitis media and resulting conductive hearing loss

fetal hydantoin syndrome disorder caused by maternal use of hydantoin (an anticonvulsant) if blood levels exceed safe levels, characterized by cognitive impairment, growth deficiency, cleft palate and lip, short nose, flat philtrum, hyoplastic distal phalanges and nails of hands and feet, low anterior hairline, cardiac anomalies, genital anomalies; associated with chronic otitis media with possible conductive hearing loss

FFR (1) fixed frequency response; a compression circuit that can be adjusted so that desired gain can be achieved for a variety of inputs without exceeding the patient's loudness discomfort level; (2) frequency following response; an auditory evoked potential obtained using a continuous tone stimulus; the periodic waveform of the response is at the same frequency as the stimulus

FFS failure of fixation suppression; an inability to suppress nystagmus during caloric testing when visually fixating on an object; finding in electronystagmographic vestibular assessment

FFT fast Fourier transform; a computerized technique, named after the French physicist and mathematician, for separating a complex waveform consisting of multiple frequencies into its individual frequency components; see also **Fourier analysis**

FG functional gain; the difference in a patient's performance between aided and unaided threshold measures obtained in a sound field; a behavioral measure; the behavioral counterpart to **insertion gain**

FG syndrome X-linked disorder characterized by cognitive impairment, macrocephaly, plagiocephaly, upsweeping anterior hairline, downslanting palpebral fissures, strabismus, micrognathia, cleft palate, imperforate anus, genital anomalies, umbilical hernia; associated with sensorineural hearing loss and possible conductive component secondary to middle ear effusion

fiberscope flexible fiberoptic viewing instrument with flexibility of shaft allowing viewing of previously inaccessible body areas; specialized instruments include bronchoscope, endoscope, and gastroscope; see also **endoscopy**

fibrodysplasia ossificans progressive autosomal dominant disorder characterized by progressive ossification and calcification of connective tissues; associated with both conductive and sensorineural hearing loss, conductive more common secondary to advancing calcification of the ossicles and connective tissues, onset usually in early childhood

field effect transistor (FET) element of an impedance converter that converts electrical impedance so that there is a relatively low-resistance output at the external microphone terminals; used in hearing aid microphones

figure-ground tasks in which an individual must discriminate some sensory input (figure) amidst a competing background (ground); e.g., auditory figure-ground requires perception of an auditory signal from competing background noise; see also **auditory figure-ground**

filter a hardware device or software program that provides a frequency-dependent transmission of energy; used to exclude energy at certain frequencies while passing on the energy at other frequencies; a **low-pass filter** passes the frequencies below a certain cutoff frequency; a **high-pass filter** passes the frequencies above a certain cutoff frequency; a **band-pass filter** passes the energy between a lower and upper cutoff frequency, and a **band-reject** filter attenuates signal frequencies within a specified frequency band between high and low extremes

filter, adaptive filter that automatically alters a designated incoming electrical signal optimally with the overall objective of improving the electrical signal-to-noise ratio; e.g., nonlinear automatic signal processing used in **bass increase at low levels (BILL) and treble increase at low levels (TILL) circuits**

filter, band-pass a filter that passes energy in a specifiable band of frequencies between a lower cutoff frequency and an upper cutoff frequency

filter, band-reject a filter that rejects energy for frequencies between an upper and lower cutoff frequency

filter, high-cut a low-pass filter that attenuates high frequencies

filter, high-pass a filter that passes electrical energy above a specific cutoff frequency and eliminates (attenuates, filters out) energy below that frequency

filter, low-cut a high-pass filter that attenuates low frequencies

filter, low-pass a filter that passes electrical energy below a specific cutoff frequency and eliminates energy above that frequency

filter, narrow-band a band-pass filter that passes energy in a narrow band of frequencies between a lower cutoff frequency and an upper cutoff frequency

filter, octave band (1) a band-pass filter that measures the sound pressure level of each octave band in a complex sound; (2) filter in which the upper cutoff frequency is twice that of the lower cutoff frequency

filter, passive type of filter in which the response is constant; unaffected by amplifier gain

filter, sintered material placed in the tone hook and/or tubing of a hearing instrument to control its maximum output; can provide an effective form of quasi-compression limiting

filter skirt practical cutoff effect of the rate of attenuation of a filter measured in dB per octave; see also **roll-off rate**

filtered speech speech that has been passed through filter banks for the purpose of removing, alternating, or amplifying frequency bands in the signal

fingerspelling a kind of manual communication in which words are spelled letter by letter using standard hand configurations; see also **manual alphabet**

fistula an abnormal opening or passage from within the body to the surface; often occurs in the inner ear labyrinthine systems; see also **perilymphatic fistula**

fistula test diagnostic test used to determine if a fistula is present; air pressure is varied in the external auditory canal to determine if nystagmus is present; the presence of nystagmus during this test indicates the possibility of a fistula

fitting in hearing aids, the process of selecting and incorporating appropriate hearing aid characteristics for successful verification and benefit; see also **hearing aid fitting**

5-dB rule rule used in hearing conservation based on a time-intensity trade-off; for every 5 dB increase in intensity, the time of exposure must be cut in half; see also **time-intensity trade-off**

fixation (1) immobility of the ossicular chain; (2) in vestibular assessment, eye movement that keeps the eyes in one position relative to the head

fixed frequency response (FFR) a compression circuit that can be adjusted so that desired gain can be achieved for a variety of inputs without changing the frequency response of the hearing aid and without exceeding the patient's loudness discomfort level

flat audiogram hearing loss configuration in which the loss of sensitivity is essentially the same as a function of frequency

Fletcher-Munson curves curves plotted as a function of frequency showing the sound pressure level required to produce a given loudness level for a typical listener; see also **equal loudness contours**

Fletcherian average a two-frequency pure-tone average; the arithmetic average of the two best hearing threshold levels for 500, 1000, and 2000 Hz, or the speech frequency region of the audiogram; typically used to check the accuracy of the speech recognition threshold when the configuration of the hearing loss is sloping; can be used instead of the three-frequency pure-tone average in these situations; the Fletcherian average should agree with the speech recognition threshold within ± 7 dB

floating footplate fragments of the stapes footplate that are dislodged during stapedectomy surgery and can potentially cause damage to inner ear structures

F

Flowers-Costello Test of Central Auditory Abilities a central auditory processing test that consists of two subtests: low-pass filtered speech and competing messages

fluctuating hearing loss hearing loss that varies in magnitude over time

fluency uninterrupted production of speech; an absence of stuttering

fluent speech speech characterized by the continuity or blending of words within phrases and a rapid rate that in adults is about 15 sounds per second

FM frequency modulation; (1) alteration of the frequency of transmitted waves in accordance with the sounds or images being sent; (2) form of sound transmission via radio waves in FM systems

FM auditory trainer an assistive listening device consisting of a microphone, transmitter, and receiver; the signal is transmitted by frequency-modulated radio waves

FM boot a small bootlike device worn on the bottom of a user's hearing aid that contains an FM receiver; used to couple the hearing aid for FM transmission

FM microphone transmitter a type of microphone that allows an individual to use an FM system, including lavaliere, lapel, or boom microphones

FM system an assistive listening device that conveys sound from a sound source to a listener by means of a sinusoidally varying carrier wave; designed to enhance signal-to-noise ratios; see also **assistive listening device (ALD)**

foil term for each of the response choices used in conjunction with the targeted stimulus item in a multiple-choice format

FOG full-on gain; an electroacoustic characteristic that assesses the amount of gain available in a hearing instrument with the gain control(s) in their full-on (maximum) positions

Fonix 6500 real ear measurement system instrumentation capable of conducting probe microphone measurements and hearing aid electroacoustic analysis; manufactured by Frye Electronics

Food and Drug Administration (FDA) U.S. government regulatory agency that stipulates and enforces standards regarding the sale and use of drugs, food, and cosmetics; purpose is to inhibit the sale and use of dangerous substances

footplate flat base of the stapes that articulates with the oval window of the cochlea; see also **stapes, stapes footplate**

foramen an opening or hole in bone or tissue

foramen magnum large opening in the center of the base of the skull through which the spinal cord passes

force (F) the product of mass and acceleration; force (F) = mass × acceleration (F = ma)

forced vibration any vibration that is imposed on a system by an external force and for which frequency is controlled; see also **free vibration**

forensic audiology subspecialty of audiology related to the legal aspects of hearing health care

formant a resonance in the vocal tract that results in specific energy regions in the acoustic spectrum; often displayed on a spectrogram; represents resonances in the vocal tract

formant 1 (F1) the first frequency band above the fundamental frequency that demonstrates high energy in the speech signal; represents resonances in the vocal tract; see also **formant**

formant 2 (F2) the second frequency band above the fundamental frequency that demonstrates high energy in the speech signal; represents resonances in the vocal tract; see also **formant**

formant 3 (F3) the third frequency band above the fundamental frequency that demonstrates high energy in the speech signal; represents resonances in the vocal tract; see also **formant**

formant 4 (F4) the fourth frequency band above the fundamental frequency that demonstrates high energy in the speech signal; represents resonances in the vocal tract; see also **formant**

formant frequency a resonance in the vocal tract that results in specific energy regions in the acoustic spectrum; often displayed on a spectrogram

formant transition segment in the speech signal that displays a rapid change in the frequency or spectral composition of the formants; important for the perception of phonemes

40 Hz response an auditory evoked potential in which the response waveform approximates the rate of stimulation; periodic auditory evoked response to a stimulus repetition rate of approximately 40 per second that normally is of greater amplitude than the response to any single stimulus

forward masking the condition in which the masking sound appears before the masked sound and results in a threshold shift; the amount of threshold shift is directly related to the interstimulus interval; see also **backward masking, masking**

fossa a depression or hollow, groove, or furrow often on a bone tip

fossa incudis depression in the middle ear for the alignment of the short process of the incus

fossa triangularis a triangular indention on the anterior superior portion of the external ear; also known as **triangular fossa**

fountain syndrome autosomal recessive disorder characterized by coarse facial appearance, swollen lips, cognitive impairment, skeletal thickening; often associated with profound sensorineural hearing loss for all frequencies except 250 and 500 Hz where there may be very low levels of hearing

4k notch hearing loss measured at 4000 Hz indicative of noise-induced hearing loss; the audiogram config-uration often reflects normal hear-ing through 2 kHz with a dip at 4 kHz and rising back to normal at 6 kHz and 8 kHz; also known as **noise notch**

Fourier analysis the process of de-composing any complex waveform to determine the amplitudes, fre-quencies, and phases of the sine waves that make up the complex wave; see also **discrete Fourier trans-form, fast Fourier transform, Fouri-er's theorem**

Fourier's theorem the degree of com-plexity of a complex sound wave depends on the number of sine waves that are combined and on their specific dimensional values (amplitude, frequency, and phase); see also **Fourier analysis**

Fpz refers to the electrode location at the frontoproximal (Fp) midline (z) according to the International 10-20 Electrode System; also referred to as the forehead

free field a free sound field; a sound field in a homogeneous, isotropic medium that is free from boundaries

free vibration once energy is impart-ed to a body that has a low damping

factor, it vibrates freely for some considerable period of time and no additional outside force is required to urge the continued vibrations; see also **forced vibration**

frenal term used to describe the indescribable

Frenzel lenses specially designed eyeglass-type lenses that magnify the eyes for easy observation of eye movements by the examiner while preventing the patient from fixating the eyes during vestibular assess-ment; a small light within the frame of the frenzel lenses permits clear view of the eyes by the examiner

frequency (f) the number of cycles occurring per unit of time, or which would occur per unit of time if all subsequent cycles were identical with the cycle under consideration; reciprocal of the period; also known as **cycles per second (cps), Hertz (Hz)**

frequency, characteristic (CF) the frequency at which the threshold of a given single neuron is lowest (i.e., the frequency at which it is most sensitive)

frequency, crossover (CF) the fre-quency or frequencies representing the cutoff frequencies of the filters that divide the frequency range into separate bands; used in filters and some hearing aids

frequency, fundamental (F₀, f₀) fun-damental frequency; the lowest component frequency of a periodic wave or quantity; represents resonance in the vocal tract

frequency, natural resonant the frequency at which a system's vibrating element will vibrate after the external force displacing it from its normal position has ceased to act; measured in cycles per second

frequency, Nyquist the highest frequency that can be sampled in digital signal processing without aliasing or distortion; frequency equal to one-half of the sampling rate

frequency analyzer a sound level meter option that measures the sound pressure level of each octave band in a complex sound using band-pass filters

frequency band a particular range of wavelengths in electromagnetic transmission

frequency boundaries the frequency spectrum passed by the speech feature-extraction device in a cochlear implant or by a frequency band in a hearing aid or amplification device

frequency counter a device that counts the number of cycles per second of a pure tone; used to calibrate equipment

frequency discrimination perception of individual frequencies in a signal; determining the perceptual difference among various frequencies

frequency following response (FFR) an auditory evoked potential

obtained using a continuous tone stimulus; the periodic waveform of the response is at the same frequency as the stimulus

frequency modulation (FM) (1) alteration of the frequency of transmitted waves in accordance with the sounds or images being sent; (2) form of sound transmission via radio waves in FM systems

frequency range the range of frequencies of a signal that a transducer or signal processing device will effectively pass

frequency resolution the ability to detect a signal of given frequency in the presence of other frequency components of the signal

frequency response (1) the output of an acoustic transducer (usually in dB) across time as a function of stimulus frequency; most transducers have an unique frequency response; (2) the output of an amplification device that plots gain as a function of frequency; displays the frequency range that is amplified by the device

frequency response shaping an advantage of digital technology that enables hearing aids to implement a variety of frequency responses for different listening situations

frequency selectivity the ability of a hearing aid or the hearing mechanism to respond differentially or selectively as a function of frequency; also known as **frequency specificity**

frequency shifting transposing the frequency of the input signal to a slightly lower or higher frequency before it reaches the hearing aid receiver in amplified form

frequency specificity the ability of a hearing aid or the hearing mechanism to respond differentially or selectively as a function of frequency; also known as **frequency selectivity**

frequency transposition hearing aid a hearing aid in which sound frequencies from one band are shifted to another (usually lower) band within the range of the individual's hearing; high-frequency energy is converted into low-frequency signals to take advantage of residual hearing in the low frequencies

frequency tuning curve (FTC) the recorded changes in the discharge rate of a single auditory neuron or hair cell as a function of fluctuating stimulus intensities across a frequency spectrum; performed in order to determine the characteristic frequency of a single auditory unit or hair cell

frequency-dependent compression (FDC) a single-channel, automatic gain control (AGC) circuit having some form of low-frequency gain reduced via a tone control located prior to the AGC sensor

frequency-modulated (FM) tone a tone that alters its frequency at a fixed rate

frequent signal signal that occurs with a larger probability than a target signal and is generally to be ignored during recording of endogenous late potentials

fricative a consonant speech sound made by forcing air through a constriction; e.g., /f, s/

friction the opposition or resistance to motion

Friedreich ataxia autosomal recessive disorder mapped to the long arm of chromosome 9, characterized by ataxia with onset at approximately 10 years of age, peripheral neuropathy, scoliosis, optic atrophy, cardiac arrhythmias beginning in the third decade of life, nystagmus, occasional diabetes; associated with mild to moderate sensorineural hearing loss

frontal (1) anterior; pertaining to the front; (2) anatomical division splitting a structure into front and back halves

frontometaphyseal dysplasia X-linked recessive disorder characterized by prominent supraorbital ridge, pointed chin, enlarged foramen magnum, generalized skeletal dysplasia; associated with progressive mixed hearing loss

F$_{SP}$ an algorithm used to estimate the statistical likelihood of the presence of a response, based on the F distribution of the variance of the response divided by the variance of a single point (SP) in time across successive samples; used in evoked potential measurement to enhance the signal-to-noise ratio

FTC frequency tuning curve; the recorded changes in the discharge rate of a single auditory neuron or hair cell as a function of fluctuating stimulus intensities across a frequency spectrum; performed in order to determine the characteristic frequency of a single auditory unit or hair cell

full-dynamic range compression (FDRC) feature of a hearing aid or amplification device that compresses amplified output levels into a narrower range than the range of input levels; the compression occurs over an input range from about 40 to 90 dB SPL; see also **wide-dynamic range compression**

full-on gain (FOG) an electroacoustic characteristic that assesses the amount of gain available in a hearing instrument with the gain control(s) in their full-on (maximum) positions

functional disorder dysfunction in the absence of any known organic cause; a patient could have a functional hearing loss

functional gain (FG) the difference in a patient's performance between aided and unaided threshold measures obtained in a sound field; a behavioral measure; see also **real-ear insertion gain (REIG)**

functional hearing impairment a hearing problem with no physiologic basis; see also **inorganic hearing loss, pseudohypacusis**

functional hearing loss a hearing problem with no physiologic basis

fundamental frequency (F_0, f_0) fundamental frequency; the lowest component frequency of a periodic wave or quantity; represents resonances in the vocal tract; see also **formant**

funiculus small, cordlike structure

furosemide loop diuretic also known as **lasix** used in the treatment of congestive heart failure and pulmonary edema; can be ototoxic

furuncle a localized infection of the skin that usually arises from a gland or hair follicle; characterized by edema, redness, and pain; can be found on the external ear

fusiform spindle-shaped

G

G conductance; reciprocal of resistance; refers to the ease of flow of energy

gain (1) increase in amplitude or energy of an electrical signal with amplification; difference between the input signal and the output signal; (2) in vestibular assessment, the ratio of actual eye movement to desired eye movement; (3) in electrophysiology, the amount of amplification used with the input electroencephalogram (EEG); see also **acoustic gain**

gain-by-frequency response formula a series of reference tables used to determine the maximum gain requirements necessary to provide optimal amplification for a specific hearing loss at each frequency

galvanic skin response audiometry a change in the response of the skin to a conditioned stimulus; used in pseudohypacusis by measuring the skin response to sound after pairing the sound with a mild electric shock during conditioning; see also **electrodermal audiometry**

ganglio- prefix: knotlike

ganglion/ganglia a collection of neural cell bodies outside of the brain or spinal cord

gap-detection a temporal resolution/integration task in which listeners have to detect the presence of a temporal gap in a burst of noise

Gardner high-frequency word lists an open-set monosyllabic word-identification test designed to provide an accurate measure of the effects from earmold modifications for those with high-frequency sensorineural hearing loss

GASP Glendonald Auditory Screening Procedure; a test of speech perception used with children who are profoundly deaf

gating the process of turning a signal on and off in a specified manner

Gaussian noise white noise; noise in which the amplitudes of the multiple frequencies follow a Gaussian distribution

gaze nystagmus type of nystagmus that occurs during gaze testing; can occur to one or both sides

gaze test the portion of the electronystagmography test battery in which patients must fix their eyes on a point for a period of 20 to 30 seconds; the purpose is to identify the presence of spontaneous eye motion during visual fixation; see also **electronystagmography (ENG)**

Gelfoam absorbable gelatinous sponge material used in otologic surgical wounds; promotes tissue growth

gene the functional unit of heredity occupying a specific place on a chromosome and capable of directing the formation of proteins

generator (1) source of electrical activity in the brain; (2) device that converts mechanical energy into electrical energy

genetic counseling providing information to prospective parents about the likelihood of an inherited condition or disorder in their children

genetic disorder any defect caused by a person's specific genotype; disorder due to hereditary factors

genetic hearing loss any type or degree of hearing loss associated with genetic abnormality; caused by hereditary factors

-genic suffix: producing

genome the completed set of genes

genotype the variations of a gene at any given locus; the genetic constitution of an individual

gentamycin aminoglycoside antibiotic used to treat severe infections; known to be ototoxic

geotropic nystagmus type of positional nystagmus that beats toward the ground; if the patient's head is positioned so that the left side is down (toward the ground), then the nystagmus beats toward that side

German measles viral infection that can cause multiple developmental anomalies of the fetus if contracted during the first trimester of pregnancy; can result in central nervous system damage, hearing loss, cardiac problems; associated with a cookie bite audiogram configuration resulting from degeneration of the membranous labyrinth

gestational age the age of a newborn infant, determined by evaluation of physical (specifically neurologic) maturity after birth and comparison to normative data for different ages after birth (usually in weeks)

Glendonald Auditory Screening Procedure (GASP) a test of speech perception used with children who are profoundly deaf

glial cells connective tissue neural cells that support central nervous system function

glioma tumor found in the brain composed of malignant **glial cells**

glissade a slow portion of the saccade movement of the eye that may be either in the same direction as the fast portion or a backward drifting; see also **dysmetria**

glomus jugulare tumor growth on the jugular bulb comprised of a small group of veins having a rich blood supply; often accompanied by a pulsatile tinnitus; can affect middle ear function

glossopharyngeal nerve cranial nerve IX responsible for the sense of taste and secretion from certain glands

glossopharyngeal schwannoma tumor of the Schwann cells surrounding the glossopharyngeal nerve; see also **glossopharyngeal nerve**

glucocorticoids steroid hormones that have an anti-inflammatory effect; can cause ototoxicity if taken in large doses

glue ear serous otitis media or otitis media with effusion; fluid is very thick and viscous with the consistency of glue

glycerol test a diagnostic test used for Ménière's disease in which auditory function is assessed before and after ingestion of glycerol

go/no go a paradigm in which there are two warning stimuli and the subject must select which stimulus response is required; commonly used in the study of the contingent negative variation but has also been used in the study of the P300

Goldberg-Shprintzen syndrome autosomal recessive disorder characterized by cleft palate, lower lip pit or mound, short stature, cognitive impairment, long curled eyelashes; associated with conductive hearing loss caused by otitis media

Goldenhar syndrome syndrome characterized by facial asymmetry, spine anomalies, microtia, ocular anomalies, dermoid cysts, cleft lip and palate, facial paresis; occasional cognitive deficiency, kidney anomalies, heart anomalies, and limb anomalies; associated with unilateral conductive hearing loss ranging from mild to severe or infrequent sensorineural hearing loss of varying degree; also known as **oculo-auriculo-vertebral syndrome**

Goldman-Fristoe-Woodcock Auditory Skills Battery a central auditory test battery that measures several auditory perceptual skills including attention, discrimination, memory, sound mimicry, recognition, analysis, blending, sound symbol association, reading of symbols, and spelling of sounds

Goldman-Fristoe-Woodcock Test of Auditory Discrimination portion of the Goldman-Fristoe-Woodcock Auditory Skills Battery that assess the patient's ability to distinguish between sounds; see also **Goldman-Fristoe-Woodcock Auditory Skills Battery**

Goode T-tubes a type of long-term ventilation tube for middle ear problems

gradient the width of a tympanogram quantified by a calculation in which a horizontal line is extended 50 daPa on either side of another line drawn vertically down from the peak pressure point; abnormal gradient can be indicative of middle ear dysfunction; see also **tympanometric width**

granuloma chronic inflammatory lesion that is an accumulation of dead epithelial cells that form into a discrete granule

grapheme-phoneme conversion a top-down reading strategy

graphic equalizer an equalizer that graphically reveals adjustment to the frequency response by varying the amplitudes of various frequency components in a signal

graphic level recorder an instrument that graphically records the intensity level at each frequency as a pure-tone oscillator sweeps across a range of frequencies

grommet a tube that is inserted in the eardrum of individuals suffering from otitis media; used to help ventilate and equalize pressure within and outside the middle ear; see also **pressure equalization tube**

ground (1) an electrical connection to the ground so electricity dispels into it; (2) to connect an electrical wire to the ground so electricity passes into it

ground electrode the electrode in an electrophysiologic set-up that attaches the patient to the ground

gyrus (pl. gyri) outfolding of tissue in the cerebral cortex

H

HA hearing aid; an electronic device for amplifying sound delivered to the ear consisting minimally of a microphone, amplifier, and receiver (e.g., behind-the-ear (BTE), completely-in-the-canal (CIC), in-the-canal (ITC), in-the-ear (ITE))

HA-1 coupler standard direct access 2-cc coupler for connecting in-the-ear and in-the-canal hearing aids to electroacoustic analysis equipment for analysis; uses putty to seal the shell of the hearing aid to the coupler

HA-2 coupler standard 2-cc coupler for connecting hearing aids that are not integrated into an ear piece (e.g., behind-the-ear and body hearing aids) to electroacoustic analysis equipment for analysis; earhook of hearing aid fits into tubing for direct connection; includes a standard earmold simulator

HA-3 coupler standard 2-cc coupler for connecting hearing aids that do not have nubs (e.g., insert receivers, earphones, and modular in-the-ear hearing aids) to electroacoustic analysis equipment for analysis

HA-4 coupler standard 2-cc coupler for connecting hearing aids to electroacoustic analysis equipment for analysis that is a modification of the HA-2 coupler; used to couple eyeglass hearing aids and some behind-the-ear hearing aids using special tubing

Haas effect reflected sound arriving at the ear within 30 ms of the direct sound is integrated with the direct sound; results in increased loudness and a pleasant change in the character of the sound

habenulae perforata openings in the osseous spiral lamina through which auditory nerve fibers travel; afferent auditory nerve fibers course from the inner and outer hair cells to the modiolus of the cochlea and efferent auditory nerve fibers course from the modiolus to the inner and outer hair cells

habilitation instructional activities designed for the initial teaching of particular skills (e.g., auditory, speech, and language); appropriate for individuals who are prelingually deafened; see also **auditory habilitation**

HAE hearing aid evaluation; procedure wherein an appropriate hearing aid is selected for an individual and its performance is verified to determine an adequate fit; see also **fitting, hearing aid fitting**

HAIC Hearing Aid Industry Conference; association for hearing aid manufacturers and companies in the hearing industry; early version of the Hearing Industries Association

hair cell (HC) the initial sensory receptor unit in the auditory system; ciliated epithelial cells located within the organ of Corti, subdivided into the inner hair cells and the outer hair cells; see also **inner hair cells, outer hair cells**

half wavelength resonator a resonator with a wave guide or tube that is either open at both ends or closed at both ends; see also **quarter wavelength resonator**

half-gain rule prescription for hearing aid fitting that states that the amount of amplification used should be about half of the hearing loss as described by the audiogram; used as the basis for several linear prescriptive methods

half-wave rectified average a metric that states that the negative half of each cycle is eliminated rather than flipped to become positive

Hallpike maneuver brisk movement of the patient's head by the examiner into hanging right or hanging left positions; used in electronystagmography (ENG) testing to determine the presence of nystagmus after a positioning movement; also known as **Dix-Hallpike maneuver**

hammer outdated term for the first middle ear bone in the chain known as the malleus; see also **malleus**

handicap the effect of an impairment or disability on an individual's life (e.g., social withdrawal)

handle refers to the long process of the malleus (middle ear ossicle); extends from the head of the malleus inferiorly and attaches to the tympanic membrane; also known as the **manubrium**

Hannover Hearing Test a determinant of baseline performance for cochlear implant users that is presented in aided and unaided conditions

HAO hearing aid orientation; (1) process of instructing a patient (and patient's family members) to handle, use, and maintain a new hearing aid; (2) process of providing hearing aid options to patients, selecting appropriate hearing aids and accessories, and making ear impressions

HAPI Hearing Aid Performance Inventory; a self-assessment scale measuring hearing aid benefit

hard-of-hearing (HOH) hearing poorer than the level of a person with normal hearing, but hearing better than a person who is deaf

hardwired tethered by a wire or cord; refers to some assistive listening devices and coupling options

hardwired cochlear implant system a cochlear implant system that utilizes a percutaneous plug and battery power sources that process sound and transmit it directly to the stimulating electrodes

hardwired induction loops an FM system set up in a large area that operates with an induction loop that encircles an area or room like an oversized neck loop

harmonic an integer multiple of the fundamental frequency in voiced sounds; ideally, the voice spectrum can be conceptualized as a line spectrum in which energy appears as a series of harmonics; harmonics of a fundamental are equally spaced in frequency; also known as **partial** in a spectrum in which the frequency of each partial equals n times the fundamental frequency, n being the number of the harmonic; see also **overtone, aural harmonic**

harmonic distortion additional spurious frequencies (nonlinearities) in the output signal that were not present in the input signal but that are related to the fundamental frequency; in a hearing aid expressed as a percentage of the total signal at the point of measurement; measured at 500, 800, and 1600 Hz

harmonic motion continuous periodic motion of a sound; simple harmonic motion; also known as **simple harmonic motion (SHM)**; see also **sinusoidal motion**

harmonic series series of frequencies in a harmonic relation existing among frequency components in a complex sound; see also **aural harmonic, harmonic**

Harvard PB-50 word lists word-identification lists that were developed in 1948 that are highly sensitive to differences in hearing loss

among patients; see also **Rush-Hughes recordings**

Hawthorne effect degree to which the setting of research interferes with the independent variable in determining a subject's performance on the dependent variable; i.e., a subject's performance may be influenced simply by knowing that he or she is participating in a research experiment

HC hair cell; the initial sensory receptor unit in the auditory system; ciliated epithelial cells located within the organ of Corti, subdivided into the inner hair cells and the outer hair cells

HCP hearing conservation program; program implemented in excessively noisy occupational environments with the goal of preventing permanent hearing loss associated with exposure to industrial noise; must be initiated whenever employee noise exposures equal or exceed an 8-hour time-weighted average sound level of 85 dBA according to the Occupational Safety and Health Administration; includes qualification (measurement of environmental sound levels); abatement of excessive noise, regular monitoring of hearing sensitivity, education, and the provision of hearing protection; can be implemented in industry, schools and the military

head baffle effect the auricle and head join to form a baffle that results in diffraction effects of low frequencies, causing an increase in sound pressure level; see also **body baffle effect, head shadow effect**

head shadow effect decrease in signal intensity presented to one side of the head when it is measured at the opposite side of the head; the opposite (far) ear is in the shadow of the head; see also **head baffle effect**

head trauma insult to the head, such as a blow or fall, that can cause traumatic brain injury and/or possible temporal bone fractures

headband hearing aids air- or bone-conduction hearing aids that are worn mounted on a headband

headphone a device for presenting a sound stimulus to the ear that consists of an acoustic transducer for converting an electrical signal into an acoustic one and a cushion that couples the transducer to the ear; also known as **earphone**; see also **insert earphone, supra-aural earphones**

headroom difference in SPL between the intensity of the sum of the average incoming signal (speech) to a hearing aid and its gain at user settings and the intensity that produces hearing aid saturation; the amount of room left for amplification between the user's volume control setting and the maximum power output of the hearing aid

head-turn conditioning a technique used to test an infant's discrimination of speech sounds between the ages of 6 and 12 months of age; the infant sits on a parent's lap and

watches an assistant located on the right play with silent toys; at the same time a loudspeaker located on the infant's left plays a background sound over and over; the infant is trained to produce a head-turn response when the background sound is changed to a comparison sound; if the infant does so when the sound changes, he or she is reinforced with a visual stimulus; see also **visual reinforcement audiometry (VRA)**

health maintenance organization (HMO) a type of health care practice that provides basic and supplemental health care to its members; members pay a set fee regardless of the amount and kind of services received

hear to perceive sound

HEAR Hearing Education and Awareness for Rockers; an organization of professional musicians that focuses on eliminating noise exposure through music

hearing the perception of sound; also known as **acusis, audition**; see also **hearing sensitivity**

hearing aid (HA) an electronic device for amplifying sound delivered to the ear consisting minimally of a microphone, amplifier, and receiver (e.g., behind-the-ear (BTE), completely-in-the-canal (CIC), in-the-canal (ITC), in-the-ear (ITE))

hearing aid, analog a hearing aid with conventional circuitry that processes the signal in a continuous fashion in the time domain

hearing aid, behind-the-ear (BTE) hearing aid that sits completely behind the ear over the pinna and is typically coupled to the ear canal by an earmold

hearing aid, BI-CROS an amplification arrangement consisting of a complete hearing aid on one ear with an additional microphone connected via a thin cable or FM transmission to the contralateral ear; used for individuals with normal or better hearing in one ear and no hearing in the other

hearing aid, body a hearing aid in which the microphone, amplifier, and fitting controls are in a housing carried on the body or in a pocket and the receiver is inserted in the ear and connected to the main unit by a cord

hearing aid, bone-anchored a hearing aid with a direct contact, through a percutaneous coupling, between a screw-shaped implant placed in the bone of the mastoid process and the transducer

hearing aid, bone-conduction a hearing aid in which the transducer is positioned over the mastoid process and vibrations are transmitted through the skin of the skull

hearing aid, canal hearing aid that fills the entire ear canal, but does not extend as deeply in the canal as completely-in-the-canal hearing aids, nor does it fill the concha portion of the external ear

hearing aid, completely-in-the canal (CIC) extremely small hearing aid that fits deeply in the ear canal; usually appropriate for mild-to-moderate hearing losses

hearing aid, CRISCROS binaural contralateral routing of signals (CROS) hearing aid arrangement for bilateral severe sensorineural hearing loss in which the microphone on each ear transmits the signal to the opposite ear (side) allowing for considerable increase in gain without feedback

hearing aid, CROS a hearing aid arrangement originally developed for patients with unilateral hearing losses; a microphone is located at the poorer ear and the signal is routed to the better ear and delivered through an "open" earmold; allows for improved localization of sounds

hearing aid, CROS-plus the typical contralateral routing of signals (CROS) amplification arrangement for the good ear combined with a second hearing aid for direct amplification to the poorer ear; the hearing aid on the poorer ear is a power in-the-ear hearing aid

hearing aid, custom hearing aids such as in-the-ear (ITE), in-the-canal (ITC), and completely-in-the-canal (CIC) that are made for specific individuals from an ear impression

hearing aid, digital hearing aid utilizing digital technology to process the signal; see also **digital signal processing (DSP) hearing aid**

hearing aid, digital signal processing hearing aid that utilizes digital signal processing; the signal is converted from an analog to a digital signal, it is manipulated according to a processing algorithm, and then the signal is converted back into an analog signal

hearing aid, digitally controlled analog (DCA) a hearing aid that has analog components but is controlled digitally; commonly referred to as programmable

hearing aid, directional amplification device that employs directional microphones to improve reception of signals at the front relative to those from the rear

hearing aid, eyeglass style of hearing aid in which the hearing aid is housed in the temple piece of a pair of eyeglasses

hearing aid, frequency transposition a hearing aid in which sound frequencies from one band are shifted to another (usually lower) band within the range of the individual's hearing; high-frequency energy is converted into low-frequency signals to take advantage of residual hearing in the low frequencies

hearing aid, HICROS a hearing aid arrangement using high-frequency **contralateral routing of signals (CROS)**; the patient wears a microphone on the "dead ear" and a high-frequency emphasis hearing aid on the better ear

hearing aid, in-the-canal (ITC) custom-fit hearing aid that fits in the external ear canal, with only a partial filling of the concha

hearing aid, in-the-ear (ITE) custom-fit hearing aid that fits entirely in the concha of the ear

hearing aid, IROS monaural hearing aid fitting for a mild hearing loss incorporating a mild gain high-frequency emphasis hearing aid using an open earmold fitting; uses **ipsilateral routing of signals (IROS)**

hearing aid, linear a hearing aid that produces equivalent gain for all input levels up until the maximum output of the device, at which point the signal saturates

hearing aid, master a hearing aid with a wide variety of fitting capabilities; older technique used to fit hearing aids

hearing aid, multiple-memory programmable hearing aid that contains several different frequency responses for use in varying listening environments; often accessed by using a remote control

hearing aid, nonlinear a hearing aid that does not provide a one-to-one correspondence between input and output at all input levels; incorporates some form of compression

hearing aid, over-the-ear (OTE) a behind-the-ear hearing aid; hearing aid that sits completely behind the ear and is typically coupled to the ear by way of an earmold

hearing aid, postauricular a behind-the-ear hearing aid; hearing aid that sits completely behind the ear and is typically coupled to the ear by way of an earmold

hearing aid, power CROS monaural hearing aid fitting with a power hearing aid that uses contralateral routing of signals (CROS); the microphone is placed on the opposite ear (side) to reduce feedback

hearing aid, programmable a hearing aid with analog circuitry that is controlled digitally; capable of being programmed to compensate for different hearing losses or different listening conditions

hearing aid, transcranial CROS unilateral hearing aid fitting using **contralateral routing of signals (CROS)**; a power in-the-ear hearing aid is placed on the poorer ear for transmission of sound via bone conduction to the better ear's cochlea

hearing aid, transpositional hearing aid fitting in which high-frequency energy is converted into low-frequency signals to take advantage of residual hearing in the low frequencies

hearing aid, vibrotactile an assistive listening device that converts acoustic energy into vibratory patterns that are delivered to the skin; different systems are available that can be single or multichannel and that have different processing strategies

hearing aid adjustment (1) varying the controls of a hearing aid or the acoustics of an earmold to improve their capability to assist a specific person with a particular hearing impairment; (2) a gradual personal-adjustment process experienced by new hearing aid users to get used to the hearing aid

hearing aid analyzer a device that automatically determines the electroacoustic measurements of a hearing aid; also known as **hearing aid test box**

Hearing Aid Compatibility Act legislation passed in 1988 requiring the telephones manufactured or used in the United States be hearing-aid compatible

hearing aid dispenser an individual qualified and licensed to sell amplification devices (e.g., hearing aids and assistive listening devices)

hearing aid effect term used to describe the negative attitudes attributed to hearing aid users based on the visual presence of hearing aids

hearing aid evaluation (HAE) procedure wherein an appropriate hearing aid is selected for an individual and its performance is verified to determine an adequate fit

hearing aid fitting the process related to a hearing aid orientation and hearing aid evaluation in which the audiologist verifies the fit of the hearing aid(s) and instructs the patient on proper use and care of the instruments

Hearing Aid Industry Conference (HAIC) association for hearing aid manufacturers and companies in the hearing industry; early version of the Hearing Industries Association

hearing aid orientation (HAO) (1) process of instructing a patient (and patient's family members) to handle, use, and maintain a new hearing aid; (2) process of providing hearing aid options to patients, selecting appropriate hearing aids and accessories, and making ear impressions; see also **hearing aid evaluation (HAE)**

Hearing Aid Performance Inventory (HAPI) a self-assessment scale measuring hearing aid benefit

hearing aid specialist an individual qualified and licensed to sell amplification devices (e.g., hearing aids and assistive listening devices); also known as a **hearing aid dispenser**

hearing aid stethoscope an instrument that allows one to listen to the output of a hearing aid or an assistive listening device to detect a malfunction

hearing aid test box a device that automatically determines the electroacoustic measurements of a hearing aid; also known as **hearing aid analyzer**

hearing aid trial period a trial period, typically lasting 30 days, in which a patient may use new hearing aids to determine their benefit in his or her home environment; if the patient is unhappy with the hearing aids, he or she can return them and receive a refund

hearing conservation prevention or reduction of hearing loss through a program of identifying and minimizing risk, monitoring hearing sensitivity, education, and providing protection from noise exposure

hearing conservation program (HCP) program implemented in excessively noisy occupational environments with the goal of preventing permanent hearing loss associated with exposure to industrial noise; must be initiated whenever employee noise exposures equal or exceed an 8-hour time-weighted average sound level of 85 dBA according to the Occupational Safety and Health Administration; includes qualification (measurement of environmental sound levels); abatement of excessive noise, regular monitoring of hearing sensitivity, education, and the provision of hearing protection; can be implemented in industry, schools and the military

hearing conservationist an individual who has certification from the **Council for Accreditation in Occupational Hearing Conservation (CAOHC)** and is qualified to perform a variety of hearing conservation services as part of a hearing conservation program

hearing disability the functional limitations imposed on an individual as consequence of an impairment in hearing (e.g., difficulty hearing in noisy places as a result of a hearing impairment)

hearing disorder a disturbance of auditory structures and/or auditory functioning

hearing dog specially trained dog who assists an individual with hearing loss; dog accompanies the individual at home and away from the home and alerts the person with the hearing loss about the presence of sounds in the environment (e.g., telephone ringing, doorbell ringing, etc.)

Hearing Education and Awareness for Rockers (HEAR) an organization of professional musicians that focuses on eliminating noise exposure through music

hearing fluctuation a continual change in hearing sensitivity

hearing handicap difficulties in everyday functioning that arise as a result of hearing loss

Hearing Handicap Inventory for Adults (HHIA) a self-assessment scale of perceived hearing loss for adults

Hearing Handicap Inventory for the Elderly (HHIE) a self-assessment scale of perceived hearing loss for older adults

Hearing Handicap Inventory for the Elderly-Screening version (HHIE-S) a screening version of the HHIE

Hearing Handicap Scale (HHS) a self-assessment scale of communicative function

hearing impaired a descriptor for an individual with any degree of hearing loss; see also **hard-of-hearing (HOH)**

hearing impairment a problem with hearing that is characterized by decreased sensitivity to sound in comparison to normal hearing; see also **hearing loss**

Hearing in Noise Test (HINT) an open-set sentence test designed to measure speech recognition thresholds in quiet or noise

Hearing Industries Association (HIA) national trade association of firms that manufacture and distribute hearing health care products; established in 1954

hearing instrument an electronic device for amplifying sound delivered to the ear consisting minimally of a microphone, amplifier, and receiver (e.g., behind-the-ear (BTE), completely-in-the-canal (CIC), in-the-canal (ITC), in-the-ear (ITE)); also known as **hearing aid (HA)**

hearing level (HL) a decibel scale of sound intensity in which the reference, or zero point, is the intensity corresponding to average normal hearing for the particular acoustic signal under consideration; the threshold of an individual relative to the average threshold of normal young adults; similar to hearing threshold level (HTL); see also **hearing threshold level (HTL)**

hearing loss (1) abnormal or reduced hearing sensitivity; (2) measured as the number of decibels that the intensity of a tone must be raised beyond the normal threshold value for that tone to be detected; (3) the percentage of hearing loss at a given frequency is 100 times the ratio of the hearing loss in decibels to the number of decibels between the normal thresholds of audibility and of feeling at that frequency; also known as **hearing impairment**

hearing loss, acquired hearing loss that occurs after speech and language have developed; hearing loss due to nonhereditary factors

hearing loss, adventitious hearing loss that occurs after speech and language have developed; hearing loss due to nonhereditary factors

hearing loss, bilateral hearing loss affecting both ears

hearing loss, bilaterally symmetrical hearing loss that is identical in type, degree, and configuration for both ears

hearing loss, central the impairment of hearing that occurs when there is damage in the auditory pathways or the auditory centers of the brain; results in auditory processing difficulty; often occurs when peripheral hearing is normal or near normal; also known as **central deafness**

hearing loss, conductive type of hearing impairment resulting from an interruption of sound transmission through an abnormal outer and/or middle ear

hearing loss, congenital a hearing impairment that occurs prior to the development of speech and language, usually before or at birth; also known as **prelingual hearing loss**

hearing loss, fluctuating hearing loss that varies in magnitude over time

hearing loss, functional a hearing problem with no physiologic basis

hearing loss, genetic any type or degree of hearing loss associated with genetic abnormality; caused by hereditary factors

hearing loss, high-frequency a configuration of hearing loss that begins with normal or essentially normal hearing in the low- and mid-frequencies, then slopes to a variable degree of loss in the high frequencies

hearing loss, iatrogenic a hearing loss caused by treatment or diagnostic procedures occurring in the ear

hearing loss, idiopathic hearing impairment of unknown cause

hearing loss, low-frequency a configuration of hearing loss that begins with variable degree of loss in the low frequencies rising to normal or essentially normal hearing in the mid- and high-frequencies

hearing loss, mid-frequency a configuration of hearing loss with normal or essentially normal hearing in the low- and high-frequencies with variable degree of loss in the mid-frequencies; see also **cookie bite**

hearing loss, mild loss of hearing sensitivity resulting in thresholds between 15 and 40 dB HL

hearing loss, mixed hearing loss with both conductive (outer and/or middle ear pathology) and sensory (cochlear or auditory nerve pathology) components; the audiogram shows a bone-conduction deficit plus an air-bone gap

hearing loss, moderate peripheral loss of hearing sensitivity resulting in thresholds between 41 and 60 dB HL

hearing loss, moderately severe peripheral loss of hearing sensitivity resulting in thresholds between 61 and 70 dB HL

hearing loss, noise-induced (NIHL) the cumulative permanent hearing loss that is due to repeated exposure to intense noise; also known as **permanent threshold shift (PTS), noise-induced permanent threshold shift (NIPTS)**; see also **permanent threshold shift (PTS)**

hearing loss, nonorganic a variety of hearing deficits for which there is no apparent anatomic and/or physiologic explanation; see also **pseudohypacusis; malingering**

hearing loss, nonsyndromal recessive a loss of hearing due to recessive hereditary transmission that is not accompanied by any other abnormalities

hearing loss, occupational noise-induced hearing loss incurred on the job

hearing loss, postlingual the loss of hearing after the normal development of speech and language (usually age 5 years or older)

hearing loss, precipitous sensorineural hearing loss characterized by a steeply sloping audiometric configuration

hearing loss, prelingual the loss of hearing before the development of speech and language; may include congenitally deaf and those deafened before the age of 2 years

hearing loss, profound a hearing loss of 90 dB HL or poorer across the frequencies; categorized as deafness

hearing loss, progressive sensorineural cochlear hearing loss that is advancing; getting worse over time

hearing loss, pure-tone loss of hearing sensitivity characterized by a reduced ability to hear pure tones as measured on an audiogram

hearing loss, sensorineural (SNHL) type of hearing loss stemming from a lesion in the cochlea and in adjacent parts of the auditory nerve

hearing loss, severe hearing loss ranging between 71 and 90 dB HL

hearing loss, severe-to-profound hearing loss ranging between 71 and 90 dB HL to poorer than 90 dB HL

hearing loss, ski-slope an audiogram configuration characterized by progressively increasing high-frequency hearing loss that appears to "drop off" at or after some mid-frequency

hearing loss, sudden hearing loss that is incurred with an acute and rapid onset

hearing loss, symmetric hearing loss that is essentially the same in both ears

hearing loss, unilateral a patient with some degree and type of hearing loss in one ear and better or normal hearing in the other

Hearing Measurement Scale a self-assessment scale of seven sections that is designed to probe the disability of hearing impairment

Hearing Performance Inventory (HPI) a comprehensive self-assessment tool that probes six areas involving communication abilities

Hearing Problem Inventory (HPI) a self-assessment scale of communication function

hearing protection general term referring to devices and techniques used to reduce the harmful effects of noise

hearing protection device (HPD) ear plugs or ear muffs that attenuate sound to minimize the risk of noise-induced hearing loss; can use active or passive forms of attenuation; also known as **hearing protectors**

hearing protectors ear plugs or ear muffs that attenuate sound to minimize the risk of noise-induced hearing loss; can use active or passive forms of attenuation; also known as **hearing protection device (HPD)**

hearing screening a limited puretone assessment designed to identify whether a problem requiring further testing exists

hearing sensitivity sound pressure level required for audibility by a patient; see also **audibility, threshold**

hearing test an assessment of an individual's hearing sensitivity; see also **audiometric test battery**

hearing therapist a trained professional who works specifically in the realm of rehabilitation of hearing-impaired adults in the full context of their family, work, educational, social, and emotional needs

hearing threshold level of intensity at which a sound is just audible to an individual; see also **absolute threshold, threshold**

hearing threshold level (HTL) the faintest intensity level (in dB hearing level) that a person can hear for a sound of a particular test frequency; normal HTL is 0 dB; see also **dB HL**

heart rate response audiometry a type of nonbehavioral test used with infants that observes temporary wavelike alterations of the electrocardiogram in the presence of brief, moderately loud pure tones

helicotrema a passage at the apical end of the cochlea connecting the perilymph of the scala vestibuli with that of the scala tympani

helix outer curved portion of the pinna (auricle)

Helmholtz resonator a reactive, tuned, sound-absorbing cavity, such as a bottle

Helwweg-Larsen syndrome autosomal dominant disorder characterized by anhidrotic ectoderal dysplasia with near complete absence of sweating, hypodontia; associated with late-onset progressive sensorineural hearing loss with high frequencies most severely affected

hemisphere asymmetry difference in function between the two halves of the brain

hemispheric dominance dominant function of one half of the brain over the other

hemispheric specialization the concept that one cerebral hemisphere is more highly specialized for a given task or function (e.g., language) than the other hemisphere

hemo-, hema- prefix: pertaining to blood

hemotympanum collection of blood in the middle-ear space, behind the eardrum, usually resulting from head trauma in the temporal bone region

Hennebert's sign nystagmus that is induced by increasing pressure inside a sealed external auditory canal; often a result of labyrinthine fistula

Hensen cells several rows of supporting cells lying on the outward (lateral) side of the Deiter's cells in the organ of Corti

Hensen's stripe a dark band on the under surface of the tectorial membrane within the organ of Corti

hepatitis an inflammatory condition of the liver characterized by liver dysfunction, jaundice, gastric discomfort, etc.; may be caused by bacterial or viral infection, alcohol and drugs, toxins, etc.

hereditary hearing loss hearing loss caused by any of more than 400 hereditary syndromes

hermetic seal an airtight seal; necessary for conducting immittance tests appropriately

herpes zoster oticus virus that can produce facial paralysis; may also af-fect both the vestibular and auditory portions of cranial nerve VIII; also known as **Ramsay Hunt syndrome**

Herrmann syndrome mitochondrial disorder characterized by late onset (onset after age 30) light-induced myoclonic seizures, progressive neurologic degeneration, ataxia, dementia, diabetes, kidney disease; associated with cochlear degeneration resulting in sensory hearing loss

Hertz (Hz) the unit of frequency of a sound; cycles per second; also known as **frequency, cycles per second (cps)**

Heschl's gyrus the primary auditory cortex region of the brain, located on the superior gyrus of the temporal lobe; named for Richard L. Heschl (1824-1881)

heterozygous a heterozygote is an individual who has two different alleles at the same locus on a pair of homologous chromosomes

HFA high-frequency average; an electroacoustic characteristic that assesses the average response values of a hearing aid in dB by measuring the maximum gain at 1000, 1600, and 2500 Hz (according to ANSI standard S3.22)

HFE high-frequency emphasis; (1) use of various acoustic and electronic modifications in hearing aids to enhance perception of high frequencies (e.g., belled bore, venting, tone controls, etc.); (2) placement of musicians so that short wavelengths acoustically reflect while long wavelength sound energy does not view the floor as a reflective obstruction and is thereby lost to the audience

HHIA Hearing Handicap Inventory for Adults; a self-assessment scale of perceived hearing loss for adults

HHIE Hearing Handicap Inventory for the Elderly; a self-assessment scale of perceived hearing loss for older adults

HHIE-S Hearing Handicap Inventory for the Elderly–Screening version; a screening version of the HHIE

HHS Hearing Handicap Scale; a self-assessment scale of communicative function

Hi-Pro a computer interface coupled to a computer that allows access to hearing instrument software for programming digital and programmable hearing aids; see also **Noah**

HIA Hearing Industries Association; national trade association of firms that manufacture and distribute hearing health care products; established in 1954

hiatus opening, aperture, gap

HICROS hearing aid a hearing aid arrangement using high-frequency contralateral routing of signals; the patient wears a microphone on the "dead ear" and a high-frequency emphasis hearing aid on the better ear; see also **contralateral routing of signals (CROS)**

high-amplitude sucking paradigm used to evaluate infant perception; changes in an infant's sucking pattern and intensity are monitored through the use of a non-nutritive sucking device; such changes in sucking reflect the infant's perception of speech and nonspeech signals

high-cut filter a low-pass filter that attenuates high frequencies

high-frequency audibility the ability of the hearing mechanism or assistive listening device to convey high-frequency information

high-frequency audiometer a clinical audiometer with a wide range of frequencies available, generally above 8000 Hz and ranging as high as 20,000 Hz

high-frequency audiometry the study of hearing thresholds for frequencies within the 10,000 to 20,000 Hz range

high-frequency average (HFA) an electroacoustic characteristic that assesses the average response values of a hearing aid in dB by measuring the maximum gain at 1000, 1600, and 2500 Hz (according to ANSI standard S3.22)

high-frequency emphasis (HFE) (1) use of various acoustic and electronic modifications in hearing aids to enhance perception of high frequencies (e.g., belled bore, venting, tone controls, etc.); (2) placement of musicians so that short wavelengths acoustically reflect while long wavelength sound energy does not view the floor as a reflective obstruction and is thereby lost to the audience

high-frequency hearing loss a configuration of hearing loss that begins with normal or essentially normal hearing in the low- and mid-frequencies, then slopes to a variable degree of loss in the high frequencies

high-frequency spondees 10 high-frequency spondaic words designed for use with individuals with high-frequency sloping sensorineural hearing loss

high-gain hearing aid high-fidelity hearing aid operating at unity insertion gain for high-level signals

high-level compression system a system that limits the maximum output of the hearing aid but operates as a linear amplifier for commonly occurring inputs that fall below the compression threshold; see also **compression**

high-level short increment sensitivity index a test that requires discrimination of 1-dB increments of intensity superimposed on a carrier tone presented above 70 dB HL; see also **low-level short increment sensitivity index, short increment sensitivity index (SISI)**

high-pass filter a filter that passes electrical energy above a specific cutoff frequency and eliminates (attenuates, filters out) energy below that frequency; see also **filter**

high-resolution computed tomography specialized X-ray scan that produces thin (usually 10-mm thick) cross-sectional reconstructions of the body using computer back-projection techniques; highly sophisticated, computer-intense process for measuring and analyzing multi-plane (multicut) X-rays; also known as **CAT scan** (obsolete usage); see also **computerized axial tomography, positron emission tomography (PET)**

high-risk hearing register a list of factors that place a neonate and an infant at risk for hearing loss

high-risk populations populations of individuals who are at risk for hearing loss

high-risk register a list of factors that place a neonate and an infant at risk for hearing loss; also known as **high-risk hearing register (HRHR)**

hindbrain embryological portion of the brain that eventually develops into the pons, cerebellum, and medulla oblongata

HINT Hearing in Noise Test; an open-set sentence test designed to measure speech recognition thresholds in quiet or noise

Hiskey-Nebraska Test of Learning Aptitude a test of intelligence that has normative data on how individuals with hearing impairment should perform

hit the event that occurs in a signal detection situation during a specified observation interval when a "signal-plus-noise" stimulus (output) follows a "signal-plus-noise" stimulus (input); the patient indicates correctly that a stimulus was present when it was actually there

HIV human immunodeficiency virus; a retrovirus that causes acquired immunodeficiency syndrome (AIDS);

it affects the function of the immune system and can be transmitted through blood, cerebrospinal fluid, semen, cervical secretions, and breast milk

HL hearing level; a decibel scale of sound intensity in which the reference, or zero point, is the intensity corresponding to average normal hearing for the particular acoustic signal under consideration; the threshold of an individual relative to the average threshold of normal young adults; similar to hearing threshold level (HTL)

HMC syndrome autosomal recessive disorder characterized by *H*yper-telorism, *M*icrotia, *C*left lip and palate, heart anomalies, renal anomalies, small stature; associated with conductive hearing loss caused by microtia of varying degree

HMO health maintenance organization; a type of health care practice that provides basic and supplemental health care to its members; members pay a set fee regardless of the amount and kind of services received

HOH hard-of-hearing; hearing poorer than the level of a person with normal hearing, but hearing better than a person who is deaf

homeo- prefix: sameness or similarity

homologous chromosomes that correspond in structure, position, origin, and so on; allogenic

homophene words that sound different but look identical on the mouth

homozygous a homozygote is an individual who has a pair of identical alleles at a given locus on homologous chromosomes

Hood plateau method a masking technique for obtaining ear specific air- or bone-conduction thresholds; see also **masking, plateau method**

Hoosier Auditory-Visual Enhancement Test a speech perception test consisting of homophenes presented in an auditory-plus-visual modality; developed to assess the integration of auditory and visual information

horizontal semicircular canal the more horizontally placed semicircular canal, sensing movement in the transverse plane of the body; part of the vestibular labyrinth; also known as the **lateral semicircular canal**

horn horn-shaped tubing (flared at one end) that enhances the high-frequency gain of hearing aids; see also **Libby horn**

Hotchkiss otoscope specially designed otoscope used in the removal of cerumen

HPD hearing protection device; ear plugs or ear muffs that attenuate sound to minimize the risk of noise-induced hearing loss; can use active or passive forms of attenuation

HPI (1) Hearing Performance Inventory; a comprehensive self-assessment tool that probes six areas involving communication abilities; (2) Hearing Problem Inventory; a self-assessment scale of communication function

HRHR high-risk hearing register; a list of factors that place a neonate and an infant at risk for hearing loss; also known as **high-risk register (HRR)**

HRR high-risk register; a list of factors that place a neonate and an infant at risk for hearing loss; also known as **high-risk hearing register (HRHR)**

HTL hearing threshold level; the faintest intensity level (in dB hearing level) that a person can hear for a sound of a particular test frequency; normal HTL is 0 dB

human immunodeficiency virus (HIV) a retrovirus that causes acquired immunodeficiency syndrome (AIDS); it affects the function of the immune system and can be transmitted through blood, cerebrospinal fluid, semen, cervical secretions, and breast milk

Hunter syndrome X-linked recessive disorder characterized by mucopolysaccharidosis II with growth deficiency, cognitive deterioration, coarse facial features, macrencephaly, enlarged liver, chronic nasal discharge, chronic middle ear disease, and delayed dental eruption; usually results in early death (childhood) when onset is early; associated with progressive conductive hearing loss, with mixed hearing loss in more severe cases

Hurler syndrome autosomal recessive disorder characterized by mucopolysaccharidosis I–H with growth deficiency, cognitive impairment, facial distortion with very coarse features, chronic mucus discharge from mouth and nose, macroencephaly, enlarged liver, chronic otitis, and respiratory disease; results in early death usually by 10 years of age; associated with progressive conductive hearing loss

Hurler-Scheie syndrome autosomal recessive disorder characterized by mucopolysaccharidosis I–H/S with growth deficiency, hernias, enlarged liver, clouding of the cornea, thickened skin, eventual congestive heart failure with death before 30 years; associated with progressive conductive hearing loss caused by mucous secretion in the middle ear

Hx history

hyaline membrane disease a condition that appears in preterm neonates with respiratory distress associated with reduced amounts of lung surfactant

hydrocephalus an abnormal accumulation of cerebrospinal fluid causing increased pressure in the cephalon

hydrops abnormal accumulation of clear, watery fluid in different tissue structures; see also **cochlear hydrops, endolymphatic hydrops, Ménière's disease**

hygiene the principles followed in the preservation of health and the prevention of disease; see also **universal precautions**

hyper- prefix: above; increased, or too much of something

hyperacusis an increased sensitivity for sound perception, subjective in nature

hyperbilirubinemia the presence of a large amount of bilirubin in the blood that, at sufficiently high concentrations, results in clinically apparent jaundice; a high-risk factor for hearing loss

hypermetric saccades condition in which the eyes overshoot the target during saccadic testing or calibration of electronystagmography testing

hyperpolarization the condition wherein the threshold for depolarization is elevated, requiring increased stimulation to discharge

hypo- prefix: below; decreased, or too little of something

hypoacusis a reduction in hearing sensitivity

hypoglossal nerve cranial nerve XII responsible for swallowing and moving the tongue

hypoglossal nucleus one of the cranial motor nuclei with motor neurons that innervate the extrinsic and intrinsic muscles of the tongue; only one muscle protrudes the tongue, with most motor neurons innervating muscles that retract the tongue or alter its shape

hypometric saccades condition in which the eyes undershoot the target during saccadic testing or calibration of electronystagmography testing

hyponasality voice characteristic that is devoid of nasality

hypoplasia defective or incomplete development of a body part

hypoxia lack of sufficient oxygen at the cellular level

hysterical deafness psychogenic hearing disorder caused by emotional trauma; severe anxiety becomes the physical appearance of deafness; hearing loss of no physiologic origin; also known as **conversion deafness**

Hz Hertz; the unit of frequency of a sound; **cycles per second (cps)**

I

I/O function input/output function; a plot of output as a function of input displaying the level of output produced based on the input level of a signal; used to display input/output information for hearing aids

IA interaural attenuation; the reduction in the intensity of a tone as it travels to the nontest ear; not all the sound from the test ear is transmitted to the nontest ear; the distance and mass between the ears attenuate the signal; the amount of interaural attenuation is frequency dependent, i.e., it increases slightly as frequency increases; interaural attenuation also varies for different people and is greater for air conduction than for bone conduction

IAC internal auditory canal; the tube-like channel through the temporal bone leading from the inner ear to the middle cranial fossa of the skull; cranial nerves VII and VIII course through the internal auditory canal

IAM internal auditory meatus; opening to the internal auditory canal; passageway of the internal auditory canal housing cranial nerves VII and VIII; also known as **internal acoustic meatus (IAM)**

iatrogenic a disorder or side effect caused by treatment or diagnostic procedures; illness or adverse effect resulting from a medical or surgical test or treatment

iatrogenic hearing loss a hearing loss caused by treatment or diagnostic procedures occurring in the ear

IC (1) inferior colliculus; a major and complex nucleus located in the upper brainstem (midbrain) in the central auditory system; all auditory pathways pass through the inferior colliculus en route to the lower brainstem to the cerebrum; (2) integrated circuit; a group of small transistors built into one circuit designed to provide power to an amplification device such as a hearing aid

icon an image that represents an object, concept, or message

ICM ipsilateral competing message; a central auditory processing test in which nonmeaningful sentences are presented to one ear while a meaningful story is presented in the same ear; the patient must repeat the meaningful story and ignore the nonmeaningful information

ICRA noise International Colloquium of Rehabilitative Audiologists'

recommended type of random noise used in electroacoustic analysis of digital hearing aids (e.g., Widex Senso) to distinguish what an aid perceives as noise versus what it perceives as speech

icterus another name for jaundice; considered a high-risk factor for sensorineural hearing loss

ICU intensive care unit; area within a hospital for patients needing comprehensive monitoring and support

IDEA Individuals with Disabilities Education Act; U.S. Public Laws 94-142 and 99-457, which mandate free, public, and appropriate education for all children with disabilities over the age of 3 years, and encourages services for children below 3 years of age

identification audiometry the process of applying simple measures to large numbers of individuals to identify those with a high probability of hearing disorders; intended to be a screening procedure rather than diagnostic; guidelines are available for hearing screening failures that identify people who are at risk for hearing loss

idio- prefix: peculiar

idiopathic a condition that appears without evident cause

idiopathic hearing loss hearing impairment of unknown cause

IDL intensity difference limen; the just-noticeable difference in the intensity of a signal; the SISI procedure is based on a patient's ability to detect small changes in the intensity of a pure tone

IEP Individualized Educational Plan; federally mandated plan for providing education to children with disabilities; updated once a year

IFSP Individual Family Service Plan; federally mandated plan for the education of preschool children with an emphasis on family involvement; updated annually

IHAFF Independent Hearing Aid Fitting Forum; hearing aid fitting procedure utilizing growth of loudness functions and hearing aid fitting software called VIOLA (visual input/output locator algorithm)

IHC inner hair cell; the inner row of hair cells of the cochlea, numbering approximately 3,500, maintaining the primary role of auditory signal transduction

IHS International Hearing Society; association of hearing instrument specialists and other hearing professionals

IID interaural intensity difference; the difference between signal intensity arriving at the left and right ears of a listener; used as a cue for localizing high-frequency sounds

IL intensity level; the intensity level of a sound in dB is 10 times the logarithm to the base 10 of the ratio of the intensity of this sound to the reference for intensity; the number of decibels that a sound is above the reference intensity

ILD interaural latency difference; the difference in latency of an auditory evoked potential component (usually ABR wave V) for right versus left ear stimulation; a measure of the degree of asymmetry reported in milliseconds; an upper limit for normal ILD of 0.40 ms often is used clinically

Illinois Test of Psycholinguistic Abilities an assessment of receptive language and auditory processing skills

immittance (1) a term representing energy flow through the middle ear including admittance, compliance, conductance, impedance, reactance, resistance, and susceptance; (2) a battery of tests including static admittance, tympanometry, and acoustic reflex thresholds and decay; provides an assessment of middle ear function

immittance audiometry battery of tests used to assess middle ear function, including tympanometry, static admittance, and acoustic reflex thresholds and decay

immittance meter instrumentation used to perform an immittance test battery

immittance screening rapid assessment of middle ear function via tympanometry and obtaining an acoustic reflex threshold at 1000 Hz

impact noise unwanted high-intensity sound that occurs when one moving body strikes against or collides with another body; can cause noise-induced hearing loss

impacted cerumen ear wax in the external auditory canal that causes a complete blockage

impairment reduced or abnormal function resulting from physiologic, anatomic, or psychologic abnormalities (e.g., elevated auditory thresholds); see also **disability, handicap**

impedance (Z) (1) a measure of total opposition to energy (current) flow in an electrical circuit; (2) interelectrode impedance in evoked response measurement is the opposition to current flow between a pair of electrodes, reported as electrical resistance in ohms

impedance bridge an outdated apparatus used for measuring impedance; see also **immittance meter**

impedance match efficient transfer of energy from one circuit or component to another in a sound system

impedance mismatch the mismatch of impedance between the air of the middle ear and the cochlear fluids of the inner ear; see also **middle ear transfer function, middle ear transformers**

impression a mold made from a patient's external auditory canal and concha for the purposes of ear plugs, earmolds, and hearing aids

impulse (1) the electrochemical process involved in an action potential for neural transmission; (2) a sudden action taken as the result of an irresistible urge or desire

impulse noise noise of a transient nature due to the impact of explosive bursts; has an instantaneous rise time and short duration; high peak sound pressures from impulse noise are often the cause of acoustic trauma

in phase condition in which the compressions and rarefactions of two sound waves are identical

in situ frequency response measurement of frequency response performance made within the actual ear; see also **real-ear aided response (REAR), real-ear unaided response (REUR)**

in utero not yet born (i.e., in the womb)

in vitro process or activity happening within an artificial environment, as in a culture media or test tube; outside the body

in vivo in the living body

in-service a program of training or instruction provided by an outside organization or agency; often used to educate other professionals who work with individuals having hearing loss (e.g., school administrators, teachers, nurses, etc.) about hearing health care

in-the-canal (ITC) hearing aid custom-fit hearing aid that fits in the external ear canal, with only a partial filling of the concha

in-the-ear (ITE) hearing aid custom-fit hearing aid that fits entirely in the concha of the ear

incidence the frequency of occurrence of a condition or a disease, or the rate at which it occurs, thereby distinguished from prevalence; see also **prevalence**

incident sound sound waves that strike a boundary surface as contrasted to sound waves that reflect from it; the angle of incidence is equal to the angle of reflection

inclusive education the education of deaf children with their hearing peers supported by special education services in the classroom setting

incomplete recruitment high-intensity signals in the normal ear are loudness matched to signals of lesser intensity in the poorer ear, however, the disparity is not as great as the asymmetry in threshold would predict; see also **complete recruitment, recruitment**

incudectomy surgical removal of the incus (middle ear ossicle)

incudomalleolar joint juncture between the malleus and the incus in the ossicular chain of the middle ear

incudostapedial joint juncture between the incus and the stapes in the ossicular chain of the middle ear

incus an ossicle in the middle ear; consists of a body, long process, short process, and lenticular process; the second of three ossicles connecting the tympanic membrane to the cochlea; see also **anvil**

Independent Hearing Aid Fitting Forum (IHAFF) hearing aid fitting procedure utilizing growth of loudness functions and hearing aid fitting software called VIOLA (visual input/output locator algorithm); see also **VIOLA**

indeterminate presbycusis the 25% of cases of presbycusis (hearing loss due to aging) that show no characteristics of sensory, neural, conductive, or strial presbycusis; see also **presbycusis**

Indiana University Speech Perception Test Battery an assessment battery used to evaluate the speech perception performance of children with profound hearing loss who use a sensory aid

indifferent electrode usually the second electrode in an electrode pair in evoked response measurement; also referred to as inactive, reference, or inverting electrode; also known as **inverting electrode**

individual transition plan the part of the individualized educational plan (IEP) that states that the addition of transition services to the IEP for students in speech education must occur no later than age 16; see also **Individualized Educational Plan**

Individualized Educational Plan (IEP) federally mandated plan for providing education to children with disabilities; updated once a year

Individualized Family Service Plan (IFSP) federally mandated plan for the education of preschool children with an emphasis on family involvement; updated annually

Individuals with Disabilities Education Act (IDEA) U.S. Public Laws 94-142 and 99-457, which mandate free, public, and appropriate education for all children with disabilities over the age of 3 years, and encourages services for children below 3 years of age

inductance the property of an electric circuit by which an electromotive force is induced in it or in a nearby circuit

induction form of energy transmission either electrically or magnetically as a result of the proximity to a different source of electricity or magnetism

induction coil a coil built into nearly all behind-the-ear hearing aids and some in-the-ear hearing aids that picks up electromagnetic signals and converts them into an electrical voltage which is then amplified when the hearing aid is switched to the "T" setting; useful for coupling to telephone and assistive listening devices; see also **induction loop, t-coil, telecoil**

induction loop loop of wire in the ceiling portion or all of a room designated as an assistive listening area; sound is transmitted by electromagnetic (inductive) energy, along with an amplifier and a microphone for the primary speaker(s); speech signals are amplified and circulated through the loop wire, with the resulting signal adapted by telecoil circuits of many hearing aids, vibrotactile devices, cochlear implant systems, or headphone induction loop receivers; also known as magnetic loop; see also **induction coil**

inductive coupling (1) use of an induction coil or loop to set up an electromagnetic field for signal transmission; (2) a transformer technology that provides a single point source for a mid/base driver and a high-frequency tweeter of a loudspeaker; see also **induction coil, induction loop**

inductive inference reasoning from the particular facts to a general conclusion

inductive reactance the reactive component of the impedance of an electric circuit that comes from its inductance

industrial audiology subspecialty of audiology that focuses on qualification of noise levels in the work setting, abatement of that noise, and hearing protection; consists of development and management of hearing conservation programs that include monitoring hearing function; see also **hearing conservation, hearing conservation program (HCP)**

inertia the tendency for a body at rest to remain at rest, and for a body in motion to remain in motion; see also **elasticity**

inertial bone conduction type of bone conduction in which the ossicular chain lags behind the bones of the skull with vibration due to inertia; the movement of the stapes in and out of the oval window causes bone conduction

infantile cochleosaccular degeneration degeneration of the cochlea during infancy resulting in unilateral or bilateral profound sensorineural

hearing loss; utricle and cristae are usually preserved; etiology is either viral or idiopathic

infantile meningogenic labyrinthitis inflammation of the labyrinthine structures as a complication from meningitis; spread of infection occurs from the subarachnoid space through the cochlear aqueduct to the inner ear; results in bilateral profound sensorineural hearing loss and vestibular problems

inferior the lower point; nearer the feet; also known as **caudal**

inferior colliculus (IC) a major and complex nucleus located in the upper brainstem (midbrain) in the central auditory system; all auditory pathways pass through the inferior colliculus enroute from the lower brainstem to the cerebrum

inferior vestibular nerve inferior portion of the vestibular branch of cranial nerve VIII; its neurons innervate the cristae of the posterior semi-circular canal and the macula of the saccule

inflation test an inflation-deflation procedure consisting of a pressure-swallow technique for assessment of eustachian tube function; see also **Valsalva, Toynbee**

informational counseling counseling that addresses the patients' "need to know" by providing the patient with factual information regarding hearing loss, hearing aids, intervention, etc.; see also **personal-adjustment counseling**

informed consent code of ethics guidelines designed to ensure that patients are sufficiently informed to make appropriate decisions to pursue or not to pursue service; also used for participation as subjects in a research study

infrared rays invisible beams of radiant energy in the form of electromagnetic waves having wavelengths shorter than radio waves but longer than light waves; see also **infrared system**

infrared system an assistive listening device for television viewing or use in a large area (e.g., lecture hall, movie theater); the sound is transmitted from the source via an infrared light signal to a headset receiver that is on the person who is hearing impaired; see also **infrared rays**

infrequent signal a target signal that occurs with a lesser probability than a second signal; the subject is usually asked to make some response when the signal occurs; used in the measurement of endogenous evoked potentials

inhibition in nervous system function, the process of reducing the ability of a neuron to discharge through synaptic action

inion the most prominent point of the external occipital protuberance, located at the back of the head

innate inborn; existing in an individual from birth; hereditary, congenital, inherent in the individual

inner ear the medialmost peripheral structure of the ear housing the sense organ for hearing (cochlea) and the sense organs for balance (vestibule and semicircular canals)

inner ear conductive presbycusis an increase in the stiffness of the supportive structures of the cochlear duct that causes a reduction of membrane movement and a "mechanically based" sensorineural hearing loss; see also **mechanical presbycusis**

inner hair cell (IHC) the inner row of hair cells of the cochlea, numbering approximately 3,500, maintaining the primary role of auditory signal transduction

inner pillars/rods of Corti support cells for the organ of Corti on the medial side; form the medial boundary for the tunnel of Corti

inner radial fibers radial afferent fibers of cranial nerve VIII innervating inner hair cells; many nerve fibers connect to each inner hair cells; also know as **Type I fibers**

inner spiral fibers efferent fibers from cranial nerve VIII that connect to the afferent fibers at the base of the inner hair cells

inner spiral bundle the densely packed and tangled lateral efferent fibers entering the organ of Corti

inner sulcus a shallow groove or depression in the organ of Corti formed by the medial surface of the inner hair cells, the tectorial membrane, and the spiral limbus

Inneraid device a multichannel cochlear implant device in which the incoming signal is separated into four frequency regions by four filters; see also **cochlear implant (CI)**

innervation stimulation by means of a nerve; the distribution of nerve fibers to a body part

inorganic hearing loss a functional, feigned, or hysterical hearing loss; also known as **functional hearing impairment**; see also **pseudohypacusis**

input information or signals introduced into a system

input compression type of compression in which the level detector is positioned before the gain control of the hearing aid; the degree of reduction in amplification is dependent on the input level and on the kneepoint of the input-output function; the volume setting of the hearing aid does not affect the compression threshold but does affect maximum power output; see also **output compression**

input noise level the noise level of a hearing aid that should be less than that of the ambient noise levels likely to be encountered by a user

input/output (I/O) function input/output function; a plot of output as a function of input displaying the level of output produced based on the input level of a signal; used to display input/output information for hearing aids

insert earphones type of earphone that is inserted into the ear canal; uses disposable adult-and pediatric-sized recovery foam plugs for appropriate fit; have greater interaural attenuation than supra-aural earphones

insertion gain the difference in SPL produced by the hearing aid at a point in the ear canal, and the SPL at the same point in the ear canal without the hearing aid; the difference between the two recordings (unaided versus aided frequency responses) is the insertion gain; see also **real-ear insertion gain (REIG), real-ear insertion response (REIR)**

insertion loss the disruption of the natural resonance properties of the ear canal that occurs when a hearing aid or earmold is inserted into the ear

instantaneous amplitude the amplitude of a signal at any point in time; see also **peak amplitude, peak-to-peak amplitude, rms amplitude**

integrated circuit (IC) amplifier a group of small transistors built into one circuit designed to provide power to an amplification device such as a hearing aid

integrated rehabilitation type of whole-child rehabilitation for cochlear implant users that provides comprehensive psychosocial support for all children

integrating sound level meter technologically advanced microchip equipment that allows hearing aids to sample the sound environment four times per second or more; see also **sound level meter (SLM)**

integument any bodily covering: skin, hair, teeth, nails

intelligibility the degree to which speech can be recognized

intensity the sound power transmitted through a given area in a sound field; units such as watts per square centimeter are used; relates to the amount of sound, such as amplitude, level, pressure, power, etc.

intensity coding ability of the nervous system to code intensity changes by changes in the firing rate of neurons

intensity difference limen (IDL) the just-noticeable difference in the intensity of a signal; the SISI procedure is based on a patient's ability to detect small changes in the intensity of a pure tone; also known as **difference limen for intensity (DLI)**

intensity level (IL) the intensity level of a sound in dB is 10 times the logarithm to the base 10 of the ratio of the intensity of this sound to the reference for intensity; the number of decibels that a sound is above the reference intensity

intensive care unit (ICU) area within a hospital for patients needing comprehensive monitoring and support

interaural between the ears

interaural attenuation the reduction in the intensity of a tone as it travels to the nontest ear; not all the sound from the test ear is transmitted to the nontest ear; the distance and mass between the ears attenuate the signal; the amount of inter-aural attenuation is frequency dependent, i.e., it increases slightly as frequency increases; interaural attenuation also varies for different people and is greater for air conduction than for bone conduction

interaural intensity difference (IID) the difference between signal intensity arriving at the left and right ears of a listener; cue used to help localize high-frequency sounds

interaural latency difference (ILD) the difference in latency of an auditory evoked potential component (usually ABR wave V) for right versus left ear stimulation; a measure of the degree of asymmetry reported in milliseconds; an upper limit for normal ILD of 0.40 ms often is used clinically

interaural phase difference the difference in arrival time of an auditory signal arriving at left and right ears of a listener

interaural timing difference (ITD) the difference between the temporal information arriving at the left and right ears of a listener; cue used in localizing low-frequency sounds

interdisciplinary team a group of professionals from different specialty areas working cooperatively and interdependently for assessment and intervention purposes

interhemispheric lesion a cortical lesion that affects fibers of the corpus callosum

interleave to interweave patterns of signals for processing; can be used in cochlear implant signal processing

interleave processing a cochlear implant processing strategy whereby trains of pulses are delivered across electrodes in the electrode array in a nonsimultaneous fashion

intermodulation distortion additional frequencies are produced in the output of a signal when two frequencies are presented to the ear simultaneously; the output contains the two frequencies of the input, plus arithmetic additions or subtractions of the input frequencies

intermodulation frequency a frequency produced during intermodulation distortion when two or more frequencies presented to the ear simultaneously interact

internal acoustic meatus (IAM) opening to the internal auditory canal; passageway of the internal auditory canal housing cranial nerves VII and VIII; also known as **internal auditory meatus (IAM)**; see also **internal auditory canal (IAC)**

internal auditory artery blood vessel arising from the cerebellar artery that supplies blood to the internal auditory canal; divides into the anterior vestibular artery and the common cochlear artery

internal auditory canal (IAC) the tubelike channel through the temporal bone leading from the inner ear to the middle cranial fossa of the skull; cranial nerves VII and VIII course through the internal auditory canal

internal auditory meatus (IAM) opening to the internal auditory canal; passageway of the internal auditory canal housing cranial nerves VII and VIII; also known as **internal acoustic meatus (IAM)**; see also **internal auditory canal (IAC)**

internal feedback unwanted amplification of sound (feedback) inside the casing of a hearing aid

internal noise any unwanted signal inside a hearing aid that is unrelated to the input signal; e.g., circuit noise

internal validity type of validity in which variability between the control and comparison groups may, other than sampling error, be from the effect being studied

International Hearing Society (IHS) association of hearing instrument specialists and other hearing professionals

International Phonetic Alphabet (IPA) alphabet of symbols (phonemes) that represent speech sounds

International Standards Organization (ISO) professional association comprised of specialists involved in the establishment of standards for measurement of instruments

International 10-20 Electrode System a systematic standard for uniform electrode placement that is computed as a percentage of head circumference

interoctave a frequency used in pure-tone audiometry that is in between the octave frequencies (e.g., 1500, 3000, and 6000 Hz)

interpeak interval the latency or time in milliseconds between any two waves (components) in an evoked potential waveform (e.g., I–III, III–V, I–V); also known as **interpeak latency (IPL)**

interpeak latency (IPL) the difference, in milliseconds, between two peaks of an auditory evoked potential; see also **interpeak interval**

interpreter an individual who translates between sign language and spoken English to better communication between deaf and hearing individuals; see also **oral interpreter**

interruptor switch the audiometer control that presents or interrupts the signal delivered to the patient; this switch can be continuously on or continuously off

interstimulus interval (ISI) the time interval between two successive stimuli; the interstimulus interval generally decreases as the rate of stimulation increases and vice versa

intersubject between or among subjects

interval scale an arbitrary, quantitative scale that has no true zero; quantification relates to a particular reference; the decibel scale is an interval scale

intervention the process followed to prevent disease or complications from disease; a plan of treatment or (re)habilitation to avoid consequences subsequent to a disorder

interview an assessment procedure to assess conversational fluency and communication handicap in which individuals talk about their conversational problems and they consider possible reasons as to why communication breakdowns happen

interwave interval the latency or time in milliseconds between any two waves (components) in an evoked potential waveform (e.g., I–III, III–V, I–V); also known as **interpeak latency (IPL)**

interwave latency the difference, in milliseconds, between two peaks of an auditory evoked potential; see also **interpeak interval**

intonation variations in pitch patterns (melody) and stress in an utterance that add meaning to the message; see also **suprasegmentals**

intra- prefix: within

intra-aural reflex contraction of the middle ear muscles (intra-aural muscles) in response to loud acoustic stimulation; the stapedius muscle provides the dominating response

intra-axial originating or located within the central nervous system, (e.g., a brainstem glioma arising from within the pons); see also **extra- axial**

intracellular within the cell

intracellular potential the negative internal polarizations of cells with respect to the surrounding tissue fluids; intracellular potentials within the cochlea are from -20 to -80

mV with respect to the perilymph within the scala tympani

intracochlear electrodes electrodes placed within the cochlea for cochlear implantation

intraoperative monitoring continuous assessment of neural integrity during surgical procedures; an interactive process consisting of on-line interpretation of change in consecutively obtained electrophysiological responses, their correlation with surgical events, and the communication of significant changes to the surgical team to help protect neural structures that may be at risk during surgery

intrasubject within a subject

intravestibular schwannoma a tumor of the Schwann cells that grows within the vestibular portion of cranial nerve VIII; see also **schwannoma, auditory nerve tumor**

intrinsic inherent; originating within

intrinsic redundancy superfluous information inherent in the central auditory processing system as a result of its extensive capacity that assists in successful speech understanding even if some speech information is distorted or missing

intro- prefix: into or within

intrusive noise noise that escapes over the boundary line of one person's property into neighboring properties

inverse filtering phonation method used for recovering the transglottal

airflow; the technique implies that the voice is fed through a computer filter that compensates for the resonance effects of the supraglottic vocal tract, especially the lowest formants

inverse-square law a law stating that the intensity of sound at a given location varies inversely with the square of the distance between the sound source and the location

inverting electrode usually the second electrode in an electrode pair in evoked response measurement; also referred to as inactive or **reference electrode**; also known as **indifferent electrode**

ion a particle carrying positive or negative charge

Iowa Medial Consonant Recognition Test a closed-set, 14-choice nonsense syllable identification test for adults that isolates the medial consonant in the syllable

Iowa Sentence Test an open-set sentence identification test for adults

Iowa Vowel Recognition Test a nine-choice closed-set monosyllabic word-identification test for adults

Iowa-Keaster Film Test of Lipreading an open-set 10-sentence test used to provide a basis of qualitative discriminations among speechreaders

IPA International Phonetic Alphabet; alphabet of symbols (phonemes) that represent speech sounds

IPL interpeak latency; the difference, in milliseconds, between two peaks of an auditory evoked potential

ipsi- same; itself

ipsilateral pertaining to the same side

ipsilateral acoustic reflex presentation of the acoustic reflex activating signal in the same ear that contains the probe unit; see also **acoustic reflex**

ipsilateral competing message (ICM) a central auditory processing test in which nonmeaningful sentences are presented to one ear while a meaningful story is presented in the same ear; the patient must repeat the meaningful story and ignore the nonmeaningful information; see also **synthetic sentence identification (SSI)**

ipsilateral masking presenting the test signal and the masking noise to the same ear simultaneously; see also **masking**

ipsilateral routing of signals (IROS) (1) term commonly used to identify a hearing aid or earmold with a large vent; (2) monaural hearing aid fitting for a mild hearing loss incorporating a mild gain high-frequency emphasis hearing aid using an open earmold fitting

IROS ipsilateral routing of signals; (1) term commonly used to identify a hearing aid or earmold with a large vent; (2) monaural hearing aid fitting for a mild hearing loss incorporating a mild gain high-frequency emphasis hearing aid using an open earmold fitting

IROS hearing aid monaural hearing aid fitting for a mild hearing loss incorporating a mild gain high-frequency emphasis hearing aid using an open earmold fitting

irrigation, caloric process of injecting warm or cool water into the external auditory canal during caloric testing as part of the electronystagmography test battery; three types include: closed-loop, open-loop, and air calorics

irrigation, closed-loop process of injecting warm or cool water into the external auditory canal during caloric testing in which the water enters an expandable, silastic balloon in the ear canal

irrigation, open-loop process of injecting warm or cool water into the external auditory canal during caloric testing in which water is injected directly into the ear canal

irrigator (1) instrumentation used in cerumen management that inserts water into the ear canal to flush out cerumen; (2) instrumentation used during caloric testing as part of the electronystagmography test battery that directs water toward the tympanic membrane to stimulate the horizontal semicircular canal

ISI interstimulus interval; the time interval between two successive stimuli; the interstimulus interval generally decreases as the rate of stimulation increases and vice versa

ISO International Standards Organization; professional association comprised of specialists involved in the establishment of standards for measurement of instruments

iso- prefix: equal

isophonic contours plots of frequency versus intensity with the tonal attributes as parameters (e.g., contours of equal pitch, equal loudness); gives the values of frequency and intensity of a pure tone that produces a sensation, one of whose attributes is a constant value, equal volume, and equal density

isthmus a narrow passageway between cavities; juncture between bone and cartilage in the outer ear canal and eustachian tube

ITC in-the-canal; custom-fit hearing aid that fits in the external ear canal, with only a partial filling of the concha

ITD interaural timing difference; the difference between the temporal information arriving at the left and right ears of a listener; cue used in localizing low-frequency sounds

ITE in-the-ear; custom-fit hearing aid that fits entirely in the concha of the ear

itinerant educational audiologist an audiologist who works in the public schools and specializes in the assessment and management of hearing impairment as it relates to children's education; see also **educational audiologist**

-itis suffix: inflammation or irritation

Iwashita syndrome autosomal recessive disorder characterized by progressive motor deterioration with onset in childhood, decreased sensation, bilateral optic atrophy (onset in second decade); associated with progressive sensorineural hearing loss beginning in the second decade of life

J

J joule; unit of energy expended in 1 second by an electric current of 1 ampere against a resistance of 1 ohm

JAAA Journal of the American Academy of Audiology; a research journal of clinical research published by the American Academy of Audiology

jack an electrical device that can receive a plug to make a connection in a circuit (e.g., an amplifier that has a specific place where earphones can be attached to other equipment)

jargon specialized vocabulary or distinctive idiom of an activity or group; in language development, infant sound production of syllable strings produced with adultlike intonation; spoken words may or may not contain "real" words; even when parts are recognizable, strings may be incomprehensible; unintelligible fluent utterance produced by individuals with aphasia

JASA Journal of the Acoustical Society of America; a research journal of acoustics published by the Acoustical Society of America

jaundice a yellowish coloring to the skin caused by an excessive amount of bilirubin in the blood; one of the high-risk factors for hearing loss; see also **hyperbilirubinemia**

JCAHO Joint Commission on Accreditation of Health Care Organizations; private nongovernmental organization that establishes guidelines for the functioning of health care organizations, especially hospitals

JCIH Joint Committee on Infant Hearing; a group of specialists on infant hearing who make recommendations regarding audiology services for infants

Jena method an outdated, traditional approach to lipreading therapy that emphasized analytic training techniques and kinesthesia

jerk nystagmus back and forth movement of the eyes with different velocities in the two directions; can be rotatory, horizontal, and vertical

Jervell and Lange-Nielsen syndrome autosomal recessive disorder characterized by profound sensorineural hearing loss bilaterally, accompanied by cardiovascular disorder; leads to unexplained death in children; strongly linked with consanguinity

Jewett bumps an early and somewhat slang term for wave components in the auditory brainstem response, named after Don Jewett, the co-discoverer of the auditory brainstem response in 1970

jitter an index of instability in the laryngeal waveform, usually measured as the cycle-to-cycle variation in the fundamental period; often perceived as hoarseness

jnd just-noticeable difference; the smallest increment of stimulus change in which the stimulus can be perceived as different; difference limen

Johanson-Blizzard syndrome autosomal recessive disorder characterized by growth deficiency, microcephaly, scalp defects, sparse hair which is upswept, pinched alar base with hypoplastic cartilages, hypothyroidism, micropenis, pancreatic dysfunction, cognitive impairment in many cases; associated with bilateral severe or profound sensorineural hearing loss common due to Mondini type anomaly, absent vestibular function

Johnson-McMillin syndrome autosomal dominant disorder characterized by micrognathia, facial asymmetry, small male genitalia, auricular anomalies, occasional cognitive impairment, occasional cleft palate, occasional dental anomalies; associated with conductive hearing loss secondary to middle ear fluid and/or external and middle ear anomalies

Joint Commission on Accreditation of Health Care Organizations (JCAHO) private nongovernmental organization that establishes guidelines for the functioning of health care organizations, especially hospitals

Joint Committee on Audiology and Education of the Deaf committee made up of members of the American Speech-Language-Hearing Association and the conference of executives of American schools for the deaf in 1964 to make recommendations regarding audiology services for children

Joint Committee on Infant Hearing (JCIH) a group of specialists on infant hearing who make recommendations regarding audiology services for infants

joule (J) unit of energy expended in 1 second by an electric current of 1 ampere against a resistance of 1 ohm

Journal of Speech and Hearing Disorders (JSHD) a research journal of speech, language, and hearing disorders published by the American Speech-Language-Hearing Association

Journal of Speech, Hearing, and Language Research (JSLHR) a research journal of speech, language, and hearing research published by the American Speech-Language-Hearing Association

Journal of the Acoustical Society of America (JASA) a research journal of acoustics published by the Acoustical Society of America

Journal of the American Academy of Audiology (JAAA) a research journal of clinical research published by the American Academy of Audiology

JSHD Journal of Speech and Hearing Disorders; a research journal of speech, language, and hearing disorders published by the American Speech-Language-Hearing Association

JSLHR Journal of Speech, Language, and Hearing Research; a research journal of speech, language, and hearing research published by the American Speech-Language-Hearing Association

jugular bulb bulbous portion of the jugular vein located below the middle ear space

jugular fossa depression that holds the jugular vein in the inferior portion of the middle ear cavity

jugular wall floor or inferior wall of the middle ear space

just-noticeable difference (jnd) the smallest increment of stimulus change in which the stimulus can be perceived as different; difference limen; see also **difference limen, Weber fraction**

K

k kilo; symbol for 1000, as in 1 kHz for 1000 Hz

K⁺ potassium; element that makes up the majority of intracellular fluid that helps regulate neuromuscular excitability and muscle contraction

K-Amp automatic signal processing hearing aid circuitry developed by Mead Killion; provides significant high-frequency gain with low input levels and progressively less high-frequency gain as input levels increase; uses **treble increase at low levels (TILL)** circuitry to improve audibility of weak high-frequency consonants

kabuki make-up syndrome autosomal dominant disorder characterized by cognitive impairment, wide palpebral fissures showing some conjunctiva at outer canthus, protuberant large ears, superiorly positioned eyebrows, short stature, cleft lip and palate, scoliosis, short fifth fingers, heart anomalies, hip dislocation; associated with conductive hearing loss secondary to chronic otitis media and/or malformed ossicles

Kallmann syndrome disorder with multiple causes including autosomal dominant, autosomal recessive, and X-linked recessive, characterized by hypogonadism, anosmia, cleft lip and palate; approximately one third of cases have mild bilateral sensorineural hearing loss; conductive hearing loss may also occur in cases with clefts

kanamycin an aminoglycoside antibiotic used in the treatment of certain severe infections that are resistant to other antibiotics; known to be ototoxic

Kartagener syndrome autosomal recessive disorder characterized by chronic sinusitis, male infertility, ciliary anomalies of the mucous membranes, occasional eye anomalies; associated with mild conductive hearing loss secondary to chronic serous otitis

karyotype the complete set of chromosomes of an individual

kbyte kilobyte; one thousand bytes

Kearns-Sayre syndrome mitochondrial disorder characterized by short stature, heart block, cardiomyopathy, ataxia, dementia, cognitive impairment, seizures, generalized myopathy, diabetes, renal dysfunction, retinitis pigmentosa, optic atrophy, ptosis, onset of neurologic, eye, and heart disorders before 20 years of age; associated with progressive high-frequency sensorineural hearing loss with onset just after ocular findings

Keipert syndrome autosomal recessive disorder characterized by hypertelorism, short large bulbous nose, downturned oral commissures, macrocephaly, broad distal phalanges of toes and fingers, cognitive impairment; associated with sensorineural hearing loss with varying severity and laterality

Keutel syndrome autosomal recessive disorder characterized by chronic upper and lower respiratory infections, pulmonic stenosis; calcification of nasal, tracheal, and auricular cartilages; small nose with depressed nasal root, short distal phalanges of hands, occasional cognitive impairment, relatively small stature; associated with sensorineural hearing loss more severe in high frequencies; conductive component secondary to chronic respiratory infections may also occur

keloid an overgrowth of scar tissue; often occurs on the earlobe or outer ear; common in the African-American population; can also occur following trauma or surgery

KEMAR *K*nowles *E*lectronics *M*anikin for *A*coustic *R*esearch; head and torso manikin incorporating the Zwislocki occluded ear simulator in its ear canal; used for in situ hearing aid performance measurements that closely approximate hearing aid performance during real life

Kent State University Speech Discrimination Test a closed-set speech perception test consisting of 150 sentences; 750 key words are presented in groups of five and embedded within sentences

keratosis obliterans a rare disorder of the external ear consisting of a cholesteatoma of the ear canal; see also **cholesteatoma**

kernicterus a grave form of jaundice (i.e., icterus) of the newborn that may lead to neurosensory and neuromotor disability as well as hearing loss

kg kilogram; unit of mass; 1000 grams

kHz kiloHertz; 1000 cycles per second; kilo = 1000, Hz = frequency (e.g., 1 kHz = 1000 Hz)

KID syndrome *K*eratitis, *I*chthyosis, *D*eafness; autosomal dominant disorder characterized by skin anomalies including keratitis on face, sparse hair, thick nails, photophobia, vascular keratitis of eyes, contracture of knees and heels, lesions of oral mucosa, small stature; associated with sensorineural hearing loss of variable severity which may be severe

kilo symbol for 1000, as in 1 kHz for 1000 Hz

kilobyte (kbyte) one thousand bytes

kilogram unit of mass; 1000 grams

kiloHertz (kHz) 1000 cycles per second; kilo = 1000, Hz = frequency (e.g., 1 kHz = 1000 Hz)

K

Kindergarten Phonetically Balanced Word List (PB-K) phonetically balanced (PB) lists of monosyllabic words used to test speech recognition by young children; see also **phonetic balancing**

kinemes 11 or 12 signals used to accompany lipreading

kinesthesia the perception of the state of one's own body parts and positions

kinesthetic relating to the perception of movement, position, and tension of body parts

kinocilium a long cilium (hair) located on Type I and Type II hair cells in the vestibular organs; also located on the cochlear inner hair cells during embryonic development that usually disappears after birth; see also **stereocilia**

Kinzie method an outdated, traditional approach to lipreading therapy that emphasized synthetic training techniques

Klippel-Feil syndrome autosomal dominant disorder that involves the neck vertebrae and the ears; fusion of the cervical (neck) vertebrae that restricts mobility resulting in possible middle ear problems including ossicular malformations as well as possible sensorineural and mixed hearing loss; also known as **oto-cervical** or **cervico-oculoacoustic dysplasia**

kneepoint compression threshold; the point on an input/output curve where the slope alters from unity (a one-to-one relation between input and output); indicates the point at which nonlinearity begins; also known as **compression threshold (CT), compression kneepoint**

Kniest syndrome autosomal dominant mutation disorder characterized by short stature, barrel-shaped chest, joint enlargement and stiffness, kyphoscoliosis, inguinal and umbilical hernias, short clavicles, tracheomalacia, myopia, round face; associated with both sensorineural and conductive hearing loss with conductive component secondary to otitis media

Knowles Electronics Manikin for Acoustic Research (KEMAR) head and torso manikin incorporating the Zwislocki occluded ear simulator in its ear canal; used for in situ hearing aid performance measurements that closely approximate hearing aid performance during real life

L

labyrinth intricate passageways within the temporal bone containing components of the inner ear including the cochlea, semicircular canals, and vestibular apparatus; types include bony, cochlear, membranous, and vestibular; see also **bony labyrinth, cochlear labyrinth, membranous labyrinth, vestibular labyrinth**

labyrinthectomy surgical removal of the inner ear labyrinth

labyrinthine fistula a hole in the labyrinth causing sensorineural deafness coupled with vertigo; also known as **fistula**

labyrinthine hydrops excessive accumulation of endolymph in the scala media; may cause fluctuating sensorineural hearing loss and vertigo; also known as **endolymphatic hydrops**

labyrinthine wall lateral portion of the inner ear which is the medial wall of the middle ear; contains the promontory and oval and round windows

labyrinthitis inflammation and irritation of the labyrinth caused by degradation of the tissues and fluid environment of the inner ear

LADD syndrome autosomal dominant disorder characterized by acrimal (tearing) problems, uricular anomalies, ental anomalies, igital anomalies; associated with conductive hearing loss secondary to external and middle ear anomalies, with occasional sensorineural hearing loss

laddergram a plot of the results from an alternating binaural loudness balancing test or a monaural loudness balancing test indicating the presence of no recruitment, complete recruitment, partial recruitment, or decruitment

lag a difference in time between one point and another

lag effect a phenomenon observed when dichotic stimuli are presented with an interaural delay and the lagging signal causes backward masking of the lagging signal; see also **backward masking**

lamina a thin, flat layer of membrane or tissue that may be part of another structure; see also **osseus spiral lamina**

lamina, spiral thin shelf of bone arising from the medial end of the cochlea near the modiolus; auditory nerve fibers travel through the spiral lamina to and from the hair cells

laminar flow a type of airflow in which the air moves in smooth layers; contrasts with turbulence

laminectomy surgical removal of the lamina to relieve compression of structures

Langer-Giedion syndrome autosomal dominant deletion disorder characterized by bulbous nose, vertical maxillary excess, small stature, microcephaly, protuberant ears, sparse hair, loose skin in infancy, multiple exostoses (bony projections) of long bones, hypotonia, cognitive impairment; associated with progressive sensorineural hearing loss that is moderate to severe

language complex system of arbitrary sounds, gestures, or marks arranged in a conventional code employed as a social tool of mutual understanding to communicate ideas and or feelings within a specific group or community; useful sound delivered by the vocal mechanisms; means by which species other than humans communicate

language delay later than normal acquisition of language

language disorder any difficulty with the production and/or reception of linguistic units ranging from minor variances in syntax to total absence of speech; see also **language learning disorder**

language learning disorder a disorder in one or more of the basic psychological processes involved in understanding or using language, spoken or written, that may manifest itself in an imperfect ability to listen, think, speak, read, write, spell, or do mathematical calculations; see also **language disorder**

Language, Speech, and Hearing Services in the Schools (LSHSS) a clinical research journal on school-based speech-language pathology and audiology published by the American Speech-Language-Hearing Association

laryngology the study of disorders of the larynx; branch of medicine that studies the causes and treatments of vocal pathology

larynx the primary organ of phonation connecting the pharynx to the trachea; sound is produced by vibration of the vocal folds

lasix loop diuretic also known as **furosemide** used in the treatment of congestive heart failure and pulmonary edema; can be ototoxic

late auditory evoked responses electrical activity evoked by sounds, that originates from portions of the auditory cortex, is measured with electrodes placed on the scalp, and occurs within 100 to 300 ms after the sound is presented; also known as **auditory late response (ALR)**

latency (1) the time interval between two events, such as a stimulus and a response; the time between the occurrence of a physiological event, usually a spike or evoked potential, and a stimulus; the time between two wave components; (2) analysis measurement used in evoked potential testing; see also **absolute latency, interpeak latency (IPL)**

latency, absolute (1) the time in milliseconds from the onset of the stimulus to the onset of the peak of a wave in any electrophysiologic response; (2) an important measurement parameter in the interpretation of the auditory brainstem response

latency, acoustic reflex the time in milliseconds between the onset of an auditory stimulus and the identification of an acoustic reflex

latency, delayed in evoked potential testing, an abnormal prolongation of the time between the stimulus onset and peak of the wave; has diagnostic significance regarding possible auditory pathology

latency, interaural the difference in latency of an auditory evoked potential component (usually ABR wave V) for right versus left ear stimulation; a measure of the degree of asymmetry reported in milliseconds; an upper limit for normal ILD of 0.40 ms often is used clinically

latency, interpeak the difference, in milliseconds, between two peaks of an auditory evoked potential

latency, interwave the difference, in milliseconds, between two peaks of an auditory evoked potential

latency-intensity (LI) function a graph of the absolute latency of wave V of the auditory brainstem response plotted as a function of stimulus level; specific patterns of L-I functions characterize different auditory disorders

lateral away from the midline of the body

lateral lemniscus (LL) a bundle of nerve fibers that is one of three major ascending fiber tracts in the central auditory pathway; provides connection between the cochlear nuclei and superior olivary complex nuclei with the inferior colliculus

lateral malleolar ligament one of the ligaments of the middle ear responsible for suspension of the ossicular chain; connects from the neck of the malleus to the lateral bony wall of the tympanic cavity

lateral nucleus of trapezoid body (LNTB) a brainstem nucleus located in the region of the superior olive, whose descending fibers contribute to the lateral efferent olivocochlear bundle; also called the posterior periolivary nucleus or lateral periolivary nucleus

lateral rectus muscle muscle of the eye responsible for eye movement away from the midline of the body

lateral semicircular canal the more horizontally placed semicircular canal, sensing movement in the transverse plane of the body; part of the vestibular labyrinth; also known as the **horizontal semicircular canal**

lateral superior olive (LSO) nuclear aggregate of the superior olivary complex involved in processing interaural intensity differences; see also **superior olivary complex (SOC)**

laterality (1) right versus left side of the brain resulting from cerebral dominance; (2) handedness preference for use of either the left or right hand due to cerebral dominance

lateralization the determination by a subject that the apparent direction of a sound is either left or right of the frontal-medial plane of the head; the localization of sounds inside the head; see also **localization**

lavaliere microphone a small microphone attached to a neck cord and resting on the chest or clipped onto a tie, shirt, or other piece of clothing

LD learning disability; one or more of a heterogeneous group of learning disorders that interfere with listening, speaking, reading, writing, reasoning, or mathematics

LDFR level dependent frequency response; type of automatic signal processing circuitry that can compensate for the degree of hearing loss in a particular frequency band; the amount of amplification for a band of frequencies is dependent on the input level of the signal; see also **bass increase at low levels (BILL), programmable increase at low levels (PILL), treble increase at low levels (TILL)**

LDL loudness discomfort level; level at which sound is perceived to be uncomfortable; a level of loudness that a patient would not want to listen to for an extended period of time; also known as **uncomfortable loudness level (UCL, ULL)**

learning disability (LD) one or more of a heterogeneous group of learning disorders that interfere with listening, speaking, reading, writing, reasoning, or mathematics; see also **language learning disorder**

LED light-emitting diode; a semiconductor that emits light when conducting a current; used in electronic equipment to display readings

left-beating nystagmus a type of horizontal nystagmus in which the fast phase angles to the left

lenticular process structure at the inferior end of the long process of the incus that connects to the head of the stapes; see also **incus**

lentigines darkly pigmented flat brown spots on the skin

LEOPARD syndrome autosomal dominant disorder characterized by multiple *l*entigines, *e*lectrocardiographic conduct abnormalities, *o*cular hypertelorism, *p*ulmonic stenosis, *a*bnormal genitalia, *r*etarded growth, sensorineural *d*eafness, and occasional cognitive impairment; associated with sensorineural hearing loss of varying severity and varying age of onset

Leq equivalent level; a time-weighted energy average that represents the total sound energy experienced over a given period of time as if the sound was unvarying; also known as **equivalent sound level (Leq)**

Lermoyez's syndrome unusual form of **Ménière's disease** characterized by fluctuations of hearing that are just the opposite of a vertiginous state (hearing is improved after a vertiginous attack); may result from endolymph pressure release with rupture of Reissner's membrane; see also **Ménière's disease**

leukodystrophy a disease of the white matter in the brain marked by demyelination; see also **adrenoleukodystrophy (ALS)**

levator veli palatini muscle in the region of the neck that contracts along with other muscles to open the eustachian tube; see also **tensor veli palatini**

level, comfort maximum level for different stimuli that does not produce an uncomfortable loudness sensation; used to determine the maximum level for a series of pulses that does not produce an uncomfortable loudness sensation for a hearing aid or cochlear implant user

level, discomfort level at which sound is perceived to be uncomfortable; a level of loudness that a patient would not want to listen to for an extended period of time

level, equivalent (Leq) a time-weighted energy average that represents the total sound energy experienced over a given period of time as if the sound was unvarying; also known as **equivalent sound level (Leq)**

level, exceedance sound measurement that describes the maximum acoustic condition allowable under certain circumstances; Lx, where L is the level in dB and x is the percentage of time that level is exceeded

(e.g., 95_{10} means that the sound level exceeds 95 dB 10% of the time)

level, hearing (HL) a decibel scale of sound intensity in which the reference, or zero point, is the intensity corresponding to average normal hearing for the particular acoustic signal under consideration; the threshold of an individual relative to the average threshold of normal young adults; similar to **hearing threshold level (HTL)**

level, hearing threshold (HTL) the faintest intensity level (in dB hearing level) that a person can hear for a sound of a particular test frequency; normal HTL is 0 dB

level, intensity the intensity level of a sound in dB is 10 times the logarithm to the base 10 of the ratio of the intensity of this sound to the reference for intensity; the number of decibels that a sound is above the reference intensity

level, loudness the subjective judgment of the loudness level of a sound in phons; numerically equal to the median sound pressure level in decibels of a 1000-Hz reference tone

level, loudness discomfort (LDL) level at which sound is perceived to be uncomfortable; a level of loudness that a patient would not want to listen to for an extended period of time; also known as **uncomfortable loudness level (UCL, ULL)**

level, noise emission the decibel level measured at a specified distance and direction from a noise source in an open environment above a specified type of surface

level, noise interference the level at which speech signals are masked by noise

level, output sound pressure (OS-PL) a test used to determine the sound pressure level obtained in an ear simulator when using an input of 90 dB SPL and the gain control in the full-on position as a function of frequency; newer, more accurate, term used instead of **maximum power output (MPO), saturation sound pressure level (SSPL)**

level, peak equivalent sound pressure (peSPL) a measure of sound intensity in which the maximum voltage of a transient stimulus (e.g., a click) is equated on an oscilloscope with the voltage of a tone stimulus of known intensity level in dB sound pressure level (SPL); click intensity level is defined in terms of **dB peSPL**

level, saturation sound pressure (SSPL) electroacoustic assessment of a hearing aid's maximum level of output signal expressed as a frequency response curve to a 90 dB signal with the hearing aid volume control set to full-on; also known as **maximum power output (MPO)**

level, sensation (SL) the intensity of a sound above or below an individual's threshold; used as a reference point for presentation levels of audiometric and speech perception testing

level, sound pressure (SPL) an absolute value measured in dB representing the physical intensity of a sound; 20 times the log of the pressure output over the pressure reference (0.0002 dyne/cm^2 or 20 micropascals)

level, speech interference (SIL) the adverse effects of noise on the intelligibility of speech communication; used originally with the articulation index when evaluating communication systems

level, uncomfortable loudness (UCL) an intensity level at which speech or a pure-tone signal is perceived as being so loud that it causes discomfort

level dependent frequency response (LDFR) type of automatic signal processing circuitry that can compensate for the degree of hearing loss in a particular frequency band; the amount of amplification for a band of frequencies is dependent on the input level of the signal; see also **bass increase at low levels (BILL), programmable increase at low levels (PILL), treble increase at low levels (TILL)**

lever advantage the benefit derived through reduction of the length of the long process of the incus relative to the manubrium of the malleus resulting in a mechanical advantage for the middle ear transformer action; see also **area-ratio hypothesis, middle ear transformers**

Lexical Neighborhood Test a speech perception test developed to assess word recognition and lexical discrimination in children with hearing loss

LI latency intensity, as in latency-intensity function for auditory brainstem response

Libby horn horn-shaped tubing (flared at one end) that enhances the high-frequency gain of hearing aids

Liden (masking) formula used to determine minimum and maximum effective masking levels; for air conduction: Mmin = At − 40 + (am − bm), Mmax = Bt + 40; for bone conduction: Mmin = Bt + (am − bm), Mmax = Bt + 40; where A = air-conduction threshold, B = bone-conduction threshold, t = test ear, m = masked ear

ligament, annular thin elastic membrane that attaches the footplate of the stapes to the oval window

ligament, anterior malleolar one of the ligaments of the middle ear responsible for suspension of the ossicular chain; connects from the anterior process of the malleus to the anterior wall of the tympanic cavity

ligament, lateral malleolar one of the ligaments of the middle ear responsible for suspension of the ossicular chain; connects from the neck of the malleus to the lateral bony wall of the tympanic cavity

ligament, posterior incudal one of the ligaments of the middle ear responsible for suspension of the ossicular chain; connects from the short process of the incus to the posterior wall of the tympanic cavity

ligament, spiral the periosteumlike outer wall of the scala media; it is attached to the outward border of the basilar membrane at the basilar crest and is covered by the stria vascularis within the cochlear duct

ligament, superior malleolar one of the ligaments of the middle ear responsible for suspension of the ossicular chain; connects from the head of the malleus to the roof of the tympanic cavity

light reflex triangular-shaped light reflex seen when a light is shone down the external auditory canal toward the tympanic membrane with an otoscope; also known as **cone of light**

light-emitting diode (LED) a semiconductor that emits light when conducting a current; used in electronic equipment to display readings

limbic system the central nervous system structures responsible for mediation of motivation and arousal, including the hippocampus, amygdala, dentate gyrus, cingulate gyrus, and fornix

limbus an extension of the osseous spiral lamina toward the scala vestibuli; near its inner edge it is attached to Reissner's membrane and on its outer edge it forms the inner spiral sulcus, which is attached to the tectorial membrane; also known as **spiral limbus**

limen threshold

Lindamood Auditory Conceptualization Test auditory processing and central auditory nervous system functioning test that focuses on auditory memory and sequencing

line spectrum a plot of a sound wave displaying amplitude as a function of frequency, the components of which occur at a number of discrete frequencies; see also **continuous spectrum**

linear a linear system that satisfies the conditions of superposition and homogeneity; an increase in one parameter results in an equal increase in another parameter

linear amplification a hearing aid or amplification device that produces equivalent gain for all input levels up until the maximum output of the device, at which point the signal saturates; see also **peak clipping (PC), linear analog circuitry**

linear analog circuitry traditional circuitry of hearing aids that provides the same gain over a range of input levels until maximum levels are reached; then it saturates and clips the signal; see also **peak clipping (PC)**

linear hearing aid a hearing aid that produces equivalent gain for all input levels up to the maximum output of the device, at which point the signal saturates

linear predictive coding (LPC) analysis that smooths the frequency spectrum by removing the fundamental frequency of the glottal pulses seen in the fast Fourier transform graphic representation; see also **fast Fourier transform (FFT)**

Ling Five Sounds Test five sounds of English /a, i, u, s, ʃ/ are used to determine a child's auditory responsiveness to speech stimuli; they are representative of a range of sounds that occur in conversational speech

Ling Six Sounds Test six sounds of English /a, i, u, s, ʃ, m/ are used to determine a child's auditory responsiveness to speech stimuli; they are representative of a range of sounds that occur in conversational speech

linguistic competence demonstration of a speaker's or listener's implicit knowledge of the underlying rules of language

linguistic deprivation not having exposure to verbal language and unable to develop language normally as a result (e.g., without intervention a congenitally deafened child may have linguistic deprivation)

lipreading deriving meaning from a person's speech by observing the speaker's lips, gestures, and facial expressions; see also **speechreading**

Lipreading Discrimination Test a test used to assess lipreading performance in individuals with hearing impairment; also used to assess viseme perception; see also **viseme**

listening understanding speech and environmental sounds by attending to auditory cues or to auditory and visual cues

listening check informal assessment of whether a listening device is functioning appropriately

listening strategies ways to improve detection, discrimination, identification, and comprehension of various auditory signals

live voice presentation of a speech signal through an audiometer by means of a microphone; the intensity of the voice is monitored visually by means of a VU meter; also known as **monitored live voice**

living ear a real world, real ear conceptualization that emphasizes the importance of considering the movement of the ear canal and its effects on the fitting of hearing aids

LL lateral lemniscus; a bundle of nerve fibers that is one of three major ascending fiber tracts in the central auditory pathway; provides connection between the cochlear nuclei and superior olivary complex nuclei with the inferior colliculus

LNTB lateral nucleus of the trapezoid body; brainstem nucleus located in the region of the superior olive, whose descending fibers contribute to the lateral efferent olivocochlear bundle; also called the posterior periolivary nucleus or lateral periolivary nucleus

lobulus auriculae ear lobe; landmark of the auricle

localization the determination by a subject of the apparent direction and/or distance of a sound source presented in a sound field; see also **lateralization**

log logarithm; the exponent (power) to which a base number is raised to equal a given number; e.g., 2 is the logarithm of 100 to the base 10 ($10^2 = 10 \times 10 = 100$); also known as **logarithm**

logarithm the exponent (power) to which a base number is raised to equal a given number; e.g., 2 is the logarithm of 100 to the base 10 ($10^2 = 10 \times 10 = 100$); also known as **log**

Lombard test a test used in the evaluation of a person suspected of malingering; based on the **Lombard voice reflex**, which is the increase in a person's vocal intensity when listening to a loud noise

Lombard voice reflex an inadvertent increase in a person's vocal intensity when talking in a background of noise; see also **Lombard test**; also known as Lombard effect

long process (1) an extension from a bony structure in the body; (2) an extension from the body of the incus toward the stapes; (3) an extension from the head of the malleus; also known as the **handle, manubrium**

long-latency auditory evoked potentials an evoked potential that occurs between approximately 90 and 200 ms having mean peaks in adults at approximately p60, n100, p160, n200; see also **auditory late response (ALR)**

L

long-term average speech spectrum (LTASS) (1) the overall level and configuration of speech energy representing everyday speech; (2) a measure of hearing aid performance as determined in the sound field versus amplified in the ear canal; see also **desired sensation level (DSL)**

long-term memory final stage of memory consisting of two broad types: episodic memory, which is personal, and semantic memory, which entails the general organized structure of knowledge

longitudinal fracture fracture of the temporal bone resulting in possible hearing loss; spares the inner ear from damage and primarily affects the outer and middle ear structures

longitudinal wave a pressure wave that moves in a medium in the direction that the sound wave travels; motion is parallel to wave movement

longitudinal wave motion the movement of particles in a medium that oscillate in the direction of travel of the sound wave, passing their motion on to adjacent particles

loop, induction loop of wire in the ceiling portion or all of a room designated as an assistive listening area; sound is transmitted by electromagnetic (inductive) energy, along with an amplifier and a microphone for the primary speaker(s); speech signals are amplified and circulated through the loop wire, with the resulting signal adapted by telecoil circuits of many hearing aids, vibro-tactile devices, cochlear implant systems, or headphone induction loop receivers; also known as magnetic loop

loop diuretics type of diuretic commonly used in patients with congestive heart failure and pulmonary edema; may cause ototoxicity; drugs include **furosemide (lasix)**, **ethacrynic acid**, and **bumetanide**

loop FM system an FM system that features loop induction and telecoil reception; see also **FM system, induction loop**

lop ears autosomal dominant disorder characterized by micrognathia, overfolded ears with large lobes, and ossicular anomalies; associated with maximum conductive hearing loss in many cases, although a mild loss is also possible

loudness that aspect of auditory sensation in which sounds may be ordered on a scale running from soft to loud; a function of the intensity of a sound that is also dependent on its frequency and composition; see also **intensity, sone**

loudness adaptation the reduction in the loudness percept of suprathreshold continuous pure tones; see also **auditory adaptation**

loudness balance perceived equality of loudness stimulation across the frequency range; see also **alternate binaural loudness balancing (ABLB), equal loudness contours**

loudness discomfort level (LDL) level at which sound is perceived to be uncomfortable; a level of loudness that a patient would not want to listen to for an extended period of time; also known as **uncomfortable loudness level (UCL, ULL)**

loudness growth function a graph charting a patient's perceived loudness as a function of stimulus intensity; the steeper the curve, the faster the growth of loudness; indicates the possibility of recruitment

loudness level the subjective judgment of the loudness level of a sound in phons; numerically equal to the median sound pressure level in decibels of a 1000-Hz reference tone; see also **phon, loudness**

loudness level contour a curve that shows the related values of sound pressure level and frequency required to produce a given loudness level for the typical subject for a stated manner of listening to the sound; see also **equal loudness contour**

loudness matching psychoacoustic procedure consisting of presenting an external signal to the patient and having the patient match its loudness to that of another signal; can be used in the evaluation of tinnitus

loudness recruitment abnormally rapid growth of loudness; a person's perception of the relative intensity of sound as intensity increases; also known as **recruitment**

loudness summation an increase in loudness when the bandwidth of a complex sound is increased so that it exceeds a critical bandwidth even

when the sound pressure level of the complex sound is kept constant; see also **critical band**

loudspeaker an electroacoustic transducer that changes electrical energy to acoustical energy at the output stage of a sound system allowing amplified sound to be heard by many persons simultaneously

low birth weight refers to a neonate weighing less than 1500 grams (3.3 lbs.) at birth; a high-risk factor for hearing loss

low-cut filter a high-pass filter that attenuates low frequencies

low-frequency hearing loss a configuration of hearing loss that begins with variable degree of loss in the low frequencies rising to normal or essentially normal hearing in the mid- and high frequencies

low-level short increment sensitivity index a test that requires discrimination of 1-dB increments of intensity superimposed on a carrier tone presented at 20 dB above threshold; test used to identify individuals with active neural pathology; see also **high-level short increment sensitivity index; short increment sensitivity index (SISI)**

low-pass filter a filter that passes electrical energy below a specific cutoff frequency and eliminates energy above that frequency; see also **bandpass filter, filter, high-pass filter**

low-pass filtered speech speech that has been passed through filter banks, leaving the lower, but not the higher, frequencies

Low-Pass Filtered Speech (LPFS) Test test of central auditory processing consisting of monosyllabic words that have been filtered above approximately 800 Hz

low-redundancy speech tests tests of central auditory processing that use speech signals that are degraded by modifying or distorting the frequency, temporal, or spectral characteristics of the signal

LPC linear predictive coding; analysis that smooths the frequency spectrum by removing the fundamental frequency of the glottal pulses seen in the fast Fourier transform graphic representation

LSHSS Language Speech and Hearing Services in the Schools; a clinical research journal on school-based speech-language pathology and audiology published by the American Speech-Language-Hearing Association

LSO lateral superior olive; nuclear aggregate of the superior olivary complex involved in processing interaural intensity differences; see also **superior olivary complex (SOC)**

LTASS long-term average speech spectrum; (1) the overall level and configuration of speech energy representing everyday speech; (2) a measure of hearing aid performance as determined in the sound field versus amplified in the ear canal; see also **desired sensation level (DSL)**

Lucae ear hook an instrument used for retracting cerumen lodged in the ear canal; consists of a hook with a blunt and rounded head

lucite a transparent or translucent plastic; type of material used in earmolds

luetic pertaining to syphilis

luetic labyrinthitis labyrinth infected by syphilis resulting in sensorineural hearing loss; also known as luetic deafness

Lumi-view headworn microscope for viewing ear canals; frees both hands for procedures such as cerumen management

Lybarger earmold type of nonoccluding earmold designed to enhance high-frequency amplification; contains a tube with two diameters that results in a resonance above 4000 Hz

M

MA mental age; age level at which an individual functions intellectually as determined by standardized psychological tests

MAA minimal audible angle; the smallest difference in localization that a listener can determine when two successive sounds originate from the same direction

MAC Minimal Auditory Capabilities battery; a comprehensive set of tests that yields a general profile of an individual's speech reception abilities ranging from awareness and identification of environmental sounds to open-set speech recognition; designed for individuals with minimal auditory capabilities; provides consistency in the evaluation of cochlear implant patients

macrocephaly a congenital abnormality resulting in an unusually large head and brain

macrotia abnormally large external ears (pinnae)

macula/maculae vestibular sensory organ of the saccule and utricle

macula, saccular vestibular sensory epithelia on the anterior wall of the saccule

macula, utricular vestibular sensory epithelia on the lateral wall of the utricle

MAF minimal audible field; minimum auditory field; the sound pressure level of a tone at the threshold of audibility measured in a free sound field for a subject facing the sound source

magnetic microphone an input transformer introduced in 1946 that was used between the microphone and the grid circuit of the first tube of a hearing aid; its advantage was that temperature or humidity conditions that were normally encountered did not damage the microphone

magnetic receiver a receiver used with carbon hearing aids that were either bipolar or monopolar

magnetic resonance imaging (MRI) a diagnostic radiological procedure using a noninvasive magnetic technique and computer for imaging the anatomy; records high-resolution magnetic fields produced in the cortex from the scalp following polarization through the use of a magnet; used to visualize soft tissue

magnitude estimation psychophysical method of measurement used primarily to scale sensations; the subject assigns numbers to a set of stimuli that are proportional to some subjective dimension of the stimuli

mainstreaming the education of deaf children in general school settings with their hearing peers

MAIS Meaningful Auditory Integration Scale; scale completed by parents used to assess a child's meaningful listening skills in everyday situations

malformation failure of normal, correct, or complete development of a body structure

malignant otitis a progressive necrotizing *Pseudomonas* infection of the ear

malignant schwannoma a malignant neoplasm of nerve sheath origin (e.g., Schwann cells) that locally infiltrates and also metastasizes

malignant tumor a growth of tissue in the body that invades and destroys neighboring tissue as well as metastasizes and spreads to distant sites in the body

malingerer an individual who feigns or exaggerates a hearing impairment

malingering feigning or exaggerating a hearing impairment; also referred to as **pseudohypacusis, functional hearing loss, nonorganic hearing loss**

malleoincudal joint joint between the malleus and the incus

malleolar fold prominent section of the tympanic membrane designed for articulation with the malleus

malleolar ligaments middle ear ligaments attaching to the malleus that help to suspend the ossicular chain in the middle ear cavity; include anterior, lateral, and superior

malleolar stripe whitish appearance on the tympanic membrane observed during otoscopy where the manubrium of the malleus is positioned; see also **manubrium**

malleus the first and largest of the three ossicles connecting the tympanic membrane to the inner ear; its shape resembles a club; the handle of the malleus (manubrium) is attached to the tympanic membrane, and the head is attached to the body of the incus; see also **hammer**

managed care health care reimbursement plan in which an organization intercedes between patient and provider and determines the kind and extent of services that will be provided

Manchester Jr. Monosyllabic Word Lists a speech perception test that consists of four sets of monosyllabic phonetically balanced word lists considered to be within the vocabulary of children 6 years of age or older

mandible a U-shaped bone forming the lower jaw

mandibulofacial dysostosis condition often associated with Treacher Collins syndrome in which cheek bones are poorly developed, there is no facial prominence, and there is a very small mandible; may be associated with aural atresia and hearing loss; see also **Treacher Collins syndrome**

mannosidosis autosomal recessive gene disorder characterized by coarse facies, progressive ataxia, hypotonia, enlarged liver and spleen, macroglossia; associated with high-frequency sensorineural hearing loss, often severe

manometer device for producing and measuring changes in air pressure

manual alphabet series of hand configurations that correspond to each letter in the alphabet; used to fingerspell words in manual communication; see also **fingerspelling, manual communication**

manual communication use of hand signals (fingerspelling, gestures, or signs) to communicate; used by some deafened persons; see also **fingerspelling, manual alphabet, manually coded English, American Sign Language (ASL)**

manually coded English any of several systems where signs represent the more important aspects of English; see also **American Sign Language (ASL)**

manubrium the long process of the malleus that rests against the tympanic membrane; see also **handle, malleus**

MAP minimal audible pressure; minimum auditory pressure; the sound pressure of a tone at the threshold of audibility that is presented by an earphone and measured or inferred at the tympanic membrane

mapping the process of setting or adjusting the speech processor for cochlear implant devices; the dynamic range of each electrode and electrode pair is determined by establishing threshold and loudness discomfort levels for electrical stimuli; also known as **cochlear implant mapping**

marginal perforation perforation or hole in the posterior-superior marginal area of the tympanic membrane; as opposed to a **central perforation**

Maroteaux-Lamy syndrome autosomal recessive disorder characterized by mucopolysaccharidosis VI with growth deficiency, coarse facies, corneal opacity, joint stiffness, hernias, macroglossia, macrocephaly, occasional hydrocephalus, chronic respiratory infections, early death from early childhood to teen years with two subtypes (A and B), A being more severe; associated with chronic middle ear fluid that leads to conductive pathology and hearing loss

Marshall syndrome autosomal dominant disorder characterized by short stature, short nose with severely depressed nasal root, myopia, cataracts, strabismus, skeletal anomalies, occasional cleft palate, maxillary and mandibular hypoplasia; associated with sensorineural hearing loss of varying severity

M

Maryland CNC lists monosyllabic word-recognition test used to discriminate among different populations with hearing impairment

masked threshold the threshold of audibility for a specified sound in the presence of another (masking) sound; see also **masker, masking**

masker (1) constant level of background noise presented to the non-test ear in an audiometric procedure; (2) type of noise used in the process of masking (e.g., narrowband noise, white noise, speech noise, multitalker babble); (3) an electronic listening device that delivers low-level noise to the ear for the purpose of masking the presence of tinnitus; see also **masked threshold, masking, tinnitus**

masker, tinnitus electronic hearing instrument designed to emit low-level noise to mask the presence of tinnitus

masking (1) the process by which the threshold of audibility for one sound is raised by the presence of another (masking) sound; (2) the amount by which the threshold of audibility of a sound is raised by the presence of another (masking) sound; see also **effective masking (EM), masked threshold, masker**

masking, backward the condition in which the masking sound appears after the masked sound and results in a threshold shift; the amount of the threshold shift is affected by the interstimulus interval

masking, binaural release from a measure of the improvement in the detectability of a signal that can occur under binaural listening conditions

masking, central masking that occurs in the higher auditory pathways of the brain when a masked sound is presented to one ear and a masking sound to the other

masking, contralateral type of masking in which a masking noise is presented to the ear opposite the test ear

masking, downward spread of the masking of low-frequency components in a signal as a result of a spread of energy from intense high-frequency components

masking, effective (EM) the least amount of narrowband noise that is theoretically required to eliminate cross hearing; the hearing threshold level to which an ear will be shifted by a given amount of noise (i.e., refers to amount of threshold shift provided by a given level of noise); refers to the level of the test signal that a masker will just-mask; does not refer to the intensity level of the masker itself

masking, forward the condition in which the masking sound appears before the masked sound and results in a threshold shift; the amount of threshold shift is directly related to the interstimulus interval

masking, maximum the highest level of masking that can be used in clinical audiometry before over-masking occurs

masking, minimum the beginning level of masking used to initiate a plateau in clinical audiometry

masking, minimum effective the lowest intensity level of a noise that just masks a signal

masking, remote downward spread of masking; situation in which low-frequency signals are masked by high-level high-frequency signals

masking, temporal obscuring the perception of a sound by pre- or poststimulatory presentation of a masker

masking, upward spread of the effect of masking that spreads from low-frequency sounds to high-frequency sounds; often occurs in speech where weaker high-frequency consonants are masked by stronger low-frequency phonemes such as vowels

masking dilemma a problem encountered in audiometric assessment of persons with moderate-to-severe conductive hearing loss; the level of noise necessary to overcome the hearing loss and to mask the nontest ear adequately exceeds interaural attenuation levels causing the masking noise to cross over to the test ear and mask the signal; see also **masking**

masking level difference (MLD) improvement in the binaural masked thresholds when the noise phase relationship is altered as compared to

stimuli that are identical in both ears; also known as **binaural release from masking**; see also **binaural masking level difference (BMLD)**

masking of tinnitus the use of an electronic listening device that delivers low-level noise to the ear for the purpose of covering (masking) the presence of tinnitus

masking tone tone used in the process of masking to eliminate the audibility of another tone or sound

mass that characteristic of matter that gives it inertia

mass reactance the acoustic analog to inductive reactance; it is greatest at high probe frequencies and is reduced with decreases in probe frequencies

master hearing aid a hearing aid with a wide variety of fitting capabilities; older technique used to fit hearing aids

mastoid the portion of the temporal bone located behind the external ear; used for bone-conduction stimulation; see also **artificial mastoid, mastoid process**

mastoid air cells air-filled spaces in the mastoid portion of the temporal bone

mastoid antrum posterior-superior region of the middle ear space containing the head of the malleus and greater part of the incus; communicates upward and backward to the mastoid antrum

mastoid cavity an air-filled tympanic space within the mastoid portion

M

of the temporal bone that contains the three auditory ossicles; communicates with the eustachian tube and the mastoid air cells

mastoid process portion of the mastoid bone that extends inferiorly and posteriorly from the external auditory meatus; see also **mastoid**

mastoidectomy surgical removal of the mastoid bone; often used to eliminate any disease process in the middle ear; see also **modified mastoidectomy, radical mastoidectomy**

mastoiditis inflammation of the mastoid; complication of otitis media that infects the mastoid bone

matrix hearing aid specifications provided by manufacturers that can be used to order hearing aids; contains desired levels of maximum output, gain, and slope

matrix, confusion a visual representation of the stimulus-response paradigm in which the stimuli are listed down the side of the matrix and the responses are represented across the top in the same order as the stimuli; may also be called a symmetric matrix; useful tool for analyzing phonemic perceptual errors

maximum comfort level the maximum intensity level of a sound that is perceived as comfortable; see also **most comfortable level (MCL)**

maximum length sequence (MLS) a signal processing technique that permits presentation of stimuli at rapid rates and subsequent deconvolution of interleaved patterns into their component responses

maximum masking the highest level of masking that can be used in clinical audiometry before overmasking occurs; see also **overmasking**

maximum power output (MPO) the maximum output limit for a hearing aid or assistive listening device that cannot be exceeded regardless of how high the volume control is raised or how loud the input sound becomes; serves as a safety feature that prevents amplification devices from emitting uncomfortably loud or harmful sounds; see also **output sound pressure level (OSPL), saturation sound pressure level (SSPL)**

May-White syndrome autosomal dominant disorder characterized by progressive ataxia beginning in the second or third decade of life, myoclonus, seizures; associated with progressive sensorineural hearing loss preceding the onset of the neurological deterioration, usually in the moderate range

McCarthy-Alpiner Scale of Hearing Handicap a self-assessment scale of self-perceived handicap imposed by a hearing loss

MCL most comfortable loudness; the intensity level of a sound that is perceived as comfortable

MCR message-to-competition ratio; relationship between the level of the desired signal (message) and the noise (competing signal) at the listener's ear; commonly reported as the difference in decibels between the intensity of the signal and the intensity of the background noise; also known as **signal-to-noise ratio (S/N, SNR)**

MCT minimal contact technology; an earmold designed to reduce the occlusion effect by only making limited contact with the cartilaginous portion of the ear canal and sealing around the perimeter at its medial tip

ME middle ear; an air-filled tympanic cavity within the mastoid portion of the temporal bone that contains the three auditory ossicles; communicates with the eustachian tube and the mastoid air cells

mean average; statistical measure of central tendency; obtained by adding the number of values and then dividing by the number of values to provide an average of all the data

mean length of utterance (MLU) use of morphemes to provide a simple index of linguistic maturity, particularly in the early stages of development

Meaningful Auditory Integration Scale (MAIS) scale completed by parents used to assess a child's meaningful listening skills in everyday situations

meatus a passageway; in the auditory system there is an external meatus (external auditory canal) and an internal meatus (internal auditory canal)

mechanical coupler the unit to which vibratory force levels are transmitted

on a bone conductor when the vibrator is excited electrically

mechanical presbycusis type of hearing loss due to aging (presbycusis) that results from changes in cochlear mechanics, often called cochlear conductive presbycusis; results in a loss of sensitivity manifested by a descending audiometric curve; see also **presbycusis**

medial toward the midline of the body

medial geniculate body (MGB) a portion of the posterior thalamus that contains major nuclei in the central auditory system

medial rectus muscle adductor muscle of the eye responsible for eye movement toward the midline of the body

medial superior olivary body nucleus in the lower brainstem where some second-order neurons synapse with third-order neurons of the ascending auditory pathways; important region for comparing inputs from the two ears; also known as **medial superior olive (MSO)**

medial superior olive (MSO) nuclear aggregate of the superior olivary complex involved in processing interaural time (phase) differences; also known as **medial superior olivary body**

median statistical measure of central tendency; determined as the midpoint of several values that are ranked

median plane localization the sensation that acoustic signals of identi-

M

cal frequency and phase presented to both ears are perceived in the middle of the head

medulla the lowest (most caudal) part of the brainstem, between the spinal cord and the pons, just above the foramen magnum; also known as the medulla oblongata

megaHertz (MHz) one million Hertz (cycles per second)

mel a unit of pitch; the pitch of a sound that is judged to be *n* times that of a 1000 mel tone is *n* thousand mels; 1000 mels is the pitch of a 1000-Hz pure tone for which the loudness level is 40 phons

membrane pliable, thin layer of tissue lining body cavities, dividing spaces, or binding structures

membrane, basement delicate noncellular layer on the bottom of the epithelium of Reissner's membrane that separates cell layers of the scala vestibuli from those of the scala media

membrane, basilar fibrous plate extending from the osseous spiral lamina to the spiral ligament on the outer wall of the cochlea; separates the scala media from the scala tympani and supports the organ of Corti

membrane, cell boundary of all body cells that controls permeability for cell entry and exit

membrane, mucous thin sheets of tissue lining body cavities or canals that open to the exterior, such as the mouth, digestive tube, and respiratory passages

membrane, otolithic membranous covering over the utricular macula;

made of small particles of mostly calcium carbonate

membrane, Reissner's membrane separating the scala media and the scala vestibuli; attached at one end to the inner part of the spiral limbus and at the other to the spiral ligament

membrane, round window thin membrane covering the round window; separates the fluid of the scala tympani from the air of the middle ear space

membrane, Scarpa's round window membrane

membrane, Shrapnell superior anterior thin portion of the tympanic membrane (near the epitympanum); also known as **pars flaccida**; does not contain the fibrous layer making it more slack than the pars tensa portion

membrane, tectorial a cellular fibrous structure in the scala media that is attached on its inner edge to the spiral limbus and is connected to the reticular lamina on its undersurface; consists of three regions: limbal, middle, and marginal zones and is superior to the organ of Corti

membrane, tympanic (TM) the membranous separation between the outer and middle ears; responsible for initiating the mechanical impedance-matching process of the middle ear; has three layers: cutaneous, fibrous, mucous

membrane, vestibular structure separating the cochlear duct from the vestibular canal

membranous labyrinth membranous sac housed within the bony labyrinth of the inner ear that contains the receptor organs for hearing and vestibular senses; filled with endolymph; see also **osseous labyrinth**

Ménière's disease pathology affecting the inner ear and resulting in sensorineural hearing loss; characteristic signs are tinnitus, vertigo, sensation of ear fullness, and a fluctuating, low-frequency sensorineural hearing loss; see also **endolymphatic hydrops**

meninges membranous sheets (dura mater, arachnoid, pia mater) surrounding the brain and spinal cord

meningioma slow-growing, vascular tumor of the membranes (meninges) surrounding the brain and spinal cord

meningitis an infection of the meninges (coverings of the brain); can be viral or bacterial; can destroy cochlear function if left untreated

mental age (MA) age level at which an individual functions intellectually as determined by standardized psychological tests

mercury battery power cell that can be used in hearing aids; inexpensive but lasts only about half as long as a zinc-air battery; approximate shelf life is year; see also **zinc-air battery**

mesencephalon referring to the midbrain just rostral to the pons

mesial toward the midline of the body or subpart, especially of the dental arch

message-to-competition ratio (MCR) relationship between the level of the desired signal (message) and the noise (competing signal) at the listener's ear; commonly reported as the difference in decibels between the intensity of the signal and the intensity of the background noise; also known as **signal-to-noise ratio (S/N, SNR)**

metabolic presbycusis loss of hearing due to physiologic aging that affects cochlear metabolism resulting in a sensorineural hearing loss; see also **presbycusis**

metacognition awareness and appropriate use of knowledge; awareness of the task and strategy variables that affect performance and the use of that knowledge to plan, monitor, and regulate performance, including attention, learning, and the use of language

metalinguistic to think about and attend to the use of language

meter, otoadmittance old instrumentation used to measure the efficiency of the middle ear system; primarily measured susceptance and conductance components

meter, sound level (SLM) an electronic instrument for measuring the RMS level of sound in accordance with an accepted national or international standard

meter, volume unit (VU) a device that records the exact output level produced in order to permit precise presentation of auditory signals in decibels

M

method of adjustment a psychophysical method of measurement used primarily to determine thresholds; the subject varies some dimension of a stimulus until that stimulus appears equal to or just noticeably different from a reference stimulus

method of constant stimuli a psychophysical method of measurement used primarily to determine thresholds; several stimuli are presented one at a time at varying intensities; the subject responds to each presentation

method of limits a psychophysical method used primarily to determine thresholds; some dimension of the stimulus, or of the difference between two stimuli, is varied incrementally until the subject changes his response; the clinician/experimenter controls the stimulus

Metz test a test that indirectly measures recruitment by determining the sensation levels at which acoustic reflex thresholds are obtained compared to pure-tone thresholds; see also **recruitment**

mg milligram; one-thousandth of a gram

MGB medial geniculate body; a portion of the posterior thalamus that contains major nuclei in the central auditory system

mho unit of measure of admittance, the reciprocal of impedance (ohm); the word is ohm spelled backward

MHz megaHertz; one million Hertz (cycles per second)

Michel dysplasia complete failure of inner ear development resulting in complete absence of the vestibule, cochlea, and internal auditory meatus; most severe form of congenital inner ear aplasia (dysplasia); see also **Mondini dysplasia, Scheibe dysplasia**

microbar one-millionth of a bar; unit of pressure

micrognathia underdevelopment of the mandible

μPa microPascal; a unit of pressure equivalent to 1 newton per square meter

microPascal (μPa) a unit of pressure equivalent to 1 newton per square meter

microphone an electronic device for converting an acoustic signal into an electrical signal; an input transducer; types include: **boom, carbon, ceramic, condenser, directional, electret, environmental, lavaliere, noise-canceling, nondirectional, omnidirectional, piezoelectric, probe, reference, unidirectional**

microphone, boom microphone used with some FM systems that is suspended out from the speaker's head

microphone, carbon early microphone that converted acoustic energy into electrical energy using carbon granules

microphone, ceramic type of piezoelectric microphone in which electric current is produced by applied mechanical emphasis

microphone, condenser a microphone with a diaphragm separated from a back plate by a small volume of air and a preamplifier

microphone, directional a microphone that is more sensitive to sound coming from one direction than from another direction; also known as **DMic**

microphone, electret a type of condenser microphone with a diaphragm made of a dielectric material that exhibits permanent polarity, as in a magnet

microphone, environmental microphone on an FM system that allows the user to hear sounds in the environment in addition to the FM signal; useful in the classroom if the child needs to hear the teacher (FM signal) as well as the other students in the classroom

microphone, lavaliere a small microphone attached to a neck cord and resting on the chest or clipped onto a tie, shirt, or other piece of clothing

microphone, noise-canceling a transducer that has an inlet to each side of its diaphragm and that is constructed so that ambient noise surrounding it is neutralized and voice input is allowed to dominate

microphone, nondirectional microphone that is sensitive to sound coming from all directions; also known as **omnidirectional**

microphone, omnidirectional microphone that is sensitive to sound coming from all directions; also known as **nondirectional**

microphone, piezoelectric type of microphone that uses crystallized substances, such as quartz, to exhibit a piezo (pressure) effect; see also **piezoelectric**

microphone, probe a tiny microphone often attached to a soft, small tube placed within the external ear canal to measure sound intensity level near the eardrum; used for real-ear measurements for hearing aid fitting and verification

microphone, reference an electret microphone used in the comparison method of signal calibration in probe microphone measurement; acts as a standard against which the probe signal is compared

microphone, unidirectional a microphone that is more sensitive to sound coming from one direction than from another direction

microphone location effect (MLE) an acoustic variable in hearing aid fittings; the increase in the input sound pressure level (SPL) in dB measured at the hearing instrument microphone location relative to the SPLs measured in the undistorted sound field

microphone telecoil switch switch on a hearing device that allows the wearer to determine the mode of input signal; options include a microphone that picks up air-borne signals or a telecoil that picks up electromagnetic signals for telephone or assistive listening device use

microphone tubing an acoustic modification for in-the-ear hearing instruments that can affect the frequency response of the device by changing the length or diameter of a tube extending from the microphone

microprocessor audiometer an audiometer that uses a small microprocessor (i.e., computer) to control signal creation, gating, attenuation, and response measurement for audiometric testing

μs microsecond; one one-millionth (1/1,000,000) of a second

microsecond (μsec) one one-millionth (1/1,000,000) of a second

microtia abnormally small external ears

μV microvolt; one one-millionth (1/1,000,000) of a volt

microvolt (μV) one one-millionth (1/1,000,000) of a volt

mid-frequency hearing loss a configuration of hearing loss with normal or essentially normal hearing in the low and high frequencies with variable degree of loss in the mid-frequencies; see also **cookie bite**

midbrain the portion of the brainstem above the pons containing the inferior colliculus; an important relay center in the auditory nervous system

middle ear (ME) an air-filled tympanic cavity within the mastoid portion of the temporal bone that contains the three auditory ossicles; communicates with the eustachian tube and the mastoid air cells

middle ear bones three small bones in the middle ear that transmit sound vibrations from the tympanic membrane to the oval window; see also **malleus, incus, stapes**

middle ear cavity an air-filled tympanic cavity within the mastoid portion of the temporal bone that contains the three auditory ossicles; communicates with the eustachian tube and the mastoid air cells

middle ear compliance ease with which energy flows through the middle ear system; determined by comparing the volume of the middle ear cavity under changing conditions of pressure during tympanometry testing

middle ear disease condition, disorder, or malfunction of middle ear structures with a recognizable set of symptoms; also known as **middle ear pathology**; see also **middle ear dysfunction**

middle ear dysfunction disorder of the middle ear that causes it to malfunction; often results in a conductive hearing loss; also known as **middle ear disease, middle ear pathology**

middle ear effusion the condition of fluid in the middle ear as a result of eustachian tube dysfunction; the fluid may be infected

middle ear elasticity flaccidity of the middle ear system measured through acoustic admittance

middle ear implants totally or semi-implantable hearing aids that often use magnetic induction to attach to some part of the ossicular chain or tympanic membrane; the amplifier and induction coil are usually placed in the external auditory canal

middle ear infection inflammation of the middle ear often resulting from eustachian tube dysfunction that can occur during or after an upper respiratory infection; often results in a conductive hearing loss; see also **middle ear dysfunction, otitis media (OM)**

middle ear muscle reflex the change in the tonus of the muscles of the middle ear in response to a stimulus; these contractions may be monitored as a change in tympanic membrane mobility (compliance) during acoustic immittance testing

middle ear pathology an abnormality of the middle ear; see also **middle ear disease**

middle ear pressure the level of air pressure in the middle ear space measured through acoustic admittance

middle ear transfer function the transfer of acoustic energy from the outer ear and the tympanic membrane to the oval window of the cochlea; achieved by changes in the mechanical energy produced from the ossicles of the middle ear; see also **middle ear transformers**

middle ear transformers physiologic mechanisms in the middle ear that transfer incoming sound from the tympanic membrane to the cochlea resulting in a mechanical advantage of energy that overcomes the impedance mismatch between the middle ear and the cochlea; see also **area-ratio hypothesis, catenary principle, lever advantage, middle ear transfer function**

middle latency response (MLR) an auditory evoked potential representing activity from the auditory radiations from the thalamus to the cortex and the primary auditory cortex; occurs between 12 and 80 ms; also known as **auditory middle latency response (AMLR)**

mild hearing loss loss of hearing sensitivity resulting in thresholds between 15 and 40 dB HL

Miller syndrome autosomal recessive disorder characterized by lower eyelid ectropion (notched lower lids), micrognathia, cleft palate and lip, anomalous auricles, limb anomalies, missing digits; associated with conductive hearing loss secondary to middle ear and/or external ear anomalies

milli- prefix: one thousandth

milligram (mg) one one-thousandth (1/1000) of a gram

millimeter (mm) a unit of measure equal to one thousandth (1/1000) of a meter

millimho (mmho) one one-thousandth (1/1000) of a mho

millisecond (ms) one one-thousandth (1/1000) of a second

millivolt (mV) one one-thousandth (1/1000) of a volt

MINI 22 (CI-22M) a miniaturized version of the Nucleus-22 cochlear implant system used for infants and children

MINICROS CROS system with a tube from the receiver directly to the ear rather than an earmold

minimal audible angle (MAA) the smallest difference in localization that a listener can determine when two successive sounds originate from the same direction

minimal audible field (MAF) the sound pressure level of a tone at the threshold of audibility measured in a free sound field for a subject facing the sound source

minimal audible pressure (MAP) the sound pressure of a tone at the threshold of audibility that is presented by an earphone and measured or inferred at the tympanic membrane

Minimal Auditory Capabilities (MAC) **battery** a comprehensive set of tests that yields a general profile of an individual's speech reception abilities ranging from awareness and identification of environmental sounds to open-set speech recognition; designed to be used with individuals having minimal auditory capabilities; provides consistency in the evaluation of cochlear implant patients

minimal contact technology (MCT) earmold an earmold designed to reduce the occlusion effect by making only limited contact with the cartilaginous portion of the ear canal and sealing around the perimeter at its medial tip

minimal pair words that sound alike except for a single phonetic feature (e.g., *cat* versus *bat*)

minimal pairs test a speech perception test used to assess the specific segmental features perceived by children who use cochlear implants

MiniMed device a type of cochlear implant that uses a transcutaneous transmission system that supports indirect transmission of stimulus information through a radio-frequency link

minimum auditory field (MAF) the sound pressure level of a tone at the threshold of audibility measured in a free sound field for a subject facing the sound source

minimum auditory pressure (MAP) the sound pressure of a tone at the threshold of audibility that is presented by an earphone and measured or inferred at the tympanic membrane

minimum effective masking the lowest intensity level of a noise that just-masks a signal; see also **effective masking (EM)**

minimum masking the beginning level of masking used to initiate a plateau in clinical audiometry

minimum masking level (MML) the lowest intensity level of a masking noise that is introduced into the nontest ear and keeps the nontest ear from responding

minispeech processor the signal processor used with a cochlear implant that is small and light and uses a magnet to affix and align the transmitter coil without a headband

mismatched negativity (MMN) an endogenous cortical auditory evoked response recorded using an oddball paradigm; results in a negative peak between 100 and 200 ms; reflects the discrimination ability for different features of sound

miss response in signal detection theory where a signal is present, but the subject does not respond

missing fundamental the perception of a low-frequency tone that is not actually in the original stimulus; a result of periodicity pitch; see also **periodicity pitch**

mixed hearing loss hearing loss with both conductive (outer and/or middle ear pathology) and sensory (cochlear or auditory nerve pathology) components; the audiogram shows a bone-conduction deficit plus an air-bone gap; see also **air-bone gap (ABG)**

mixer a sound system device for mixing two or more signal inputs to provide a common audio signal output

MLB monaural loudness balancing; a procedure for measuring recruitment or abnormal growth of loudness in patients with bilateral hearing loss; performed on one ear of a patient who has normal hearing at one frequency and a hearing loss at a different frequency; the growth of loudness with increasing intensity at the impaired frequency is compared with loudness growth for a frequency where hearing sensitivity is normal; see also **alternate binaural loudness balancing (ABLB)**

MLD masking level difference; improvement in the binaural masked thresholds when the noise phase relationship is altered as compared to stimuli that are identical in both ears; also known as **binaural release from masking**; see also **binaural masking level difference (BMLD)**

MLE microphone location effect; an acoustic variable in hearing aid fittings; the increase in the input sound pressure level (SPL) in dB measured at the hearing instrument microphone location relative to the SPLs measured in the undisturbed sound field

MLR middle latency response; an auditory evoked potential representing activity from the auditory radiations from the thalamus to the cortex and the primary auditory cortex; occurs between 12 and 80 ms; also known as **auditory middle latency response (AMLR)**

MLS maximum length sequence; a signal processing technique that permits presentation of stimuli at rapid rates and subsequent deconvolution of interleaved patterns into their component responses

MLU mean length of utterance; uses morphemes to provide a simple index of linguistic maturity, particularly in the early stages of development

MLV monitored live voice; presentation of a speech signal through an audiometer by means of a microphone; the intensity of the voice is monitored visually by means of a VU meter

mm millimeter; a unit of measure equal to one one-thousandth (1/1000) of a meter

mmho millimho; one one-thousandth (1/1000) of a mho

MML minimum masking level; the lowest intensity level of a masking noise that is introduced into the nontest ear and keeps the nontest ear from responding

MMN mismatched negativity; an endogenous cortical auditory evoked response recorded using an oddball paradigm; results in a negative peak between 100 and 200 ms; reflects the discrimination ability for different features of sound

mobilization of stapes a surgical treatment procedure used to loosen or set the stapes into motion; often used for patients who have otosclerosis; see also **otosclerosis**

mode (1) a room resonance or standing wave; (2) a statistical descriptor indicating the value that occurs most often in a set of values

moderate hearing loss peripheral loss of hearing sensitivity resulting in thresholds between 41 and 60 dB HL

moderately severe hearing loss peripheral loss of hearing sensitivity resulting in thresholds between 61 and 70 dB HL

modified mastoidectomy mastoidectomy (surgical removal of the mastoid) that eliminates the disease process with minimal sacrifice of the middle ear structures; see also **mastoidectomy**

Modified Rhyme Hearing Test (MRHT) a revised version of the Modified Rhyme Test (MRT), which is a phoneme recognition test that uses most of the same stimuli as in the MRT; used for standardization purposes; see also **Modified Rhyme Test (MRT)**

Modified Rhyme Test (MRT) a multiple-choice test utilizing rhyming consonant-vowel-consonant (CVC) speech stimuli in which the vowel is the same but the consonants differ

Modified Speech Transmission Index (MSTI) an acoustical index that combines some features of the articulation index and the speech transmission index; see also **speech transmission index (STI), articulation index (AI)**

modified Stenger test the modification of the Stenger test for malingering that uses speech stimuli instead of pure tones; also known as **speech Stenger test**; see also **Stenger test**

modiolus central part of the cochlea extending from base to apex; conically shaped central core of the cochlea; contains the spiral ganglia of the cochlea and forms the inner wall of the scala vestibuli and the scala tympani; see also **Rosenthal's canal**

modular instrument an in-the-ear hearing instrument that is built into a standard housing and then attached to a custom earmold

modulation any periodic alteration of a parameter of a vibratory phenomenon; modulations can be produced by varying the frequency, intensity, or phase of the wave

modulation, amplitude (AM) a stimulus type consisting of a carrier sound in which the amplitude is varied (modulated)

modulation, frequency (FM) (1) alteration of the frequency of transmitted waves in accordance with the sounds or images being sent; (2) form of sound transmission via radio waves in FM systems

modulation transfer function (MTF) the ability of a transmission system to reproduce patterns that vary in spatial frequency

Mohr syndrome autosomal recessive disorder characterized by relatively short stature, midline cleft of lip, broad nasal tip, hyperplastic frenulae, maxillary hypoplasia, cleft tongue, nodular tongue, and occasional cleft palate; associated with conductive hearing loss caused by ossicular anomalies, especially of the incus

monaural (1) the use of only one ear; (2) the use of only one hearing aid is a monaural fitting; (3) stimuli presented to one ear at a time in an audiologic test

monaural amplification the use of only one hearing aid; see also **monaural**

monaural loudness balance (MLB) test a procedure for measuring recruitment or abnormal growth of loudness in patients with bilateral hearing loss; performed on one ear of a patient who has normal hearing at one frequency and a hearing loss at a different frequency; the growth of loudness with increasing intensity at the impaired frequency is compared with loudness growth for a frequency where hearing sensitivity is normal; see also **alternate binaural loudness balancing (ABLB)**

monaural low-redundancy speech tests central auditory processing tests that consist of speech stimuli that are degraded by modifying or distorting the frequency, temporal, or spectral characteristics of the signal

Mondini dysplasia a congenital disorder of the inner ear consisting of incomplete development of the membranous and bony labyrinths; typically only one and one-half turns of the cochlea are affected; see also **Michel dysplasia, Scheibe dysplasia**

monitored live voice (MLV) presentation of a speech signal through an audiometer by means of a microphone; the intensity of the voice is monitored visually by means of a VU meter

monomere healed portion of the tympanic membrane that is thin and flaccid resulting from repeated perforations and a lack of regeneration of the fibrous layer of the membrane; also referred to as a monomeric eardrum

M

monopolar refers to a recording electrode arrangement in which one electrode of a pair is detecting the response and the second electrode is inactive; usually located distant from the response generator and not detecting the response

monopolar stimulation refers to the stimulation mode in which one electrode of a pair is detecting the response and the second electrode is inactive; usually located distant from the response generator and not detecting the response

monosyllabic word recognition one type of speech perception assessment that determines a patient's ability to identify single-syllable words presented in an open-set format; scored as a percentage correct; also known as **word recognition test**

Monosyllable-Trochee-Spondee (MTS) test a speech perception test consisting of one-syllable words (monosyllables), two-syllable words with unequal stress on each syllable (trochees), and two-syllable words with equal stress on each syllable (spondees); used to determine a child's ability to perceive the difference among the types of stimuli

monotic presenting a sound to only one ear (mono = one, otic = ears); see also **monaural**

monotic speech tests speech perception tests designed to determine how distortions of speech affect an individual's ability to understand words or sentences when presented to each ear separately

monotic tone tests nonspeech tests designed to assess a child's ability to perceive tones presented to each ear separately

montage the electrode positions used to record an evoked potential; usually referred to by the International 10-20 Electrode System

Moro reflex response of infants (birth to 3 months of life) to acoustic stimuli characterized by extension and abduction of arms, hands, and fingers

morpheme smallest unit of language that conveys meaning

morphology the qualitative features of an evoked potential; considers the "noisiness," the "smoothness," and the replicability of the recording, and how the recording compares to an ideal recording

most comfortable level (MCL) the intensity level of a sound that is perceived as comfortable

motherese a method of speaking to young children used by adults that is characterized by simplicity, consistency, redundancy, and exaggerated prosody; these features facilitate a child's acquisition of language

motility of outer hair cells movement (contraction and expansion) of outer hair cells in response to acoustic stimulation, reflecting active processes within the cochlea; related to generation of otoacoustic emissions; inner hair cells are not capable of motility; see also **outer hair cell**

motor neurons neurons that innervate muscle

motorboating term used to describe the sound produced from a hearing aid as the battery weakens

mouth-hand system the use of hand signals presented near the lips to supplement speechreading; provides information about those speech sounds that are not visible on the lips; see also **cued speech**

MPEAK cochlear implant signal-processing strategy most commonly used in the multispeak speech processor of the Nucleus-22 cochlear implant; identifies four different speech features and assigns each part to a different electrode

MPO maximum power output; the maximum output limit for a hearing aid or assistive listening device that cannot be exceeded regardless of how high the volume control is raised or how loud the input sound becomes; serves as a safety feature that prevents amplification devices from emitting uncomfortably loud or harmful sounds; see also **output sound pressure level (OSPL), saturation sound pressure level (SSPL)**

MRHT Modified Rhyme Hearing Test; a revised version of the Modified Rhyme Test (MRT), which is a phoneme recognition test that uses most of the same stimuli as in the MRT; used for standardization purposes; see also **Modified Rhyme Test (MRT)**

MRI magnetic resonance imaging; a diagnostic radiological procedure using a noninvasive magnetic technique and computer for imaging anatomy; records high-resolution magnetic fields produced in the cortex from the scalp following polarization through the use of a magnet; used to visualize soft tissue

MRT Modified Rhyme Test; a multiple-choice test utilizing rhyming consonant-vowel-consonant (CVC) speech stimuli in which the vowel is the same but the consonants differ

ms millisecond; one one-thousandth (1/1000) of a second

MSO medial superior olive; nuclear aggregate of the superior olivary complex involved in processing interaural time (phase) differences

MSP multispeak speech processor; cochlear implant signal-processing strategy most commonly used in the multispeak speech processor of the Nucleus-22 cochlear implant; identifies four different speech features and assigns each part to a different electrode

MSTI modified speech transmission index; an acoustical index that combines some features of the articulation index and the speech transmission index; see also **speech transmission index (STI), articulation index (AI)**

MTF modulation transfer function; the ability of a transmission system to reproduce patterns that vary in spatial frequency

MTS Monosyllable-Trochee-Spondee test; a speech perception test consisting of one-syllable words (monosyllables), two-syllable words with un-equal stress on each syllable (trochees), and two-syllable words with equal stress on each syllable (spondees); used to determine a child's ability to perceive the differ-ence among the types of stimuli

Muckle-Wells syndrome autoso-mal dominant disorder character-ized by nephritis, large rash over much of the body, limb pains; asso-ciated with progressive sensorineur-al hearing loss, first appearing in childhood, becomes severe in adult years

mucoid otitis media middle ear in-flammation with white, cloudy fluid resulting from cell secretion known as mucoid effusion; found in lengthy infections

mucopolysaccharidoses a group of heritable diseases characterized by a disorder of metabolism of mu-copolysaccharide, a protein found in blood groups; associated with **Hunter and Hurler syndromes**

mucosal wave undulation along the vocal fold surface traveling in the direction of the airflow

mucous membrane thin sheets of tissue lining body cavities or canals that open to the exterior, such as the mouth, digestive tube, and respira-tory passages

Muller-Zeman syndrome autoso-mal recessive disorder characterized by severe cognitive impairment, se-vere psychomotor retardation, usu-ally in infancy although in some cas-

es onset is in childhood, progressive visual impairment, progressive con-tractures; associated with progres-sive sensorineural hearing loss

multiband compression a type of nonlinear amplification that uses in-dependent automatic gain control circuits for each frequency band within a hearing aid; allows variabil-ity in the amount of reduced gain across each frequency range; see also **compression**

multichannel cochlear implants cochlear implants using multiple electrodes that result in the poten-tial use of multiple channels for stimulation

multichannel hearing aids type of hearing aid that contains several channels or bands of frequencies; al-lows considerable flexibility in mak-ing adjustments to the frequency re-sponse of the hearing aid for greater user satisfaction

multielectrode/multichannel more than one channel of information; of-ten used to describe cochlear im-plants that present different chan-nels of information to different regions of the cochlea; see also **cochlear implant (CI)**

multifrequency coding a type of sig-nal processing strategy used for both intra- and extracochlear cochlear im-plants that splits a full bandwidth into separate bands; each band is in-dependently balanced for loudness and then recombined into a single signal

multimemory hearing aid hearing aid that has the ability to store different "listening programs" for access by the user; see **digitally controlled analog (DCA) aid**

multipeak cochlear implant signal-processing strategy most commonly used in the multispeak speech processor of the Nucleus-22 cochlear implant; identifies four different speech features and assigns each part to a different electrode

multiple sclerosis (MS) a progressive disease in which nerve fibers of the brain and spinal cord demyelinate; can affect the conduction of auditory information via auditory nerve fibers resulting in retrocochlear hearing loss

multiple synostosis conductive hearing loss a conductive hearing loss resulting from a skeletal or articular syndrome

Multiple-Choice Discrimination Test a phoneme recognition test that consists of monosyllabic words presented in a multiple-choice closed-set format; yields more information regarding phoneme perception than that obtained from other monosyllabic word tests

Multiple-Choice Intelligibility Test a measure of a person's speaking efficiency as reflected by another listener's performance in communication situations; a speech perception test that determines a speaker's ability to be heard correctly; an assessment of intelligibility under quiet and noisy conditions

multiple-memory hearing aid programmable hearing aid that contains several different frequency responses for use in varying listening environments; often accessed by using a remote control

multipolar one of seven types of morphologic cell types in the auditory brain stem

multisensory approach educational approach for deaf children that emphasizes the use of vision, residual hearing, and touch to enhance communication

multispeak speech processor (MSP) cochlear implant signal-processing strategy most commonly used in the multispeak speech processor of the Nucleus-22 cochlear implant; identifies four different speech features and assigns each part to a different electrode

multitalker noise speech noise made up of several talkers, all speaking at once; may be all male, all female, or a combination of both; used in speech perception testing to simulate realistic communication environments

multitalker noise test a speech perception test presented in a background of noise; used to determine an individual's perception of speech in noise

mumps childhood infectious disease known to cause unilateral sensorineural deafness

muscle tissue of contractible fibers, generally grouped as smooth, skeletal, cardiac; supports movement of organs and body parts

muscle, auricularis muscle that inserts into the cartilage of the ear; innervated by the facial nerve; five branches include anterior, posterior, superior, transverse, oblique

muscle, lateral rectus muscle of the eye responsible for eye movement away from the midline of the body

muscle, levator veli palatini muscle in the region of the neck that contracts along with other muscles to open the eustachian tube

muscle, medial rectus adductor muscle of the eye responsible for eye movement toward the midline of the body

muscle, stapedius the smallest muscle in the human body attached to the posterior portion of the neck of the stapes and innervated by cranial nerve VII; it contracts in response to high-intensity sound; the combined action of the stapedius and tensor tympani muscles limits the motion of the auditory ossicles and thereby protects the inner ear from damage from intense sound

muscle, tensor tympani an intra-aural muscle of the middle ear whose tendon is attached to the manubrium of the malleus; its contraction increases tension on the tympanic membrane; the combined action of the tensor tympani and the stapedius muscles limits the motion of the auditory ossicles and thereby helps to protect the inner ear from damage from intense sound, especially low frequencies

muscle, tensor veli palatini muscle in the region of the neck that contracts along with other muscles to open the eustachian tube

muscle artifact signals recorded in electrophysiologic measurements that are not from the generator site but are from random muscle activity that occurs in the same time frame as the desired response; these signals typically are not included in the averaging of the response

mV millivolt; one one-thousandth (1/1000) of a volt

myasthenia gravis a defect in the conduction of nerve impulses at the myoneural junction resulting in chronic fatigability and muscle weakness, particularly in the throat and face

myelencephalon portion of the embryonic brain giving rise to the medulla oblongata

myelin fatty sheath surrounding axons of some nerves; speeds transmission of nerve impulses; see also **Schwann cell**

myogenic resulting from muscle activity (versus neurogenic)

myringitis inflammation of the tympanic membrane

myringoplasty surgical repair of the tympanic membrane with a skin graft

myringotomy a surgical procedure in which an opening is cut in the eardrum and fluid is drained from the middle ear; may also include the insertion of a pressure equalization (PE) tube

N

N Newton; unit of physical force

N/m² Newton per square meter; unit of measurement for sound pressure

N1 the first negative voltage peak of the auditory late response normally occurring approximately 90 to 110 ms after an acoustic stimulus; presumably arising from the auditory cortex; also known as **N100**

N100 the first negative voltage peak of the auditory late response normally occurring approximately 90 to 110 ms after an acoustic stimulus; presumably arising from the auditory cortex; also known as **N1**

N2 the second negative peak of the auditory late response following the middle latency auditory evoked potentials or the first negative peak following the N100 and occurring between 180 to 250 ms in adults; also known as **N200**

N200 the second negative peak of the auditory late response following the middle latency auditory evoked potentials or the first negative peak following the N100 and occurring between 180 to 250 ms in adults; also known as **N2**

N400 an endogenous response to semantic and linguistic constraints occurring about 400 to 500 ms after the end of a sentence; unlike the earlier waves, it is not necessarily the fourth negative peak in sequence

N90 the first negative peak following the middle latency auditory evoked potentials occurring between 80 and 150 ms in adults

Na the first major negative-voltage peak in the middle latency response that precedes peak Pa and normally occurs approximately 13 to 15 ms after an acoustic stimulus

Na+ sodium; chemical found in extracellular fluid

NAD National Association of the Deaf; advocacy group whose purpose is to safeguard the accessibility and civil rights of deaf and hard-of-hearing Americans in education, employment, health care, and telecommunications; established in 1880

Nager syndrome autosomal recessive disorder characterized by severe micrognathia, cleft or absent palate, absent or hypoplastic thumbs, radial anomalies, external and middle ear anomalies; associated with conductive hearing loss caused by ossicular anomalies including fixation of the footplate of the stapes

NAL National Acoustic Laboratories; acronym for hearing aid prescription formula devised by the National Acoustic Laboratories in Australia

NAL-R curve revised National Acoustics Laboratory hearing aid fitting prescriptive procedure that prescribes specific target gain values per frequency

nanovolt (nV) one billionth of a volt

narrow-band filter a band-pass filter that passes energy in a narrow band of frequencies between a lower cutoff frequency and an upper cutoff frequency

narrow-band noise (NBN) a band of noise with its sound energy concentrated around a center frequency; used in masking pure tones

nasion a location on the scalp that is midline on the forehead between the eyebrows or on the bridge of the nose where the frontal and nasal bones meet; the ground electrode for electrophysiology is often placed here

nasopharynx back of the throat that connects to the middle ear by way of the eustachian tube

National Acoustics Laboratory (NAL) procedure a linear hearing aid fitting prescriptive procedure devised at the National Acoustic Laboratories in Australia that prescribes specific target gain values per frequency

National Association of the Deaf (NAD) advocacy group whose purpose is to safeguard the accessibility and civil rights of deaf and hard-of-hearing Americans in education, employment, health care, and telecommunications; established in 1880

National Examination in Speech-Language Pathology and Audiology (NESPA) an objective, comprehensive assessment of knowledge in the field of communication sciences and disorders; a passing score on this examination satisfies one of the requirements for obtaining a certificate of clinical competence from the American Speech-Language-Hearing Association; see also **certificate of clinical competence (CCC)**

National Hearing Aid Society (NHAS) a professional organization that disseminates information about hearing aids and hearing problems to the public

National Hearing Conservation Association (NHCA) organization of hearing conservationists

National Institute for Hearing Instrument Sciences (NIHIS) branch of the International Hearing Society responsible for education

National Institute for Occupational Safety and Health (NIOSH) national organization that performs studies regarding the safety and health of various occupations; prominent organization in the development and enforcement of legislation for noise control

National Institute on Deafness and Other Communication Disorders (NIDCD) branch of the National Institutes of Health providing financial support for research on communicative disorders; established in 1988

National Student Speech-Language-Hearing Association (NSSLHA) a professional student organization under the auspices of the American Speech-Language-Hearing Association that involves undergraduate and graduate students in audiology and speech-language pathology; established in 1972

natural resonant frequency the frequency at which a system's vibrating element will vibrate after the external force displacing it from its normal position has ceased to act; measured in cycles per second (cps)

Nb the second major negative voltage peak in the middle latency response that follows peak Pa and normally occurs in the 30 to 40 ms region

NBN narrow-band noise; a band of noise with its sound energy concentrated around a center frequency; used in masking pure tones

NCC noise criterion curve; standard spectrum curves by which a given measured noise may be described by a single noise criterion number

near-field a sensory-evoked response recorded with an electrode close to or on the neural generator; results in high amplitude recordings of the response; see also **far-field**

NECCI Network of Educators for Children with Cochlear Implants; professional organization of speech and hearing professionals and educators who are involved with children who receive and use cochlear implants

neckloop a transducer worn around the neck as part of an FM assistive device system consisting of a cord from a receiver; transmits signals via electromagnetic induction to the telecoil of the user's hearing aid

necrosis the death of localized tissue resulting from some injury or disease

negative correlation inverse relationship between two parameters; as one value increases, the other decreases

negative middle ear pressure the level of air pressure in the middle ear space that is below atmospheric pressure; suggests poor eustachian tube functioning and the possibility of a retracted tympanic membrane

negativity difference wave the resulting negative wave from subtraction of one waveform from another in electrophysiologic measurement; see also **mismatched negativity (MMN)**

neomycin sterile antibacterial and anti-inflammatory solution; can be ototoxic

neonatal intensive care unit (NICU) area within a hospital for neonates who need comprehensive monitoring and support

neonatal screening identification audiometry performed on newborns utilizing behavioral and electrophysiologic techniques; used for early identification of potential hearing loss; see also **universal newborn hearing screening**

neonate a newborn infant; the first 28 days of life after term (40 weeks gestation)

neoplasia a growth or tumor (e.g., schwannoma or neoplasm)

neoplasm an abnormal growth of benign or malignant tissue

nephritis inflammation and abnormal function of the kidneys (nephrons)

nephrons the structural and functional unit of the kidneys

nephrotoxic poisoning of the kidneys; often occurs with ototoxic drugs

nerve bundle of nerve fibers outside the central nervous system that has functional utility

nerve, abducens cranial nerve VI responsible for control of eye movements

nerve, accessory cranial nerve XI responsible for speech, swallowing, and head and shoulder movements

nerve, acoustic cranial nerve VIII; consists of two sets of fibers: the anterior branch or cochlear nerve and the posterior branch or vestibular nerve; conducts neural signals from the inner ear to the brain

nerve, auditory division of cranial nerve VIII that provides the link between the cochlea and the central auditory system

nerve, cochlear cranial nerve VIII; consists of two sets of fibers: the anterior branch or cochlear nerve and the posterior branch or vestibular nerve; conducts neural signals from the inner ear to the brain; preferred terminology is auditory nerve

nerve, cranial 12 pairs of nerves originating at the base of the brain that carry messages for such functions as hearing, vision, swallowing, phonation, tongue movement, smell, eye movement, pupil contraction, equilibrium, mastication, facial expression, glandular secretion, taste, head movement, and shoulder movement; starting with the most anterior, cranial nerves are enumerated by Roman numerals; (CN I) olfactory, (CN II) optic, (CN III) oculomotor, (CN IV) trochlear, (CN V) trigeminal, (CN VI) abducens, (CN VII) facial, (CN VIII) acoustic (cochleovestibular), (CN IX) glossopharyngeal, (CN X) vagus, (CN XI) accessory, (CN XII) hypoglossal

nerve, facial cranial nerve VII that innervates facial muscles

nerve, glossopharyngeal cranial nerve IX responsible for the sense of taste and secretion from certain glands

nerve, hypoglossal cranial nerve XII responsible for swallowing and moving the tongue

nerve, oculomotor cranial nerve III responsible for movements of the eyes

nerve, olfactory cranial nerve I responsible for the sense of smell

nerve, optic cranial nerve II responsible for afferent innervation from the eyes

nerve, trigeminal cranial nerve V responsible for chewing, face sensitivity, and muscle innervation; innervates the tensor tympani middle ear muscle and muscles used to open and close the eustachian tube

nerve, trochlear cranial nerve IV responsible for efferent innervation for eye movement

nerve, vagus cranial nerve X named for its wandering course that extends through the neck, thorax, and abdomen; provides neural innervation to the external ear and the speech mechanism including the larynx, tongue, and palate

nerve, vestibular branch of cranial nerve VIII responsible for carrying balance sensations to the brain; runs alongside the auditory and facial nerves inside the internal auditory canal

nerve, vestibulocochlear cranial nerve VIII with its auditory and vestibular branches

nerve, VIIIth cranial nerve VIII, known as the **vestibulocochlear nerve** consisting of vestibular and cochlear branches

nerve deafness inappropriate term used to describe severe-to-profound hearing loss due to some pathology of cranial nerve VIII

nervous system anatomic neural pathways including the peripheral and central nervous systems with their associated ganglia, nerves, and sense organs; gathers and evaluates stimuli and sends impulses to effector organs; responsible for motion, sensation, thought, and control of various other bodily functions; includes the autonomic, central, parasympathetic, peripheral, and sympathetic nervous systems

NESPA National Examination in Speech-Language Pathology and Audiology; an objective, comprehensive assessment of knowledge in the field of communication sciences and disorders; a passing score on this examination satisfies one of the requirements for obtaining a certificate of clinical competence from the American Speech-Language-Hearing Association

netilmicin aminoglycoside antibiotic similar to kanamycin used to treat severe infections; known to be ototoxic

Network of Educators of Children with Cochlear Implants (NECCI) professional organization of speech and hearing professionals and educators who are involved with children who receive and use cochlear implants

neural density refers to the number of nerve fibers that fire in response to stimulation; the louder the stimulus, the greater the neural density

neural discharge release of a neural substance during neuronal firing; to release a burst of energy from or through a neuron

neural firing rate the rate at which individual and groups of nerve fibers fire when stimulated; neural firing rate typically increases with rapid, intense stimulation

neural generator neurologic site that is the origin of a response measured in electrophysiologic testing

neural plasticity the ability of the neural system to change and develop over time in response to sensory input

neural plate embryonic structure made up of a thick layer of ectodermal tissue; gives rise to the neural tube and subsequently structures of the brain and spinal cord as well as other tissues of the central nervous system

neural presbycusis a type of hearing loss due to physiologic aging resulting from a loss of spiral ganglion cells or their peripheral processes that is out of proportion to organ of Corti degeneration; see also **presbycusis**

neural synchrony the ability of a group of neurons to activate simultaneously; the simultaneous discharge of multiple auditory neurons that is often elicited by a loud transient stimulus (e.g., a click)

neural tinnitus tinnitus (ringing in the ears) with a neural origin or etiology

neural tube embryonic structure surrounded by ectoderm that develops from the neural groove and eventually gives rise to the structures of the central nervous system (e.g., brain, spinal cord)

neurilemma the layer of Schwann cells that forms the myelin sheath surrounding peripheral nerve fibers

neurilemmoma tumor, synonymous with schwan- noma

neurinoma a benign tumor of the nerve sheath

neuritis inflammation of a nerve that may result in paralysis, muscular atrophy, and defective reflexes

neuro-otology branch of medicine concerned with the neurological aspects of the auditory and vestibular systems; concerned with diagnosis and medical treatment of hearing and balance disorders

neuroaudiology subspecialty of audiology concentrated on the diagnosis of peripheral and central lesions of the auditory system

neurodiagnosis differentiation and localization of cochlear versus retrocochlear auditory dysfunction that can be obtained through a battery of tests including both behavioral and electrophysiologic measures; see also **differential diagnosis, site of lesion (SOL)**

neuroepithelial abnormalities defects of the sensory neuroepithelia, including the organ of Corti, leading to uncomplicated hearing loss or nonsyndromal hearing loss

neurofibroma fibrous tissue growth on nerve cells; results from abnormal proliferation of Schwann cells

neurofibromatosis a congenital nervous system disorder transmitted via autosomal dominance resulting in numerous fibrous tumors on nerve tissue; peripheral (NF1) or central (NF2) nervous system disease; also known as **von Recklinghausen's disease**

neurologic dysfunction improper function of the neural system

neurologist a medical doctor who specializes in the nervous system and its disorders

neurology the study of the nervous system

neuroma a tumor or growth along a nerve (e.g., an acoustic tumor in the internal auditory canal)

neuromaturation the process of development and growth of the nervous system in regard to processing and understanding language

neuron the basic unit of the nervous system consisting of an entire nerve cell, including cell body, axon, and dendrites; transmits information usually in the form of nerve impulses

neuronal circuitry refers to the configuration or arrangement of nerve fibers that allows for the transmission of information via neural impulses

neuronal pathway a particular route of nerves that transmits information to and from specific points of origin

neuronitis an extralabyrinthine cochleovestibular disorder that causes a paroxysmal attack of severe vertigo; due to unilateral vestibular dysfunction

neuropathy degeneration or inflammation of nerve fibers; a disorder involving the cranial nerves on the peripheral or autonomic nervous system; also known as **neuritis**

neurophysiology the manner in which individual neurons and populations of neurons respond to stimuli

neuroplasticity the ability of the nervous system to undergo organizational changes in response to internal and external deviations

neuropresbycusis a type of hearing loss due to aging that results from atrophy of the spiral ganglion and nerves of the osseous spiral lamina, mainly in the basal corridor; characterized by high-frequency sensorineural hearing loss with poor single-syllable word identification; see also **presbycusis**

neurotransmitter chemical agent released by vesicles of a nerve cell that permits synaptic transmission between neurons

Newton (N) unit of physical force

Newton's laws of motion (1) law of inertia: all bodies remain at rest or in a state of uniform motion unless another force acts in opposition; (2) law of force: the acceleration of an object is directly proportional to the net force applied to the object and inversely proportional to the object's mass; (3) law of reaction force: with every force there must be associated an equal reaction force of opposite direction

NF1 neurofibromatosis I; von Recklinghausen's disease; peripheral disorder characterized by multiple tumors that can occur on any nerve (neurofibromas)

NF2 neurofibromatosis II; central disorder characterized by bilateral vestibular schwannomas that are fast-growing

NH normal hearing; standard against which to compare hearing loss; in an audiometric test booth it is approximately 0 dB for a pure-tone test and nearly 100% for word identification

nHL decibels hearing level; a decibel scale used in auditory brainstem response measurement referenced to the average behavioral threshold for a click stimulus of a small group of normal-hearing subjects; see also **dB nHL**

NHAS National Hearing Aid Society; a professional organization that disseminates information about hearing aids and hearing problems to the public

NHCA National Hearing Conservation Association; organization of hearing conservationists

nickel cadmium battery nicad; a rechargeable storage battery having a positive plate of nickel, a negative plate of cadmium, and an electrolyte of potassium hydroxide

NICU neonatal intensive care unit; area within a hospital for neonates needing comprehensive monitoring and support

NIDCD National Institute for Deafness and Other Communicative Disorders; branch of the National Institutes of Health providing financial support for research on communicative disorders; established in 1988

NIHIS National Institute for Hearing Instrument Sciences; branch of the International Hearing Society responsible for education

NIHL noise-induced hearing loss; the cumulative permanent hearing loss

that is due to repeated exposure to intense noise; also known as **permanent threshold shift (PTS)** or **noise-induced permanent threshold shift (NIPTS)**; see also **permanent threshold shift (PTS)**

NIOSH National Institute for Occupational Safety and Health; national organization that performs studies regarding the safety and health of various occupations; prominent organization in the development and enforcement of legislation for noise control

NIPTS noise-induced permanent threshold shift; permanent decrease in an individual's hearing thresholds as a result of exposure to excessive sound levels

Nitchie method an aural rehabilitation method involving speechreading using analytic techniques

NITTS noise-induced temporary threshold shift; transient shift in an individual's hearing thresholds as a result of exposure to excessive sound levels; hearing returns to the pre-exposure levels after sufficient recovery time

nitrogen mustard antineoplastic drug used in the treatment of cancer and tumors; has significant ototoxic potential

Noah computer software package used for fitting programmable and digital hearing aids; used with the Hi-Pro computer interface

node a point, line, or plane in a vibrating body or room where minimal vibration occurs

nodes of Ranvier regions of myelinated fibers in which there is no myelin

noise (1) any undesired sound; any unwanted disturbance within a useful frequency band such as undesired electric waves in a transmission channel or device; (2) in evoked response measurement, unwanted electrical or muscular activity that interferes with detection of the response (signal); see also **electrophysiology**

noise, ambient background noise from all sources that are in the test environment

noise, background ambient noise, often in competition with a speech signal; a major complaint of hearing aid users

noise, broad-band a band of noise covering a wide range of frequencies

noise, Gaussian white noise; noise in which the amplitudes of the multiple frequencies follow a Gaussian distribution

noise, impact unwanted high-intensity sound that occurs when one moving body strikes against or collides with another body; can cause noise-induced hearing loss

noise, impulse noise of a transient nature due to the impact of explosive bursts; has an instantaneous rise time and short duration; high peak sound pressures from impulse noise are often the cause of acoustic trauma

noise, narrow-band (NBN) a band of noise with its sound energy concentrated around a center frequency; used in masking pure tones

noise, pink an irregular type of noise sometimes used in hearing science but generally irrelevant for clinical audiology; spectrum level of the noise decreases as frequency increases

noise, speech type of stimulus consisting of filtered white noise with a frequency spectrum containing the typical spectrum of speech

noise, white (WN) a broadband noise with approximately equal energy per cycle; the bandwidth is limited by the characteristics of the transducer; also known as **Gaussian noise**

noise blocker an adaptive circuit for noise reduction or speech enhancement in a hearing device; see also **zeta noise blocker**

noise box an instrument that contains a simple clockwork mechanism that produces a loud white noise; also known as **Barany box**

noise canceling microphone a transducer that has an inlet to each side of its diaphragm and that is constructed so that ambient noise surrounding it is neutralized and voice input is allowed to dominate

noise control methods and strategies that reduce the intensity of a noise or the time of noise exposure in order to minimize an individual's risk for hearing damage

noise criterion curve (NCC) standard spectrum curves by which a given measured noise may be described by a single noise criterion number

noise emission level the decibel level measured at a specified distance and direction from a noise source in an open environment above a specified type of surface

noise exposure refers to the intensity level and the length of time one is exposed to noise

noise interference level the level at which speech signals are masked by noise

noise floor the number of decibels at the bottom end of the rejection rate of a filter; corresponds to the frequency limit for energy rejection

noise notch hearing loss measured at 4000 Hz indicative of noise-induced hearing loss; the audiogram configuration often reflects normal hearing through 2 kHz with a dip at 4 kHz and rising back to normal at 6 kHz and 8 kHz; also known as **4k notch**

noise reduction the attenuation of the sound pressure level of a noise measured at two different locations

noise reduction rating (NRR) a scale used to rate the amount of sound attenuation provided by hearing protection devices

noise suppression type of signal processing for hearing aids that minimizes amplification of low-frequency noise in hearing instruments

noise transmission the propagation of noise through different media with interference

noise-induced hearing loss (NIHL) the cumulative permanent hearing loss that is due to repeated exposure to intense noise; also known as **permanent threshold shift (PTS)** or **noise-induced permanent threshold shift (NIPTS)**; see also **permanent threshold shift (PTS)**

noise-induced permanent threshold shift (NIPTS) permanent decrease in an individual's hearing thresholds as a result of exposure to excessive sound levels; see also **permanent threshold shift (PTS)**

noise-induced temporary threshold shift (NITTS) transient shift in an individual's hearing thresholds as a result of exposure to excessive sound levels; hearing returns to the pre-exposure levels after sufficient recovery time; see also **temporary threshold shift (TTS)**

nominal impedance minimum impedance of a loudspeaker

nominal operating level the signal level that provides the best operating parameters and performance from sound equipment

nominal scale a qualitative scale of measurement that categorizes the measurement of interest into appropriate groupings or classifications

nonacoustic reflex a middle-ear muscle reflex that is elicited by a nonacoustic stimulus

nondirectional microphone microphone that is sensitive to sound coming from all directions

noninverting electrode a primary or active electrode usually leading to the positive voltage input of a differential amplifier; the vertex electrode in auditory evoked response measurements

nonlinear circuitry components in a hearing device that are responsible for varying the amount of amplification depending on the input levels and maximum power output settings

nonlinear distortion interference that affects a signal such that the sound output varies from its input in a nonlinear fashion; often described as harmonic or intermodulation distortion

nonlinear hearing aid a hearing aid that does not provide a one-to-one correspondence between input and output at all input levels; a hearing aid that uses some form of compression

nonlinear hearing protection device type of hearing protection that provides selective hearing protection as a function of input levels; provides no protection for low-intensity signals; provides increasing protection as intensity levels increase

nonoccluding earmold an open earmold that markedly reduces low-frequency amplification by allowing low-frequency energy to enter the ear without being amplified; useful device for a high-frequency steeply sloping hearing loss; also useful in ears that require substantial ventilation because it does not close off the ear canal

nonorganic hearing loss a variety of hearing deficits for which there is no apparent anatomic and/or physiologic explanation; see also **pseudohypacusis, malingering**

nonsense syllable monosyllabic meaningless combination of consonants and vowels; used in speech audiometry

Nonsense Syllable Test (NST) speech perception test using nonsense syllables; Edgerton-Danhauer NST (ED-NST) utilizes bisyllabic nonsense syllables in an open-set format; Closed-Response NST (CR-NST) utilizes monosyllabic nonsense syllables in a closed-set format

nonsuppurative otitis media middle ear inflammation with effusion that is uninfected; e.g., mucoid or serous otitis media

nonsyndromal recessive hearing loss a loss of hearing due to recessive hereditary transmission that is unaccompanied by any other abnormalities

nontest ear (NTE) the ear not intended to be tested during an audiometric procedure; the ear receiving the masking noise during clinical masking

nonverbal patients individuals who are unable to use oral speech and language

Noonan syndrome autosomal dominant disorder characterized by small stature, cognitive impairment, low posterior hairline, webbed neck, pulmonary stenosis, vertebral anomalies, downslanting eyes, and occasional cleft palate (often submucous); associated with occasional sensorineural hearing loss and/or conductive impairment

normal hearing (NH) standard against which to compare hearing loss; in an audiometric test booth it is approximately 0 dB for a pure-tone test and nearly 100% for word identification

normalization standardization from a sample of the population of interest thought to represent typical values of the characteristic under study or test

normative data statistical information on normal characteristics of data; used to differentiate patients with peripheral or central auditory system dysfunction from patients without dysfunction

Northhampton charts aural rehabilitation method involving phonetic significance of the letters of the alphabet

Northwestern University Auditory Test No. 6 (NU-6) commonly used phonetically balanced monosyllabic word recognition test; see also **NU-6**

Northwestern University Children's Perception of Speech (NU-CHIPS) a pediatric speech audiometry picture identification procedure for young children

nosology the science of disease classification; any system of classification of diseases

notch filter (1) type of filter used in evoked response measurement designed to reduce interference from 60-Hz (cycle) electrical activity (power line noise); (2) a filter that at-

tenuates a given frequency band of the input signal; also known as **band-reject filter**

NR no response

NRR noise reduction rating; a scale used to rate the amount of sound attenuation provided by hearing protection devices

NSSLHA National Student Speech-Language-Hearing Association; a professional student organization under the auspices of the American Speech-Language-Hearing Association that involves undergraduate and graduate students in audiology and speech-language pathology; established in 1972

NST Nonsense Syllable Test; speech perception test using nonsense syllables; Edgerton-Danhauer NST (ED-NST) utilizes bisyllabic nonsense syllables in an open-set format; Closed-Response NST (CR-NST) utilizes monosyllabic nonsense syllables in a closed-set format

NTE nontest ear; the ear not intended to be tested during an audiometric procedure; the ear receiving the masking noise during clinical masking

NU-CHIPS Northwestern University Children's Perception of Speech; a pediatric speech audiometry picture identification procedure for young children

NU-6 a word-identification list from the Northwestern University (NU-6) test that contains consonant-nucleus-consonant (CNC) stimuli

nubbin slang term for button receivers used with body style hearing aids

nucleus (1) the part of the cell that contains the genetic material; an aggregate of neuron cell bodies within the brain or spinal cord; (2) the most prominent word in an utterance; (3) the vocalic portion of a syllable

nucleus, ambiguus one of the cranial motor nuclei of the brainstem with motor neurons that innervate laryngeal, pharyngeal, and esophageal muscles

nucleus, caudate a major deep brain cell body of gray matter that is part of the basal ganglia

nucleus, cochlear (CN) initial brainstem nucleus of the auditory neural pathway found within the pons and subdivided into anteroventral, posteroventral, and dorsal cochlear nuclei; primary origin of sources of the lateral lemniscus, or central auditory pathway

nucleus, hypoglossal one of the cranial motor nuclei with motor neurons that innervate the extrinsic and intrinsic muscles of the tongue; only one muscle protrudes the tongue, with most motor neurons innervating muscles that retract the tongue or alter its shape

nucleus, solitary tract one of the cranial sensory nuclei of the brainstem that receives sensory input from the oral, pharyngeal, and laryngeal regions; some of the sensory input is involved with taste; interneurons within discrete subdivisions of the nucleus serve multiple functions including controlling blood pressure, respiratory regularity, swallowing, and taste

Nucleus Perceptual Skills Battery a battery of tests designed to measure the perceptual skills of children between the ages of 2 and 15; see also **Test of Auditory Perception Skills (TAPS)**

Nucleus-22 channel cochlear implant a multielectrode, multichannel cochlear implant used in children and adults who have profound hearing loss and do not benefit from more traditional types of amplification; contains up to 22 electrodes that are implanted in the cochlea and provide direct electrical stimulation of auditory nerve fibers

null hypothesis the hypothesis to be tested in statistics; assumes no difference between data sets

nV nanovolt; one billionth of a volt

Nyquist frequency the highest frequency that can be sampled in digital signal processing without aliasing or distortion; frequency equal to one-half of the sampling rate

nystagmus involuntary, rhythmic, horizontal movements of the eyeballs; may result from stimulation of the vestibular (balance) system; recorded during electronystagmography; types include **ageotropic, caloric, down-beating, gaze, geotropic, jerk, left-beating, optokinetic, positional, positioning, right-beating, rotary, spontaneous, up-beat-**

ing; see also **electronystagmography (ENG)**

nystagmus, ageotropic type of positional nystagmus that beats away from the ground; if the patient's head is positioned so that the left side is down (toward the ground), then the nystagmus beats away from that side

nystagmus, caloric type of nystagmus induced by stimulation of the horizontal semicircular canal with warm or cool water

nystagmus, down-beating type of vertical nystagmus in which the fast phase beats downward; can be pathological

nystagmus, gaze type of nystagmus that occurs during gaze testing; can occur to one or both sides

nystagmus, geotropic type of positional nystagmus that beats toward the ground; if the patient's head is positioned so that the left side is down (toward the ground), then the nystagmus beats toward that side

nystagmus, jerk back and forth movement of the eyes with different velocities in the two directions; can be rotatory, horizontal, and vertical

nystagmus, left-beating type of horizontal nystagmus in which the fast phase angles to the left

nystagmus, optokinetic (OKN) repetitive eye movement with alternating fast saccadic eye movements in one direction and then slower smooth movements in the opposite direction as during head rotation or movement of a visual stimulus past the eyes

nystagmus, positional the presence of nystagmus that occurs in specific head positions

nystagmus, positional alcoholic (PAN) nystagmus that is evoked by a change in head position after the ingestion of alcohol

nystagmus, positioning the presence of nystagmus that is evoked by movement and changes in head position

nystagmus, right-beating type of horizontal nystagmus in which the fast phase angles to the right

nystagmus, rotary type of nystagmus characterized by rotation of the eyes in a clockwise or counter-clockwise direction

nystagmus, spontaneous the presence of nystagmus without an evoking stimulus

nystagmus, up-beating type of vertical nystagmus in which the fast phase beats upward; can be pathological

O symbol used to reflect unmasked, right ear, air-conduction thresholds on an audiogram

OAE otoacoustic emission; sound generated by energy produced by the outer hair cells in the cochlea and detected with a microphone placed within the external ear canal; useful technique for determining cochlear function; can be included as part of a diagnostic test battery; see also **distortion product otoacoustic emission (DPOAE), transient evoked otoacoustic emission (TEOAE)**

objective physically measurable

objective tinnitus rare form of tinnitus (ringing in the ears) that is audible to other individuals as well as the patient; see also **tinnitus**

objective vertigo the sensation that the room is spinning around the patient; see also **vertigo**

oblique diagonal

OCB olivocochlear bundle; the efferent auditory nerve fibers that originate from the periolivary nuclei, following the vestibular nerve to the cochlear nerve in the inner ear and eventually to the hair cells

occipital lobe most posterior lobe of the brain that contains the primary and secondary visual cortices

occluded ear simulator device designed to have the same acoustic impedance as the average normal adult ear; used for the evaluation of electronic or acoustic modifications of a hearing aid; see also **2-cc coupler**

occlusion effect (OE) (1) the perception of increased loudness of a bone-conducted signal when the outer ear is somehow occluded (e.g., covered with a supra-aural earphone or sealed with an insert earphone, earmold, or hearing aid); characteristic of normal hearers and patients with sensorineural hearing losses; not seen in patients with conductive losses; (2) barrel effect, a common complaint of hearing aid wearers

occupational hearing conservation program (OHCP) program implemented in excessively noisy occupational environments with the goal of preventing permanent hearing loss associated with exposure to industrial noise; must be initiated whenever employee noise exposures equal or exceed an 8-hour time-weighted average sound level of 85 dBA according to the Occupational Safety and Health Administration; includes qualification (measurement of environmental sound levels); abatement of excessive noise, regular monitoring of hearing sensitivity, education, and the provision of hearing protection

occupational hearing loss noise-induced hearing loss incurred on the job

occupational noise exposure exposure to high levels of noise as a result of one's job

Occupational Safety and Health Administration (OSHA) federal agency that established legislation (the Occupational Safety and Health Act) that was passed in 1970 that established minimum standards for worker safety and health including industrial hearing conservation regulations

occupational therapist (OT) a health-care professional who assists individuals in regaining and/or building physical, developmental, social, and emotional skills that are important for health and well-being

octave the interval between two sounds having a basic frequency ratio of two; a doubling of frequency

octave band refers to a doubling relationship existing between center frequencies of adjacent bands of sound energy rising from 31 Hz to 16 kHz or higher

octave band analyzer an instrument that electronically dissects the environment into a series of bands that have been specifically defined; allows one to identify those portions of the spectrum that contain the greatest amount of sound energy

octave band filter (1) a band-pass filter that measures the sound pressure level of each octave band in a complex sound; (2) filter in which the upper cutoff frequency is twice that of the lower cutoff frequency; see also **band-pass filter, filter, octave band**

octopus cells nerve cells in the cochlear nucleus with branching extensions; specialized to probe information from a variety of fibers corresponding to several different frequencies

ocular dysmetria abnormal eye movement resulting in the production of hypermetric saccades or hypometric saccades during calibration for electronystagmography testing; consistent with cerebellar pathology

ocular flutter abnormal eye movement similar to ocular dysmetria except that the overshoot or undershoot is spiky rather than squared off in appearance; consistent with brainstem pathology

oculomotor nerve cranial nerve III responsible for movements of the eyes

oculopharyngeal muscular dystrophy autosomal dominant disorder characterized by late onset (after age 20 years) weakness of the facial and pharyngeal muscles including the eyelids and mandible; associated with progressive sensorineural hearing loss in some cases

oculo-auriculo-vertebral spectrum heterogenous syndrome characterized by facial asymmetry, spine anomalies, microtia, ocular anomalies, dermoid cysts, cleft lip and palate, facial paresis; occasional cognitive deficiency, kidney anomalies, heart anomalies, and limb anomalies; associated with unilateral conductive hearing loss ranging from mild to severe or infrequent sensorineural hearing loss of varying degree; also known as **Goldenhar syndrome**

oculo-cerebro-cutaneous syndrome characterized by asymmetric facies, multiple accessory skin tags, microphthalmia, eyelid defects, skin lesions, and cognitive impairment; associated with conductive and sensorineural hearing loss

oculo-dento-digital syndrome autosomal dominant disorder characterized by microphthalmia, small corneas, small nose with pinched alar base, enamel hypoplasia, sparse hair with abnormal texture, broad lower jaw, minor skeletal anomalies, occasional cleft palate, occasional neuropathy; associated with occasional mild conductive hearing loss secondary to chronic otitis media

oddball paradigm task type of stimulus delivery in which the stimulus train contains two different stimuli: a frequent or standard stimulus and a rare or deviant stimulus; see also **P300**

OE occlusion effect; (1) the perception of increased loudness of a bone-conducted signal when the outer ear is somehow occluded (e.g., covered with a supra-aural earphone or sealed with an insert earphone, earmold, or hearing aid); characteristic of normal hearers and patients with sensorineural hearing losses; not seen in patients with conductive losses; (2) barrel effect, a common complaint of hearing aid wearers

off response a post (or peri) stimulus time histogram response pattern representing neural spike activity characterized by an initial transient spike beginning shortly (~5 to 8 ms) after the stimulus offset, followed by a 3- to 6-ms period composed of a few spikes or inactivity; off units either do not respond or may exhibit inhibition of spontaneous activity during the presentation of a short-duration stimulus and produce the discharges after the stimulus is terminated; see also **poststimulus onset time histogram**

OHC outer hair cell; outer three rows of hair cells of the organ of Corti, numbering approximately 34,000

OHCP occupational hearing conservation program; program implemented in excessively noisy occupational environments with the goal of preventing permanent hearing loss associated with exposure to industrial noise; must be initiated whenever employee noise exposures equal or exceed an 8-hour time-weighted average sound level of 85 dBA according to the Occupational Safety and Health Administration; includes qualification (measurement of environmental sound levels); abatement of excessive noise, regular monitoring of hearing sensitivity, education, and the provision of hearing protection

ohm impedance measure; electrical resistance between two points of a conductor when a constant difference of potential of 1 volt, applied between these points, produces in this conductor a current of 1 ampere, the conductor not being the source of any electromotive force; from German scientist Georg Simon Ohm (1782–1854)

ohm meter instrumentation that measures electrical resistance

Ohm's law an electrical law expressing the relationship between the number of ohms, amperes, and volts in a circuit; E (volts) = I (amperes) × R (ohms)

OKN optokinetic nystagmus; repetitive eye movement with alternating fast saccadic eye movements in one direction and then slower smooth movements in the opposite direction as during head rotation or movement of a visual stimulus past the eyes

olfaction the sense of smell

olfactory nerve cranial nerve I responsible for the sense of smell

olivary body, medial superior nucleus in the lower brainstem where some second-order neurons synapse with third-order neurons of the ascending auditory pathways; important region for comparing inputs from the two ears

olivary complex, superior (SOC) a major collection of nuclei in the lower portion of the brainstem in the central auditory system; the first place where there is a neural interaction to stimulation of each ear (binaural stimulation)

olive, lateral superior (LSO) nuclear aggregate of the superior olivary complex involved in processing interaural intensity differences

olive, medial superior (MSO) nuclear aggregate of the superior olivary complex involved in processing interaural time (phase) differences

olivocochlear bundle (OCB) the efferent auditory nerve fibers that originate from the periolivary nuclei, following the vestibular nerve to the cochlear nerve in the inner ear and eventually to the hair cells

OM otitis media; inflammation of the middle ear; a general term for various forms of middle ear disease such as acute or chronic serous otitis media, otitis media with effusion, and acute or chronic purulent otitis media; one of the most common childhood diseases that usually produces a conductive hearing loss caused by fluid in the middle ear space and/or perforations of the eardrum; types include **acute, adhesive, chronic, mucoid, nonsuppurative, purulent, recurrent, secretory, serous, suppurative**

OME otitis media with effusion; non-purulent (uninfected) inflammation of the middle ear, associated with an accumulation of serous or mucoid fluid, caused by obstruction of the eustachian tube; see also **otitis media (OM)**

omnidirectional characteristic of a microphone that is equally sensitive to sound coming from any direction

omnidirectional microphone microphone that is sensitive to sound coming from all directions

on-off cycle the duration of time a noise source is on versus off in a repetitive condition

1.5-cc coupler Zwislocki coupler used in the Knowles Electronic Manikin for Acoustic Research (KE-MAR) designed to be analogous to the human ear canal; see also **Zwislocki coupler**

one-third octave refers to a one-third octave relationship between center frequencies of adjacent bands of sound energy rising from 31 Hz to 16 kHz or higher; see also **octave**

onset response in auditory brainstem response measurement; the synchronous firing of neurons following rapid click stimuli

open captioning printed text or printed dialog on the screen that corresponds to the auditory speech signal from a television program or movie without the need for specific circuitry to be operational; see also **closed captioning (CC)**

open earmold an earmold fitting consisting of only a piece of tubing inserted into the ear canal to deliver sound from a hearing aid; sometimes referred to as a tube fit

open set testing or training task that does not provide a set of choices to the patient; see also **closed set**

open-canal fitting an earmold fitting consisting of only a piece of tubing inserted into the ear canal to deliver sound from a hearing aid; often used with a CROS (contralateral routing of signals) hearing aid fitting to allow sound to pass to the "good ear" without being amplified; see also **contralateral routing of signals (CROS)**

open-ear response unaided frequency response to a stimulus as measured in a human ear canal; includes the total contributions of the pinna, concha, and external ear canal resonances; also known as **external ear effects (EEE)**

open-loop irrigation process of directly injecting warm or cool water into the external auditory canal during caloric testing to stimulate the horizontal semicircular canal

open-platform digital hearing aid digital hearing aid that is capable of using many different algorithms to fit a particular patient's hearing loss

optic nerve cranial nerve II responsible for afferent innervation from the eyes

optokinetic nystagmus (OKN) repetitive eye movement with alternating fast saccadic eye movements in one direction and then slower smooth movements in the opposite direction as during head rotation or movement of a visual stimulus past the eyes

oral communication a communication methodology that emphasizes the use of speech rather than sign language for both receptive and expressive exchanges; see also **auditory-oral approach, oralism**

oral interpreter a professional who silently repeats a talker's message as it is spoken, so that a person who is hard-of-hearing may lipread the message

oral-aural communication method of auditory habilitation that emphasizes auditory and speechreading cues; manual communication is not included; also known as **auditory, auditory-verbal, aural-oral approach**

oral-facial-digital syndrome type I characterized by hyperplastic frenula, median pseudo-cleft of the upper lip, lobulated tongue, cleft palate, palatal asymmetry, digital anomalies, mild cognitive impairment, abnormal scalp hair, milia (small pimplelike lesions) of the ears, agenesis of the corpus callosum; associated with possible conductive hearing loss caused by chronic otitis secondary to cleft palate

oral-peripheral examination a preliminary evaluation of the neuromusculature of the upper articulatory tract; also known as oral-mechanism examination

oralism method of instruction for deaf children that emphasizes spoken language skills to the exclusion of manual communication; see also **auditory-oral approach, oral communication**

oralist individual who is a proponent of the oralism approach; see also **oralism, oral communication**

ordinal scale a nonquantitative scale of measurement that has nominal properties and has the ability to determine greater than or less than (ranking)

organ of Corti sense organ of hearing in the inner ear; a series of neuroepithelial hair cells (receptor cells for hearing) and their supporting structures lying against the osseous spiral lamina and the basilar membrane within the scala media of the cochlea; extends from the base of the cochlea to the apex

orientation reflex a type of conditioning audiometry used with infants in which sound and a lighted toy are presented simultaneously, one on each side of the child; after the child is conditioned, the lighted toy is used as a reinforcer; also known as **conditioned orientation reflex (COR)**; see also **orienting response**

orienting response an unconditioned response to a sound stimulus that facilitates subsequent processing; see also **orientation reflex**

oscillation the vibration, usually with time, of the magnitude of a quantity with respect to a specified reference when the magnitude is alternately greater and smaller than the reference; see also **oscillator**

oscillator a device or circuit that produces one or more pure-tone frequencies or oscillations but not simultaneously; see also **oscillation**

oscillograph a device used to record the changing currents or voltages that can be translated into electrical energy; can record a sound wave as amplitude as a function of time; see also **oscilloscope**

oscillopsia eye movements that produce blurring vision when the patient is walking or involved in other activities that move the head; indicates a vestibulo-ocular reflex abnormality and usually a bilateral vestibular disorder; see also **vestibulo-ocular reflex (VOR)**

oscilloscope an electronic device for visually displaying an electrical signal on a screen permitting measurement of the signal amplitude, frequency, or temporal characteristics; see also **oscillograph**

OSHA Occupational Safety and Health Administration; federal agency that established legislation (the Occupational Safety and Health Act) that was passed in 1970 that established minimum standards for worker safety and health including industrial hearing conservation regulations

OSHA noise standard criteria intended to protect the average worker from permanent threshold shift for 40 years of exposure, 50 weeks per year, and 8 hours per day; determines permissible exposure levels of noise; also known as **damage risk criteria (DRC)**

OSPL output sound pressure level; a test used to determine the sound pressure level obtained in an ear simulator when using an input of 90 dB SPL and the gain control in the full-on position as a function of frequency; newer, more accurate, term used instead of **maximum power output (MPO)** or **saturation sound pressure level (SSPL)**

osseotomy incision or transection of bone

osseotympanic bone conduction bone-conduction hearing produced when vibrations are transmitted from the skull to the air in the external ear canal; hearing then occurs via the usual air-conduction mechanism (through the middle ear to the cochlea)

osseous labyrinth the bony cavities of the inner ear that provide a protective covering for the membranous labyrinth that houses the sense organs for hearing and balance; filled with perilymph; see also **membranous labyrinth**

osseous spiral lamina the bony ledge that projects from and winds around the modiolus for 2 $\frac{5}{8}$ turns from the base of the cochlea to the apex; the basilar membrane is attached to the free border of the osseous spiral lamina and runs parallel to it

ossicles three small bones in the middle ear that transmit sound vibrations from the tympanic membrane to the oval window; see also **malleus, incus, stapes**

ossicular chain collective term for the malleus, incus, and stapes; see also **ossicles**

ossicular discontinuity a discontinuous or unconnected ossicular chain that may result from congenital defects, skull trauma, or middle ear disease; results in a unilateral conductive hearing loss of about 40 to 60 dB; also known as ossicular disarticulation

ossicular fixation immobilization of the ossicular chain

ossiculoplasty surgical reconstruction of the ossicular chain

ossification a conversion of tissue to bone

osteochondrodysplasia genetic disorder of the skeleton

osteogenesis imperfecta autosomal dominant disorder characterized by bone fragility, blue sclerae, and dental anomalies; associated with conductive hearing loss related to fixation of the footplate of the stapes or fracture of the ossicles; sensorineural and mixed hearing loss are also common, all of late onset; also known as **van der Hoeve disease**

osteoma a single benign tumor that resembles cortical bone; usually occurs at the tympanomastoid suture line and tends to have a narrow base

OT occupational therapist; a healthcare professional who assists individuals in regaining and/or building physical, developmental, social, and emotional skills that are important for health and well-being

otalgia ear pain (earache)

OTE over the ear; a hearing aid that sits completely behind the ear over the pinna and is typically coupled to the ear canal by an earmold; also known as **behind-the-ear (BTE)**

otic pertaining to the ear

otic capsule bony labyrinth of the inner ear that houses the membranous labyrinth; outer portion of the inner ear

otic placode thickening of ectoderm in the neural folds of the human embryo; precursor to the inner ear; also known as **auditory placode**

otic vesicle embryologic structure formed by the closing of the auditory pit; lined with ectoderm; known as the early otocyst (developing inner ear); also known as **auditory vesicle**

otitis inflammation of the ear; see also **external otitis, otitis media (OM)**

otitis externa an affliction of the external ear canal usually the result of a bacterial infection; also known as **swimmer's ear**; often develops after water immersion; also known as **otitis externa**; see also **bacterial external otitis**

otitis media (OM) inflammation of the middle ear; a general term for various forms of middle ear disease such as acute or chronic serous otitis media, otitis media with effusion, and acute or chronic purulent otitis media; one of the most common childhood diseases that usually produces a conductive hearing loss caused by fluid in the middle ear space and/or perforations of the eardrum; types include **acute, adhesive, chronic, mucoid, nonsuppurative, purulent, recurrent, secretory, serous,** and **suppurative**

otitis media, acute middle ear inflammation of recent onset accompanied by symptoms and signs of infection; generally lasts 2 to 3 weeks

otitis media, adhesive condition in which fibrous adhesions are present in the middle ear as a result of previous inflammation

otitis media, chronic slow developing and long lasting inflammation or infection of the middle ear

otitis media, mucoid middle ear inflammation with white, cloudy fluid resulting from cell secretion known as mucoid effusion; found in lengthy infections

otitis media, nonsuppurative middle ear inflammation with effusion that is uninfected; e.g., mucoid or serous otitis media

otitis media, purulent middle ear inflammation with effusion that is actively infected; e.g., suppurative otitis media

otitis media, recurrent inflammation of the middle ear that reoccurs 3 to 6 times in a 6-month period

otitis media, secretory inflammation of the middle ear with effusion that is sterile, pale yellow transudate of low viscosity; usually follows short-term illness; (e.g., serous or mucoid otitis media)

otitis media, serous inflammation of the middle ear with effusion that is sterile, pale yellow transudate of low viscosity; usually follows short-term illness

otitis media, suppurative acute and/or chronic otitis media with infected fluid (suppuration); inflammation of the middle ear with infected fluid (effusion); also known as **tubotympanic disease**

otitis media with effusion (OME) nonpurulent (uninfected) inflammation of the middle ear, associated with an accumulation of serous or mucoid fluid, caused by obstruction of the eustachian tube; see also **otitis media (OM)**

otitis prone child having more than three bouts of otitis media in the first 12 months of life; see also **otitis media (OM)**

oto-palato-digital syndrome type I X-linked recessive disorder characterized by prominent superior orbital ridge, hypertelorism, downslanting eyes, cognitive deficiency, small stature, abnormal digits with curvature spacing anomalies, cleft palate, Robin sequence, and micrognathia; associated with conductive hearing loss secondary to ossicular malformations

otoacoustic emission (OAE) sound generated by energy produced by the outer hair cells in the cochlea and detected with a microphone placed within the external ear canal; useful technique for determining cochlear function; can be included as part of a diagnostic test battery; see also **distortion product otoacoustic emission (DPOAE), transient evoked otoacoustic emission (TEOAE)**

otoacoustic emission suppression characteristic a reduction in the amplitude and/or a time change or phase shift in an otoacoustic emission; demonstrated as a change in the time of occurrence of peaks or zero crossings in the emission; see also **contralateral suppression**

otoadmittance a measure of the efficiency of the middle ear system in receiving and transmitting sound energy; the measurement of the amount of sound absorbed by the ear and how it is influenced by the pressure applied to the tympanic membrane and contraction of the middle ear muscles

otoadmittance meter old instrumentation used to measure the efficiency of the middle ear system; primarily measured susceptance and conductance components

otoblock cotton or foam ear dam with a string attached that is used to keep impression material from the eardrum when taking of an ear impression

otoconia small particles of mostly calcium carbonate found in the macula of the inner ear; same as otolith (ear dust); also known as **otolith, statoconia**

otolaryngologist an ear, nose, and throat medical doctor who performs surgery

otolaryngology a branch of medicine that deals with the study of the ear, nose, and throat and their functions

otolith small particles of mostly calcium carbonate found in the maculae of the inner ear; same as otoconia (ear dust); also known as **otoconia**

otolithic membrane membranous covering over the utricular macula; made of small particles of mostly calcium carbonate

otologic evaluation a procedure used to diagnose and assess the function of the ear and the auditory system

otologist an otolaryngologist who specializes in treatment of ear problems

otology a branch of medicine that deals with the study of the ear and its function

otomycosis infection of the ear due to fungus in the external auditory canal

otoneurology branch of medicine dealing with disorders of the auditory and vestibular nervous system

otopalatodigital syndrome a syndrome transmitted by X-linked recessive inheritance characterized by severe signs of dysplasia (e.g., wide spacing of toes, cleft palate, broad thumbs); associated with conductive hearing loss

otoplasty surgical reconstruction of the ear

otorhinolaryngologist an ear, nose, and throat physician who diagnoses and treats disorders of the ear, nose, and throat; also known as **otolaryngologist**

otorhinolaryngology a branch of medicine that deals with the study of the ear, nose, and throat and their function

otorrhagia bleeding from the external auditory canal

otorrhea any type of discharge from the ear (e.g., serous, purulent, or cerebrospinal fluid)

otosclerosis a bony degenerative disease process that can involve the stapes footplate and/or cochlea; also called **otospongiosis**; see also **cochlear otosclerosis**

otoscope instrument used for visual examination of the external ear and tympanic membrane; see also **otoscopy**

otoscopy visual examination of the external ear, the ear canal, and the tympanic membrane; provides observations that will often confirm audiological findings and may lead to a medical referral; see also **otoscope**

otospongiosis a term sometimes used to describe otosclerosis which is a bony degenerative disease process that can involve the stapes footplate and/or cochlea; otospongiosis is used to describe the consistency of the new bone growth which is spongy rather than sclerotic; see also **cochlear otosclerosis**

otosyphilis a syphilis infection that causes membranous labyrinthitis and results in sensorineural hearing loss

ototopicals commonly used medications with an acidic base to treat mi-

cro-organisms; most are combinations of several different drug types

ototoxic drugs pharmaceuticals known to be toxic to the inner ear (cochlear and vestibular) structures; also known as **ototoxins**

ototoxic hearing loss hearing loss resulting from exposure to toxic substances affecting the cochlear structures

ototoxicity the poisonous effect of toxic substances to the structures of the ear, particularly hair cells in the cochlea and vestibular organs

ototoxins pharmaceuticals known to be toxic to the inner ear (cochlear and vestibular) structures; also known as **ototoxic drugs**

outer ear peripheral part of the auditory mechanism that includes the pinna, the concha, and the external auditory canal

outer ear canal the canal of the outer ear leading from the concha to the tympanic membrane; also known as **ear canal, outer ear canal**

outer hair cell (OHC) outer three rows of hair cells of the organ of Corti, numbering approximately 34,000

outer hair cell atrophy degeneration of the outer hair cells that may be the result of physiologic aging, noise exposure, or metabolic changes in the cochlea

outer pillars of Corti the outer row of stiff rodlike structures supported by the basilar membrane; the heads of the rods are in contact with the reticular lamina and enclose the tunnel of Corti along with the basilar membrane

outer spiral fibers spiral afferent fibers of cranial nerve VIII innervating outer hair cells; each nerve fiber connects to many outer hair cells; also know as **Type II fibers**

output energy or information exiting from a listening device

output amplifier an amplifier in its final (output) stage; see also **amplifier**

output compression type of compression in which the level detector is positioned after the gain control so that the volume control setting affects the compression threshold but not the maximum power output

output distortion constant saturation of a hearing instrument to an amplified signal; often results from peak clipping; automatic gain control or compression is often used to limit output distortion

output limiting limiting the output of a listening device by means of peak clipping or compression

output sound pressure level (OSPL) a test used to determine the sound pressure level obtained in an ear simulator when using an input of 90 dB SPL and the gain control in the full-on position as a function of frequency; newer, more accurate, term used instead of **maximum power output (MPO)** or **saturation sound pressure level (SSPL)**

output-organization deficit an inability to sequence, plan, and organize responses

oval window the opening into the scala vestibuli to which the footplate of the stapes is attached

over-the-ear (OTE) hearing aid hearing aid that sits completely behind the ear over the pinna and is typically coupled to the ear canal by an earmold; also known as **behind-the-ear (BTE) hearing aid**

overamplification giving more amplification than needed from a hearing device; can potentially cause a decrease in hearing sensitivity

overmasking in clinical masking; the point at which the masker is raising the threshold in the test ear; occurs when too much masking is presented to the nontest ear; run the risk of overmasking whenever the level of effective masking presented to the nontest ear minus interaural attenuation is greater than the bone-conduction threshold of the test ear

overrecruitment abnormal growth of loudness in which the loudness of a high-intensity sound presented to the impaired ear exceeds the perceived loudness in the normal ear

overtone a partial having a frequency higher than that of the basic frequency; see also **harmonic**

Owens threshold tone decay test a test of tone decay that measures the amount of tone decay in dB and time to audibility

oxyacoia hypersenstivity to sound; occurs as a result of stapedius muscle paralysis

P

P1 the first major positive-voltage peak in the auditory late response normally occurring approximately 40 to 60 ms after an acoustic stimulus; suspected generator is the auditory cortex

P160 the second positive peak following the middle latency response; the first positive peak following the N100 occurring between 145 and 180 ms; also known as **P2**

P2 the second positive peak following the middle latency response; the first positive peak following the N100 occurring between 145 and 180 ms; also known as **P160**

P300 an event-related cognitive auditory evoked potential occurring in the 300 ms region; recorded when the patient attends to or listens for rare, oddball, or target stimuli that are presented along with frequent stimuli; also referred to as P3 as the third major positive voltage component of the waveform

Pa (1) the first major positive voltage peak of the auditory middle latency response normally occurring approximately 25 to 30 ms after an acoustic stimulus; suspected generator is the primary auditory cortex; (2) abbreviation for Pascal

pachyotia abnormally coarse and thick auricles

Paget disease chronic bone disease of one or many bones of the skull that results in disordered and active reconstruction of bone with alternating resorption of bone; can be associated with conductive and/or sensorineural hearing loss; also known as **Beethoven's deafness**

paired comparison a data collection method in which a listener compares two hearing aids (or settings or stimuli) and determines which meets the criteria defined by either the clinician or the listener

PAL Auditory Word Lists early speech audiometry word lists developed in the late 1940s and early 1950s at the Psychoacoustic Laboratory (PAL) at Harvard University

PAM postauricular muscle; one of three muscles attaching the external ear (pinna) to the scalp; located behind the ear

PAN positional alcoholic nystagmus; nystagmus that is evoked by a change in head position after the ingestion of alcohol

paracentesis procedure in which fluid is removed from a body cavity;

procedure used to remove fluid from the middle ear

paracusis hearing disorder; often affects pitch perception

paracusis willisi a feature of conductive hearing loss characterized by better understanding of speech in the presence of background noise than in quiet

paradigm a design used in clinical evaluation or research

parallel talk a language-stimulation technique in which an adult matches language to an activity a child is performing

parallel vent a bore made in an earmold or hearing aid that is parallel to the sound bore and runs from outside the mold to the external auditory meatus

paralysis loss of muscle function and/or sensation

paralysis of facial nerve loss of muscle function and/or sensation of the face and its muscles

parameter any defining or characteristic factor of a system

parasympathetic nervous system autonomic nervous system craniosacral aspect, with effects including bronchiole and pupil constriction, alimentary canal and smooth muscle contraction, heart rate moderation, and some glandular secretion

parietal bone one of the seven bones of the skull; a pair of bones forming the sides of the cranium

paroxysmal vertigo sudden, brief sensation of dizziness and spinning

often accompanied by nausea and vomiting; see also **benign paroxysmal positioning vertigo (BPPV)**

pars flaccida superior, anterior, thin portion of the tympanic membrane near the epitympanum; portion of the tympanic membrane that does not contain the fibrous layer; also known as **Shrapnell's membrane;** see also **pars tensa, tympanic membrane (TM)**

pars tensa major portion of the tympanic membrane containing all three layers (cutaneous, fibrous, and mucous); fairly rigid portion of the tympanic membrane; see also **pars flaccida, tympanic membrane (TM)**

partial in acoustics, a component of a complex tone; its frequency may be either higher or lower than that of the basic frequency and may or may not bear an integral relationship to the basic frequency; see also **harmonic**

partial recruitment possible result from loudness balance testing; abnormal growth of loudness in which the loudness of a high-intensity sound presented to the impaired ear comes close to but remains less than the perceived loudness in the normal ear

Pascal (Pa) a unit of measurement for pressure; an alternative to the newton per square meter with the MKS system; $1 \text{ Pa} = 1 \text{ Ntm}^2 = 10 \text{ dyne/cm}^2$

Pascoe High-Frequency Test monosyllabic word-recognition test composed of high-frequency stimuli; uses only three vocalic nuclei

passband the range of frequencies between the filter cutoff frequencies that are passed through the filter and not attenuated; see also **band-pass filter**

passive attention condition in which the observer is made aware that there will be a target stimulus but no response is required

passive filter type of filter in which the response is constant; unaffected by amplifier gain

patent (1) open, unoccluded; (e.g., patent pressure equalization (PE) tube or eustachian tube); (2) governmental right awarded to the inventor to manufacture, sell, or use an invention

patent eustachian tube unoccluded eustachian tube; indicates that the tube is functioning appropriately; see also **patulous eustachian tube**

patent PE tube unoccluded pressure equalization tube; indicates that the tube is functioning appropriately

pathogenic the ability to cause a disease

pathology the study of the symptoms, possible causes, and effects of disease

patient confidentiality the legal right of a patient not to have his or her clinical information revealed to persons other than the clinician

patulous eustachian tube abnormally open (patent) eustachian tube with accompanying symptoms of a stuffy sensation in the ear, tinnitus, respiratory noises in the ear, and autophony

pauser response nerve response characterized by an initial on-response followed by silence and subsequent low-level firing rate throughout stimulation

Pb the second major positive voltage peak of the auditory middle latency response normally occurring approximately 50 to 70 ms after an acoustic stimulus; suspected generator is the primary auditory cortex

PB phonetically balanced; term applied to word lists in which the sounds occur with the same frequency as they do in a representative sample of English speech

PB max the maximum percentage of words correctly repeated by a patient tested with a phonetically balanced (PB) word list; may occur at different sensation levels for different listeners; PB max occurs at lower sensation levels when the stimuli have more redundancy (e.g., sentences)

PB monosyllabic word lists monosyllabic word lists that are phonetically balanced; these lists contain all the phonetic elements of general American English speech that occur with the approximate frequency of occurrence in conversational speech; see also **phonetic balancing (PB)**

PB-K Kindergarten Phonetically Balanced Word Lists; phonetically balanced (PB) lists of monosyllabic words used to test speech recognition by young children; also known as the **Kindergarten PB Word Lists**

PB-K Monosyllabic Word Lists phonetically balanced (PB) lists of monosyllabic words used to test speech recognition by young children; also known as the **Kindergarten PB Word Lists**; see also **phonetic balancing (PB)**

PC peak clipping; common form of output limiting used in linear hearing aids; the peaks of the waveform are eliminated when the amplifier is saturated; results in distortion of the signal

PE tube pressure-equalization tube; a short polyethylene tube or grommet placed through a myringotomy incision in a tympanic membrane that permits continuous middle-ear ventilation; see also **myringotomy**

Peabody Picture Vocabulary Test–Revised (PPVT-R) test of receptive language skills

peak (1) the highest point of a wave representing its maximum amplitude (e.g., hearing aid frequency responses); (2) a component of an evoked potential waveform or the extreme amplitude for the component; describes the positive-voltage component of the wave

peak amplitude a measure of amplitude that relates to the peak amount of displacement from either the condensation (positive) component or the rarefaction (negative) component; see also **peak-to-peak amplitude**

peak clipping (PC) common form of output limiting used in linear hearing aids; the peaks of the waveform are eliminated when the amplifier is saturated; results in distortion of the signal; see also **asymmetric peak clipping, symmetric peak clipping**

peak clipping, asymmetric form of output limiting seen in linear class A amplifiers in hearing aids; the peaks of the positive portion of the waveform are eliminated when the amplifier is saturated; results in significant signal distortion; see also **peak clipping, symmetric peak clipping**

peak clipping, soft form of output limiting used in linear hearing aids; the peaks of the waveform are removed in a gradual manner when the amplifier is saturated; results in a reduction of signal distortion compared to traditional peak clipping; see also **peak clipping (PC)**

peak clipping, symmetric form of output limiting seen in linear class B amplifiers in hearing aids; the peaks of the positive and negative portions of the waveform are eliminated when the amplifier is saturated; results in less signal distortion than asymmetric peak clipping; see also **peak clipping (PC), asymmetric peak clipping**

peak equivalent sound pressure level (peSPL) a measure of sound intensity in which the maximum voltage of a transient stimulus (e.g., a click) is equated on an oscilloscope with the voltage of a tone stimulus of known intensity level in dB sound pressure level (SPL); click intensity level is defined in terms of dB peSPL; see also **dB peSPL**

peak sound pressure the maximum physical intensity of a short-duration stimulus

peak-to-peak amplitude a measure of amplitude that relates to the difference between the most positive peak and the most negative trough (i.e., the extremes of the quantity); see also **peak amplitude**

pedestal refers to a transducer that is placed through unbroken skin used in early versions of cochlear implants; also known as percutaneous plug in cochlear implants; see also **percutaneous plug, cochlear implant (CI)**

pediatric audiology area of audiology dealing with the diagnosis and management of hearing loss in children; uses a pediatric test battery including developmentally appropriate behavioral and objective hearing tests

Pediatric Speech Intelligibility (PSI) test speech audiometry procedure for assessment of peripheral and central auditory system function in children

pediatrician a medical doctor who specializes in the diagnosis, treatment, and care of infants and children

PELs permissible exposure levels; acceptable intensity levels of industrial or occupational noise specified by the Occupational Safety and Health Administration that are considered safe and unlikely to produce permanent hearing loss

Pendred syndrome autosomal recessive disorder characterized by goiter with sensorineural hearing loss; also associated with moderate to profound sensorineural hearing loss, more severe in the high frequencies with Mondini cochlear anomaly; decreased vestibular function

pendular tracking component of the electronystagmography test battery that assesses the ability of the smooth pursuit eye movement system; its purpose is to match the angular velocity of the eye with a slowly moving object; the object moves sinusoidally and the patient is to track the object visually in the horizontal and vertical plane

penetrance the frequency of phenotypical expression of a genotype; if the trait appears less than 100% of the time, it is said to have reduced penetrance; the proportion of individuals of a specified genotype who show the expected phenotype under a given set of environmental conditions

percent correct method of scoring speech perception tests that reflects the number of stimuli perceived correctly divided by the total number of stimuli presented

perception the cognition of some external object that causes a sensation; the power of acquiring knowledge through the senses

percutaneous plug a transducer that is placed through unbroken skin used in early versions of cochlear implants; the percutaneous plug was used to couple the external transmitter to the internal receiver by way of holes in the plug that went through the skin; see also **cochlear implant (CI), pedestal**

perfect pitch the ability possessed by certain people to name the musical pitch of a note without the aid of a standard reference

perforated tympanic membrane disorder of the tympanic membrane resulting from a hole through the membrane; can be marginal or central; can be caused by trauma, middle ear infection, cholesteatoma, etc.

perforation a anomalous hole or opening in tissue or structure

perforation, attic negative pressure in a portion of the tympanic membrane; often occurs in the pars flaccida portion near Prussak's space

perforation, central perforation or hole in the central area of the tympanic membrane; as opposed to a **marginal perforation**

perforation, marginal perforation or hole in the posterior-superior marginal area of the tympanic membrane; as opposed to a **central perforation**

perforation, tympanic membrane hole in the tympanic membrane; usually occurs in the attic in the pars flaccida portion of the structure

performance-intensity (PI) function a graph showing the percentage correct of speech audiometry materials as a function of intensity; performance generally improves with increasing intensity up to a maximum point and then plateaus; see also **PB max**

peri-modiolar electrodes a smooth free-fitting electrode array placed close to the modiolus where the ganglion cells are located; used with cochlear implantation

perichondrium a fibrous connective tissue covering cartilage; the auricle has perichondrium

perilinguistically deafened the loss of hearing during the period of speech and language development

perilymph pale fluid within the scala vestibuli and scala tympani of the membranous labyrinth of the cochlea; a clear, watery fluid contained within the osseous labyrinth

perilymphatic fistula abnormal communication between the perilymphatic space and the middle ear; an abnormal opening in the inner ear labyrinthine system; may be a congenital defect or caused by trauma; see also **fistula**

perilymphatic gusher a sudden, rapid eruption of perilymph from the oval window; can be spontaneous or surgically induced

perilymphatic leak leak of perilymph (fluid in the bony labyrinth) into the middle ear as a result of a perilymphatic fistula; see also **fistula, perilymphatic fistula**

perinatal around the time of birth; refers to the birthing process

perinatal cause of deafness deafness or hearing loss that occurs during the birthing process; see also **high-risk register (HRR)**

period the duration (in seconds) of one cycle of vibration; reciprocal of frequency (e.g., the period of a 1000-Hz tone is 1/1000 second)

period pulse train a repetitious series of rectangularly shaped "pulses" of some width that occur at some regular rate

periodic sound a sound whose waveform repeats itself regularly as a function of time; see also **periodic vibration**

periodic vibration an oscillatory motion whose amplitude pattern repeats after fixed increments of time; see also **periodic sound**

periodicity pitch the perception of a low-frequency tone that is not actually in the original stimulus; also referred to as **missing fundamental**

periolivary nuclei (PON) nuclei in the superior olivary complex that surround the medial and lateral superior olives; receive projections from the acoustic stria

periosteal bone bone that forms from cartilage; also known as perichondrial bone

peripheral pertaining to the surface or outside of a structure

peripheral auditory mechanism auditory structures that are not part of the central auditory system; includes the outer ear, middle ear, inner ear, and auditory nerve

peripheral nervous system (PNS) components of the nervous system that lie outside of the central nervous system, including the cranial nerves and nerves in the extremities

peripheral presbycusis degeneration of the peripheral hearing mechanism resulting in hearing loss due to physiologic aging; see also **presbycusis**

peripheral site of lesion dysfunction established in the auditory system up to but not involving the brainstem

peritympanic hearing aid a hearing instrument that terminates deeply within the bony portion of the external auditory canal (in the vicinity of the tympanic membrane); see also **completely-in-the-canal (CIC) hearing aid**

permanent threshold shift (PTS) permanent increase in the threshold of audibility for an ear at a specified frequency above a previously established reference level; expressed in decibels; see also **temporary threshold shift (TTS), compound threshold shift (CTS)**

permavent tube a pressure-equalization tube designed for long-term ventilation; see also **grommet, pressure equalization (PE) tube**

permissible noise exposure levels (PELs) acceptable intensity levels of industrial or occupational noise specified by the Occupational Safety and Health Administration that are considered safe and unlikely to produce permanent hearing loss

Perrault syndrome autosomal recessive disorder characterized by ovarian dysgenesis in females; associated with severe or profound sensorineural hearing loss

personal amplification amplification devices that are worn by an individual (e.g., hearing aids) as opposed to by a group (e.g., group auditory trainers)

personal FM system a frequency modulation radio system with individual wearable receiver units

personal-adjustment counseling counseling that assists patients and their families in the acceptance of their hearing loss from an emotional standpoint

perstimulatory occurs during stimulation

perstimulatory fatigue auditory adaptation; a reduction in the audibility of a sound during extended stimulation; perstimulatory effect, occurs during exposure to stimulation

pertubation (1) change from predicted behavior, disturbance of direction, equilibrium, or distribution; (2) in chaos theory, a minor bump

peSPL peak equivalent sound pressure level; equal to the amplitude of a 1000-Hz tone as if it were equivalent to the peak of a transient signal such as a click; used to determine the intensity level of a click

PET positron emission tomography; the imaging of body (especially brain) sections by tracking positron-emitting radionuclides; depending on the radionuclides employed, researchers can measure regional cerebral blood flow, blood volume, oxygen uptake, and glucose transport

and metabolism in addition to locating neurotransmitter receptors

petrous bone most dense portion of the temporal bone that is shaped like a pyramid; houses the inner ear auditory and vestibular structures; also referred to as the **petrous pyramid**

petrous pyramid most dense portion of the temporal bone that is shaped like a pyramid; houses the inner ear auditory and vestibular structures; also referred to as the **petrous bone**

Pfeiffer syndrome autosomal dominant disorder characterized by craniosynostosis, maxillary deficiency, exophthalmus, broad thumbs, and occasional choanal atresia or stenosis; associated with conductive hearing loss secondary to the reduced size of the middle ear and/or chronic middle ear disease

PHAB Profile of Hearing Aid Benefit; self-assessment questionnaire examining an individual's perceived benefit from hearing aid use

phalangeal process an extension of the Deiter's cells that passes next to the hair cells and up to the reticular membrane; provides support to the hair cells; see also **Deiter's cells**

PHAP Profile of Hearing Aid Performance; a self-assessment measurement tool that assesses the patient's benefit from a hearing instrument

pharmacokinetics changes in drug concentration with the body over time; the rate of removal of drug from circulation

pharynx the respiratory passageway from the larynx to the oral and nasal cavities

phase the part of the sound wave that at a given instant is part of the cycle in which the wave finds itself relative to some arbitrary reference point; measured in degrees or radians

phase angle the angle of rotation at any specified moment in time; also known as instantaneous phase

phase locking the tendency of a neuron to respond to a particular phase of an acoustic signal

phase radians the unit of measurement in degrees that indicates that portion of the wave that has been completed

phase spectrum the starting phase as a function of frequency

phenotype the total nature of an individual in biochemical, physical, and physiological terms; the result of the genotype; see also **genotype**

phenylketonuria (PKU) a deficiency of phenylalanine metabolism that results in brain damage characterized by mental retardation; autosomal recessive transmission

phon unit for measuring the loudness level of a tone; the number of phons is equal to the number of decibels that a 1000-Hz tone is above the reference intensity when judged to be equal in loudness to the tone in question; see also **loudness level**

phone an individual speech sound; see also **phoneme**

phoneme group of speech sounds with similar acoustic characteristics that corresponds to a symbol in the phonetic alphabet; the minimal unit of sound in a language that is distinct from other sounds

phoneme recognition test monosyllabic word tests designed to isolate particular phonemes within the words; typically presented in a closed-set fashion

phonemic analysis separating words or syllables into a sequence of phonemes

phonemic balancing lists in which each initial consonant, each vowel, and each final consonant appear with the same frequency of occurrence in the test list; see also **phonetic balancing (PB)**

phonemic regression decrease in word-recognition ability with relatively normal-hearing sensitivity; usually associated with aging

phonemic synthesis blending of discrete phonemes into the correctly sequenced coarticulated sound patterns

phonetic pertains to the production and transcription of speech sounds

phonetic alphabet alphabet of symbols (phonemes) that represent speech sounds; also known as **International Phonetic Alphabet (IPA)**

phonetic balancing (PB) term applied to word lists in which the sounds occur with the same frequency as they do in a representative sample of English speech; see also **phonemic balancing (PB)**

phonetic task evaluation (PTE) nonsense syllable test designed to estimate a child's speech feature discrimination abilities

phonetic transcription the written interpretation of the auditory perception of speech sounds using the International Phonetic Alphabet

phonetically balanced word lists monosyllabic word lists that are phonetically balanced; these lists contain all the phonetic elements of general American English speech that occur with the approximate frequency of occurrence in conversational speech; see also **phonetic balancing (PB)**

phonetics the science of speech sounds used in language; the study of speech sound production and perception, including transcription and analysis

phonological awareness explicit awareness of the sound structure of language, including the recognition that words are comprised of syllables and phonemes

physical volume test (PVT) the measurement of ear canal volume as part of the immittance battery

physiology the study of the function of the body and its components

PI function a performance-intensity function; a graph showing the percentage correct of speech audiometry materials as a function of intensity

PI-PB a performance intensity (PI) function for phonetically balanced (PB) word lists; procedure used to determine the presentation level revealing a patient's maximum word recognition; also used to determine if rollover is present (i.e., if a decrease in performance occurs at high stimulus intensity levels); see also **rollover, PI function**

PI-SSI a performance-intensity (PI) function using stimuli in the Synthetic Sentence Index (SSI) test

Picture Identification Task monosyllabic word-recognition test designed to estimate performance in nonverbal adults who are unable to respond orally to conventional word-recognition tests

piebaldness integumentary-pigmentary syndrome characterized by depigmentation of skin (head, hair, or chest), blue irides; associated with profound deafness in some classifications

Pierre Robin sequence autosomal dominant disorder characterized by a triad of micrognathia, cleft palate, glossoptosis; sequence is a pattern of anomalies, unlike a syndrome; results from a primary anomaly, often from fetal alcohol; associated with cranial, facial, and skeletal problems; cleft palate; small jaw and chin; low-set auricles; congenital conductive or sensorineural hearing loss

piezoelectric related to electrical polarity caused by pressure; certain crystallized substances, such as quartz, commonly exhibit a piezo (pressure) effect; used in hearing aid microphones

piezoelectric microphone type of microphone that uses crystallized substances, such as quartz, to exhibit a piezo (pressure) effect

pili torti autosomal recessive disorder characterized by twisted, brittle, short, dry hairs all over body, including hair on the head and scalp as well as the fine hair all over body; results in congenital moderate to severe sensorineural hearing loss

PILL programmable increase at low levels; a form of nonlinear amplification (automatic signal processing); level dependent frequency response that can be adjusted to provide either **bass increase at low levels (BILL)** or **treble increase at low levels (TILL)**; see also **level dependent frequency response (LDFR)**

pillar cells supportive cells of the organ of Corti around the tunnel of Corti

pillars of Corti the outer row of stiff rodlike structures supported by the basilar membrane; the heads of the rods are in contact with the reticular lamina and enclose the tunnel of Corti along with the basilar membrane

pink noise an irregular type of noise sometimes used in hearing science but generally irrelevant for clinical audiology; spectrum level of the noise decreases as frequency increases

pinna abnormalities anomalies of the pinna (outer ear) including microtia, macrotia, maldevelopment of appropriate landmarks, etc.

pinna/pinnae the outer, most obvious portion of the ear; also known as the auricle; see also **auricle/auriculae**

pip a short-duration tone that may be one or more cycles of a sinusoid, but usually not more than five; also called a **tone pip**; provides tonal information via a transient stimulus; see also **tone burst**

piston phone instrument used in the calibration of audiometric equipment; produces a tone at a specific frequency and intensity

pitch the perception of the frequency of sound with high pitches corresponding to high frequencies and low pitches corresponding to low frequencies; unit of measurement is the mel; see also **mel**

pitch discrimination the ability of the cochlear amplifier to determine changes in the fundamental frequency of complex tones

pitch distortion changes in the ability of the ear to discriminate minimum changes in frequency often as a result of inner ear pathology

pitch matching the process used to determine the frequency of an individual's tinnitus; the patient perceptually matches the pitch of a signal to the pitch of his or her tinnitus

Pitch Pattern Sequence (PPS) test a central auditory measure that requires identification of a sequence of three high or low tones presented in random configurations

pitch perception (1) the ability to distinguish the perceptual correlate of variations in frequency; (2) for cochlear implant users, it is the ability to distinguish different pitches at different electrode sites or for different rates of stimulation

pitch ranking process used in fitting cochlear implants in which patients judge whether sounds are presented in increasing or decreasing pitch when electrodes are stimulated from the basal to the apical end of the cochlea or vice versa

PKU phenylketonuria; a deficiency of phenylalanine metabolism such that it results in brain damage characterized by mental retardation; autosomal recessive transmission

PL 93-112 the Rehabilitation Act of 1973; ensured access of impaired students (including hearing impaired) from elementary school through college to federally funded programs

PL 94-142 the Education for all Handicapped Children Act of 1975; ensured access to a free, appropriate, public education for students who were hearing impaired aged 3 through 21; included mainstreaming as much as possible with the use of individualized educational plans; see also **individualized educational plan (IEP)**

PL 99-457 the Individuals with Disabilities Education Act (IDEA); an amendment to PL 94-142 in 1986 that extended federal funding for impaired children from birth to 3 years of age; see also **PL 94-142**

PL 101-336 Americans with Disabilities Act; federal law enacted to provide protection from discrimination based on disability; it was modeled after the Rehabilitation Act of 1973 and passed in 1990

place of articulation the location on the vocal tract where changes occur to produce consonants; includes lips, teeth, alveolar ridge, palate, and glottis

place pitch the perception of pitch using the place theory that suggests that frequency perception is determined by the location of the maximum displacement of the traveling wave along the basilar membrane; see also **place theory of hearing**

place theory of hearing theory of hearing that states that frequency processing of the cochlea arises primarily through differential displacement of locations along the basilar membrane, and subsequently, stimulation of the hair cells of the excited regions; see also **place pitch**

placode thickening of primordial tissues of the human embryo; precursor to organs and body structures; see also **auditory placode**

plasticity (1) malleability of the central nervous system prior to stabilization of neural function; (2) alteration of neurons to conform better to immediate environmental influences, often associated with a change in behavior

plateau (1) the time that a signal is at its maximum intensity; (2) range of effective masking (between minimum and maximum effective masking) where the masking is considered appropriate allowing accurate measurement of the threshold of the test ear

plateau method procedure used in clinical masking to determine the actual threshold in the test ear by increasing the masking level until cross hearing is prevented; the test tone and masking are increased in specified dB steps until masking levels can be raised several times without changing the level of the test tone; used to establish the true masked threshold

plateau phase a discharge rate/stimulus level function generated in response to an auditory stimulus representing the constant, saturated discharge rate of a single auditory neuron under study

plateau time the time a signal is on at its maximum intensity

play audiometry the highest level of pediatric task in hearing testing; involves the active cooperation of the child as an auditory stimulus is paired with an operant task, such as dropping a block in a bucket; see also **behavioral play audiometry, conditioned play audiometry**

plenum a space that is filled with air (e.g., a ceiling plenum that may be above two adjacent rooms) and provides a flanking path for sound transmission

PLL preferred listening level; intensity level that is most comfortable for a patient to listen to speech for long periods of time; also known as **most comfortable level (MCL)**

plosive stop-consonant speech sound that is produced by creating an oral cavity closure, building air pressure behind the closure, and then releasing it (e.g., /p, b, t, d, k, g/)

pneumatic otoscopy an otoscopic examination performed using an otoscope equipped with an air-filled bulb that releases pressure into the ear canal to visualize tympanic membrane movement

pneumotachograph instrument used to measure air flow

PNS peripheral nervous system; components of the nervous system that lie outside of the central nervous system, including the cranial nerves and nerves in the extremities

POGO prescription of gain and output; a linear hearing aid prescriptive fitting method that determines specific target gain values for amplification; the threshold at 250 Hz is multiplied by 0.5 and then 10 dB is subtracted from it; the threshold at 500 Hz is multiplied by 0.5 and then 5 dB is subtracted from it; the thresholds at 1000 through 6000 Hz are multiplied by 0.5

polar response curve the recording of sound pressure (amplification) as a function of the angle of rotation in the Knowles Electronics Manikin for Acoustic Research (KEMAR) system

polarity the voltage characteristics of a stimulus or response waveform; stimuli are of negative (rarefaction), positive (condensation), or alternating polarity; see also **rarefaction, condensation**

Politzer bag inflatable bag used to force air through the nose during politzerization; see also **politzerization**

politzerization inflation of the middle ear by forcing air through the nose and into the eustachian tube; considered a eustachian tube maneuver; also known as politzer inflation; see also **Valsalva maneuver, Toynbee maneuver**

polyotia the presence of an additional pinna on one or both sides of the head

polyp a small, benign growth on a mucoid surface; see also **aural polyps**

polytomography specialized X-ray scan that produces thin (usually 10-mm thick) cross-sectional reconstructions of the body using computer back-projection techniques; highly sophisticated, computer-intense process for measuring and analyzing multiplane (multicut) X-rays; also known as **CAT scan** (obsolete usage); see also **computerized axial tomography, positron emission tomography (PET)**

PON periolivary nuclei; nuclei in the superior olivary complex that surround the medial and lateral superior olives; receive projections from the acoustic stria

pons caudal (low) portion of the brainstem just above the medulla and below the midbrain; contains important auditory centers (e.g., cochlear nuclei, trapezoid body, inferior colliculus, and lateral lemniscus)

pontine relating to the pons

pontobulbar palsy autosomal recessive disorder characterized by facial weakness, grooved tongue, vocal cord paresis, swallowing disorder, aspiration; associated with sensorineural hearing loss with usual age of onset in childhood

popcorn noise noise that sounds like popcorn popping

porous permeable or full of pores or tiny holes; allows for absorption of sound

PORP partial ossicular replacement prosthesis; used in tympanoplasty to aid in reconstruction of the ossicular chain; see also **TORP**

positional alcoholic nystagmus (PAN) nystagmus that is evoked by a change in head position after the ingestion of alcohol

positional nystagmus the presence of nystagmus that occurs in specific head positions

positional testing component of the electronystagmography test battery designed to identify the presence of nystagmus elicited by certain head positions that do not involve head movement

positional vertigo dizziness and the sensation of spinning with specific stationary head positions

positioning nystagmus the presence of nystagmus that is evoked by movement and changes in head position

positive middle ear pressure the level of air pressure in the middle ear space that is above atmospheric pressure; suggests poor eustachian tube functioning and the possibility of a bulging tympanic membrane

positive venting valve (PVV) a type of vent used in some hearing aid earmolds that allows for changes in the size of the opening; see also **vent, venting**

positron emission tomography (PET) the imaging of body (especially brain) sections by tracking positron-emitting radionuclides; depending on the radionuclides employed, researchers can measure regional cerebral blood flow, blood volume, oxygen uptake, and glucose transport and metabolism in addition to locating neurotransmitter receptors

post stimulus onset time (PST) histogram a plot of the time course of the neural response relative to the onset of a stimulus

postauricular located behind the ear

postauricular hearing aid hearing aid that sits completely behind the ear over the pinna and is typically coupled to the ear canal by an earmold; also known as **behind-the-ear (BTE) hearing aid**

postauricular incision a surgical cut that is made behind the pinna for various operations (e.g., mastoidectomy, tympanoplasty, cochlear implantation, etc.)

postauricular muscle (PAM) one of three muscles attaching the external ear (pinna) to the scalp; located behind the ear

postauricular myogenic response postauricular (behind the pinna) muscle activity that may occur in response to sound stimulation; may interfere with middle latency response measurements

posterior toward the rear

posterior incudal ligament one of the ligaments of the middle ear responsible for suspension of the ossicular chain; connects from the short process of the incus to the posterior wall of the tympanic cavity

posterior semicircular canal one of the three canals of the vestibular system that contains the sense organ (crista ampularis) for responding to angular motion; also known as the vertical-inferior canal; see also **semicircular canals (SCCs)**

posterior ventral cochlear nucleus (PVCN) the lower brainstem nucleus into which the auditory nerve terminates; located in the rostral medulla and caudal pons

postlingual refers to the timing of an insult (hearing loss) occurring after the normal development of speech and language

postlingual deafness the profound loss of hearing after the normal development of speech and language (usually age 5 years or older)

postlingual hearing loss the loss of hearing after the normal development of speech and language (usually age 5 years or older)

postnatal after birth

poststimulatory fatigue diminution of the response from the sensory and neural receptors of the ear after prolonged exposure to intense stimulation; also known as **temporary threshold shift (TTS)**; poststimulatory effect occurs after exposure to stimulation

postsynaptic activity neural activity within the inferior colliculus that can be represented by a slow negative electrophysiologic response

posturography a type of vestibular assessment that focuses on the function of the balance system in maintaining postural stability in a variety of simulated conditions; computer-induced platform movements evaluate motor responses that include strength, symmetry, and latency of muscle response; see also **sensory organization test (SOT)**

pot abbreviation for potentiometer

potassium (K^+) element that makes up the majority of intracellular fluid that helps regulate neuromuscular excitability and muscle contraction; see also **sodium-potassium pump**

potential (1) a difference in electrical charge measured between two electrodes; (2) in evoked potential measurement, the source of electrical potentials is stimulus-evoked activity in sensory portions of the peripheral or central nervous system; (3) each cell in the body pumps ions across cell membranes to keep an electrical potential difference across the membrane: ions travel in and out of a cell through channels in the membrane; passive channels allow free move-

ment; chemically gated channels are selective; see also **electrical potential**

potential, action (AP) (1) gross neural potential; summed or averaged activity of action potentials of cranial nerve VIII in response to acoustic stimulation; (2) in auditory evoked potential measurements, it is the whole-nerve response of cranial nerve VIII; (3) the main component of the electrocochleogram and wave I of the auditory brainstem response; also known as **whole nerve action potential**

potential, auditory evoked (AEP) small electrical potential superimposed by auditory input on the steady-state electrical activity of the brain; usually detectable only by signal averaging; see also **auditory evoked response (AER)**

potential, corneoretinal an electrical potential of the eyes resulting from the positive electrical charge from the cornea and the negative electrical charge from the retina; the electrical potential is about 1 mV; the eye acts as a dipole (molecule having two equal and opposite charges); used in the measurement of eye movements during electronystagmography testing

potential, electrical (1) a difference in electrical charge measured between two electrodes; (2) in evoked potential measurement, the source of electrical potentials is stimulus-evoked activity in sensory portions of the peripheral or central nervous system; (3) each cell in the body pumps ions across cell membranes to keep an electrical potential difference across the membrane: ions travel in and out of a cell through channels in the membrane; passive channels allow free movement; chemically gated channels are selective

potential, endocochlear a type of cochlear potential that reflects the constant positive potential difference between the scala media and the peripheral scalae vestibuli and tympani

potential, endolymphatic cochlear electrical potential within the endolymph and its cells; endolymph in the scala media relative to the perilymph in the scala vestibuli and scala tympani is positive: +70 to +90 mV (±20 mV); see also **endocochlear potential**

potential, event-related (ERP) term used to describe certain evoked responses, such as the 40-Hz response or the P300 response, that are elicited with stimuli other than a simple sequence of brief duration clicks or tones; usually elicited by an endogenous stimulus representing high-level processing (e.g., cognition)

potential, evoked (EP) a series of electrical charges occurring in the peripheral and central nervous system following stimulation of an end organ or peripheral nerve

potential, receptor graded electrical potential that is always stimulus dependent; e.g., **cochlear microphonic (CM)** or **summating potential (SP)**

potential, resting (1) each cell in the body pumps ions across cell membranes to keep an electrical potential difference across the membrane: ions travel in and out of a cell through channels in the membrane; passive channels allow free movement; chemically gated channels are selective; (2) voltage potential differences that can be measured from the cochlea at rest

potential, somatosensory evoked (SEP) an evoked potential created by stimulation of the somatosensory system usually by electrical stimulation over a peripheral nerve or the spinal cord; cortical and subcortical response to repetitive stimulation of sensory fibers of the peripheral nerves that are averaged by a computer

potential, summating (SP) a sustained direct current shift in the endocochlear potential that occurs when the organ of Corti is stimulated by sound; a direct-current electrical potential of cochlear origin that can be measured using electrocochleography

potentiometer controls used in hearing aids to adjust gain, output, frequency response, etc; are often modified with external screw-set controls; also used in audiometers and sound level meters to adjust physical parameters of sound for calibration

power the rate at which energy is expended or work is done; unit of measurement is the **watt**

power amplifier an amplifier that strengthens weak signals at the input stage of a sound system

power CROS monaural hearing aid fitting with a power hearing aid that uses contralateral routing of signals (CROS); the microphone is placed on the opposite ear (side) to reduce feedback

PPDT Psychoacoustic Pattern Discrimination Test; a central auditory processing measure assessing the perception of nonspeech stimuli presented in a variety of temporal patterns

PPO preferred provider organization; group of physicians, pharmacists, and hospitals that provides discounts to its members for using its services and facilities

PPS Pitch Pattern Sequence; a central auditory measure that requires identification of a sequence of three high or low tones presented in random configurations

PPVT-R Peabody Picture Vocabulary Test–Revised; test of receptive language skills

pragmatics a language term for the development of and the set of rules for language in context; includes speaker-listener intentions and relationships

preamplifier an electronic device that receives an electrical signal and increases the strength (amplitude) of the signal before it is sent for further processing; used in hearing aid amplification and evoked response measurement

preauricular in front of or anterior to the ear

preauricular pit craniofacial anomaly characterized by a small hole or indentation that is anterior to the auricle; also referred to as a preauricular sinus

preauricular tag craniofacial anomaly characterized by a small flap or piece of skin that is anterior to the auricle

precedence effect the phenomenon that occurs during auditory fusion when two (primary) sounds of the same order of magnitude are presented dichotically and produce localization of the secondary sound toward the ear receiving the first (primary) sound stimulus

precipitous very steep

precipitous hearing loss sensorineural hearing loss characterized by a steeply sloping audiometric configuration

predictive validity the ability of a test instrument to estimate a particular type or level of behavior; measures how well the test correlates with some outside validating criterion

preferred listening level (PLL) intensity level that is most comfortable for a patient to listen to speech for long periods of time; also known as **most comfortable level (MCL)**

preferred provider organization (PPO) group of physicians, pharmacists, and hospitals that provides discounts to its members for using its services and facilities

prelingual deafness the profound loss of hearing before the development of speech and language; may include congenitally deaf and those deafened before the age of 2 years

prelingual hearing loss the loss of hearing before the development of speech and language; may include congenitally deaf and those deafened before the age of 2 years

prenatal occurring before birth

presbycusis decrease in hearing sensitivity associated with aging

presbyvertigo (PV) the experience of vertigo (sensation of spinning and dizziness) that occurs with increasing age

prescribed gain the gain and frequency response of a hearing aid that are determined by the use of a prescriptive formula

prescription method a means of predicting the electroacoustic performance of a hearing aid from audiologic and patient history data

prescription of gain and output (POGO) a linear hearing aid prescriptive fitting method that determines specific target gain values for amplification; the threshold at 250 Hz is multiplied by 0.5 and then 10 dB is subtracted from it; the threshold at 500 Hz is multiplied by 0.5 and then 5 dB is subtracted from it; the thresholds at 1000 through 6000 Hz are multiplied by 0.5

prescriptive gain targets the desired gain values as a function of frequency for a hearing aid that are

based on a particular prescriptive method; these gain values are compared to the actual output of the hearing aid to verify fitting

prescriptive hearing aid fitting strategy for fitting hearing aids by using a formula to calculate the desired gain and frequency response; formula incorporates pure-tone audiometric thresholds and usually information about uncomfortable loudness levels

prescriptive method strategy for fitting hearing aids by using a formula to calculate the desired gain and frequency response; formula incorporates pure-tone audiometric thresholds and usually information about uncomfortable loudness levels

prescriptive selection procedure strategy for fitting hearing aids by using a formula to calculate the desired gain and frequency response; formula incorporates pure-tone audiometric thresholds and usually information about uncomfortable loudness levels

pressure measure of force divided by the area to which the force is applied; usually measured in dynes per square centimeter ($dyne/cm^2$); the ear is a pressure receptor

pressure spectrum level the sound pressure level in a frequency band of unit width

pressure vent a bore made in an earmold or hearing aid that is approximately 0.06 to 0.8 mm in diameter; has no measurable effect on the frequency response but provides pressure equalization in the external auditory meatus

pressure-equalization (PE) tube a short polyethylene tube or grommet placed through a myringotomy incision in a tympanic membrane that permits continuous middle-ear ventilation; see also **myringotomy**

prevalence the total number of cases of a specific disease or disorder existing in a given population at a certain time

primary auditory cortex the auditory cortical region located on the superior plane and insula of the superior gyrus of the temporal lobe; receives information from lower portions of the brain; possible generator site for the Pa component of the auditory middle latency response

primary auditory neurons first-order auditory nerve fibers from the cochlear branch of cranial nerve VIII; relay information from the cochlear hair cells in the organ of Corti to the spiral ganglia in the modiolus to the cochlear nuclei of the central auditory system

probe (1) a slender instrument and wire for making electrical contact at various stages of a sound system; (2) a small tube placed at the end of a microphone and inserted within the external auditory canal that is used for probe microphone, immittance, and otoacoustic emission measurements

probe microphone a tiny microphone often attached to a soft,

small tube placed within the external ear canal to measure the sound intensity level near the eardrum; used for real ear measurements for hearing aid fitting and verification; also known as **probe tube microphone**; see also **probe microphone measurement**

probe microphone measurement real ear measurement taken using a probe microphone to verify aided and unaided performance at the eardrum; aided performance is often compared to different prescriptive fitting techniques to verify fit; see also **probe microphone**

probe tip a disposable or reusable tip that provides a seal to the ear for acoustic immittance and otoacoustic emission measures

probe tone steady-state stimulus used in immittance audiometry that provides a known quantity of sound pressure; used indirectly to measure changes in the mobility of the middle ear system; low-frequency probe tone is typically 226 Hz

probe tube microphone a tiny microphone often attached to a soft, small tube placed within the external ear canal to measure sound intensity level near the eardrum; used for real ear measurements for hearing aid fitting and verification; also known as **probe microphone**

processing, auditory those processes that occur within the central auditory nervous system in response to acoustic stimuli; see also **central auditory processing (CAP)**

processing, central auditory the ability to achieve sound localization and lateralization; auditory discrimination; auditory pattern recognition; temporal aspects of audition including temporal resolution, temporal masking, temporal integration, and temporal ordering; auditory performance with competing acoustic signals; and auditory performance with degraded acoustic signals; these auditory system mechanisms and processes generate electric brain waves or auditory evoked potentials (i.e., electrocochleography, auditory brainstem response, auditory middle latency response, auditory late response, and auditory event-related response) in response to acoustic stimuli

processing, compressed analog signal processing strategy used in cochlear implants in which signals are divided into frequency bands and delivered to the appropriate frequency-specific electrode pairs

processing, continuous interleaved sampling signal processing strategy used in the Clarion cochlear implant that sends the speech signal to the electrodes through a series of very rapid pulses

processing, digital signal (DSP) conversion of continuous time analog signals into sampled discrete time data points (numbers); allows for the use of multiple algorithms for processing signals

processing, signal manipulation of various parameters of the signal

processing strategy strategy used by cochlear implants to determine how the input signal is processed, including the degree of amplification of different frequency bands and the manner in which the signal is delivered by different electrodes in the electrode array; process used to transform the speech signal into a pattern of electrical stimulation

Profile of Hearing Aid Benefit (PHAB) self-assessment questionnaire examining an individual's perceived benefit from hearing aid use

Profile of Hearing Aid Performance (PHAP) a self-assessment measurement tool that assesses the patient's benefit from a hearing instrument

profound hearing loss a hearing loss of 90 dB HL or poorer across the frequencies; categorized as deafness

profoundly deaf a categorization of deafness (hearing loss) in which the audiometric thresholds are 90 dB HL or poorer

progeria disorder characterized by premature aging, deficient subcutaneous fat, brittle nails, progressive delayed dental eruption, early coronary artery disease, and atherosclerosis; results in death before age 30 in most cases

programmable CIC a completely-in-the-canal hearing aid that has analog circuitry and digital programming capabilities

programmable circuit analog circuitry in a hearing aid that can be programmed either by computer or other specialized equipment in a dispenser's office

programmable hearing aid a hearing aid with analog circuitry that is controlled digitally; capable of being programmed to compensate for different hearing losses or different listening conditions

programmable increase at low levels (PILL) a form of nonlinear amplification (automatic signal processing); level dependent frequency response that can be adjusted to provide either **bass increase at low levels (BILL)** or **treble increase at low levels (TILL)**; see also **level dependent frequency response (LDFR)**

progressive sensorineural hearing loss cochlear hearing loss that is advancing; getting worse over time

prolapsed canal a collapsed ear canal that has lost its rigidity due to occlusion by cartilaginous tissue

promontory a rounded, bony projection on the medial wall of the middle ear produced by the basal turn of the cochlea; site for transtympanic needle electrode placement in electrocochleography; used for promontory stimulation in cochlear implants; see also **promontory stimulation**

promontory stimulation a test used to measure the degree of neuron survival by placing an electrode on the promontory of the cochlea and evaluating psychophysical capabilities; used in cochlear implant evaluations; also known as promontory testing

propagation act of extending, projecting, or traveling through space

prophylaxis actions taken to prevent or protect against disease

proprioception the awareness of weight, posture, movement, and position in space

prosodic stress, rhythm, pitch, and intonation features of speech; see also **suprasegmental**

prosodic speech features variations of loudness, pitch, rhythm, stress, and intonation patterns used in speech production; also known as **suprasegmental**

prosody suprasegmental aspects of spoken language; the dynamic melody, timing, rhythm, and amplitude fluctuations of fluent speech; see also **suprasegmental**

prosthesis (1) a device that replaces a defective body part; (2) a device designed to improve function (e.g., a hearing aid)

proteus syndrome characterized by multiple hamartomas, enlarged hands and feet, bony projections on skull, large head, cognitive deficiency in about half of known cases, thought to be disease affecting Joseph Merrick (the Elephant Man); associated with conductive hearing loss resulting from bony growths in the ear canal

protocol written plan of procedures to be followed during a treatment or experiment

proximal toward the center or medial part of a structure; opposite of distal; see also **distal**

Prussak's space small space in the middle ear medial to Shrapnell's membrane and lateral to the neck of the malleus; common site for an **attic retraction pocket**

pseudohypacusis faked or exaggerated hearing loss with no known physiologic cause; also known as **malingering, functional hearing loss,** and **nonorganic hearing loss**

pseudotinnitus (1) the feigning of tinnitus (ringing in the ears); (2) the incorrect interpretation of the perception of an environmental sound as tinnitus

pseudotumor benign intracranial hypertension disorder that may produce bilateral reductions in caloric nystagmus

PSI Pediatric Speech Intelligibility Test; speech audiometry procedure for assessment of peripheral and central auditory system function

PST poststimulus onset time histogram; a plot of the time course of the neural response relative to the onset of a stimulus

Psychoacoustic Pattern Discrimination Test (PPDT) a central auditory processing measure assessing the perception of nonspeech stimuli presented in a variety of temporal patterns

psychoacoustics the science that deals with the psychological correlates of the physical parameters of acoustics; a branch of psychophysics; see also **psychophysics**

psychogenic deafness psychogenic hearing disorder caused by emotional trauma; severe anxiety becomes the physical appearance of deafness; hearing loss of no physiologic origin; also known as **conversion deafness**

psychogenic hearing loss faked or exaggerated hearing loss with no known physiologic cause; also known as **malingering, functional hearing loss, nonorganic hearing loss**

psychometric function a mathematical relationship in which the independent variable is a measure of the stimulus and the dependent variable is a measure of the response

psychophysical tuning curve a V-shaped threshold curve similar to tuning curves obtained from auditory nerve fibers; obtained with a "probe tone" of fixed frequency and intensity that is just-masked by a tone whose frequency is made to vary; see also **tuning curve**

psychophysics the science that deals with the quantitative relationship between physical and psychological events; a branch of psychology; see also **psychoacoustics**

PT pure tone; sound produced by an instantaneous sound pressure that is a simple sinusoidal function of time; a single-frequency tonal sound (e.g., 1000 Hz); a sinusoid

PTA pure-tone average; the arithmetic average of hearing threshold levels for 500, 1000, and 2000 Hz, or the speech frequency region of the audiogram; the PTA should agree with the speech recognition threshold within ±7 dB

PTE Phonetic Task Evaluation; nonsense syllable test designed to estimate a child's speech feature discrimination abilities

PTS permanent threshold shift; permanent increase in the threshold of audibility for an ear at a specified frequency above a previously established reference level; expressed in decibels; see also **temporary threshold shift (TTS), compound threshold shift (CTS)**

PTT Pursuit Tracking Test; subtest in the electronystagmography test battery for assessing the smooth following of moving objects by the eyes; the goal is to keep the image of the objects focused on the fovea of the eye; see also **optokinetic nystagmus (OKN)**

Public Law 93-112 the Rehabilitation Act of 1973; ensured access of impaired students (including hearing impaired) from elementary school through college to federally funded programs

Public Law 94-142 the Education for all Handicapped Children Act of 1975; ensured access to a free, appropriate, public education for students who were hearing impaired aged 3 through 21; included mainstreaming as much as possible with the use of individualized education plans; see also **individualized educational plan (IEP)**

Public Law 99-457 the Individuals with Disabilities Education Act (IDEA); an amendment to PL 94-142

in 1986 that extended federal funding for impaired children from birth to 3 years of age; see also **PL 94-142**

Public Law 101-336 Americans with Disabilities Act; federal law enacted to provide protection from discrimination based on disability; it was modeled after the Rehabilitation Act of 1973 and passed in 1990

pulsatile tinnitus head noise characterized by a pulsing sensation caused by a vascular disorder; often a combination of hypertension or anemia with atherosclerosis causing turbulent arterial flow; can be associated with a glomus jugulare tumor; see also **tinnitus**

pulse a brief electrical signal; usually a square wave

pure oralism method of instruction for deaf children that emphasizes spoken language skills to the exclusion of manual communication; see also **oralism**

pure tone (PT) sound produced by an instantaneous sound pressure that is a simple sinusoidal function of time; a single-frequency tonal sound (e.g., 1000 Hz); a sinusoid

pure-tone audiogram a graph expressing hearing loss (hearing sensitivity) as a function of frequency; plot of air- and bone-conduction thresholds in dB HL for the octave frequencies between 250 and 8000 Hz; also known as **audiogram**

pure-tone audiometer clinical instrumentation used to present calibrated pure-tone stimuli for the purpose of obtaining an audiogram

pure-tone audiometry the procedure most commonly used for the measurement of hearing impairment; pure tones are presented via air conduction and bone conduction and the patient's sensitivity to discrete frequencies is measured; see also **air conduction (AC), bone conduction (BC)**

pure-tone average (PTA) the arithmetic average of hearing threshold levels for 500, 1000, and 2000 Hz, or the speech frequency region of the audiogram; the PTA should agree with the speech recognition threshold within ±7 dB

pure-tone hearing loss loss of hearing sensitivity characterized by a reduced ability to hear air- and bone-conducted pure tones as measured on an audiogram

pure-tone testing the procedure most commonly used for the measurement of hearing impairment; pure tones are presented via air conduction and bone conduction and the patient's sensitivity to discrete frequencies is measured; see also **air conduction (AC), bone conduction (BC)**

pure-tone threshold the lowest level that a patient can hear a pure sinusoid that provides a direct indication of the amount of hearing loss the individual has at each frequency for both air and bone conduction

Pursuit Tracking Test (PTT) subtest in the electronystagmography test battery for assessing the smooth following of moving objects by the eyes; the goal is to keep the image of the objects focused on the fovea of the eye; see also **optokinetic nystagmus (OKN)**

purulence the condition of discharging or producing pus; case of infection

purulent otitis media middle ear inflammation with effusion that is actively infected; e.g., **suppurative otitis media**

push-pull circuitry a hearing aid amplifier circuit that contains two amplifiers: one that acts on the positive phase of the incoming signal and the other that acts on the negative phase; results in an increase in the power of the device while minimizing distortion; used in class B circuits

PV presbyvertigo; the experience of vertigo (sensation of spinning and dizziness) that occurs with increasing age

PVCN posterior ventral cochlear nucleus; the lower brainstem nucleus into which the auditory nerve terminates; located in the rostral medulla and caudal pons

PVT physical volume test; the measurement of ear canal volume as part of the immittance battery

PVV positive venting valve; a type of vent used in some hearing aids or earmolds that allows for changes in the size of the opening; see also **vent, venting**

pyramidal eminence structure in the posterior wall of the middle ear cavity that houses the stapedius muscle

Q

Q directivity factor; a loudspeaker characteristic that can be calculated from its directivity index; log Q = DI/10; see also **directivity index (DI)**

quadra-, quadri- prefix: four

quality term used in psychoacoustics to determine the perceptual correlate to a physical sound; the perceptual impression of the spectrum of a sound (e.g., tonality, density, brightness, consonance, dissonance, etc.); the psychological correlate of spectrum

quantization the assignment of discrete values to the amplitude dimension of an analog signal; process by which a continuous variation in amplitude is represented as a sequence of discrete values; necessary to represent the signal in a digital computer

quantization noise a signal distortion resulting from an inadequate number of quantization levels in digitizing a signal

quarter wavelength resonator the fundamental resonance of an air-filled tube that is closed at one end and open at the other that is four times the length of the tube; see also **quarter-wave frequency**

quarter-wave frequency one of the lowest frequency standing wave frequencies possible for a specific tube; the length of the ear canal equals one quarter of the wavelength of the resonance; see also **quarter wavelength resonator**

quasiperiodic (1) a behavior that has at least two frequencies in which the phases are related by an irrational number; (2) form of motion that is recurrent, but never exactly repeating

quinine a drug used to fight malaria that is known to be ototoxic; can cause temporary or permanent hearing loss; see also **ototoxicity**

R

R acoustic resistance; the in-phase component of impedance; opposition to the flow of energy via dissipation

R-HPI Revised Hearing Performance Inventory; an assessment of self-perceived handicap imposed by hearing loss

radical mastoidectomy surgical removal of all middle ear structures to eliminate middle ear disease completely; see also **mastoidectomy**

radio frequency hearing aid a hearing instrument with a radio microphone transmitter that improves the signal-to-noise ratio; see also **FM system**

radio receiver device that picks up a transmitted radio signal, demodulates the audio frequency signal from it, preamplifies the audio signal, and delivers it to an amplifier; see also **FM system**

radio transmitter device that modulates the frequency of a radio signal with an audio frequency signal and broadcasts the modulated signal; see also **FM system**

Radioear (B71 & B72) widely used bone vibrators that comply with the standard of a plane circular arriving face with an area of 150 to 200 mm^2; used in bone-conduction audiometry; see also **bone conduction (BC)**

radiography the use of radiation to produce shadow images on photographic emulsion; the image is a result of the reduction in radiation as it passes through the object being radiographed

radiology (1) branch of medicine that examines body structures using X-rays; (2) type of examination of the cochlea using a high-resolution computed tomography (CT) scan; procedure is used to determine the status of the structures of the ear prior to any surgery; is a necessary procedure prior to cochlear implant surgery

ramp the onset or rise portion of a stimulus, usually a tone, that is shaped or modified in some way, rather than immediately rising to the maximum (peak) amplitude within the first portion of a cycle of the stimulus

Ramsay Hunt syndrome herpes zoster virus infection of the ganglia of cranial nerve VII; includes lesions of the external ear and mastoid with severe pain; see also **herpes zoster oticus**

255

random noise noise whose instantaneous amplitude is not specified at any instant of time; can only be defined statistically by an amplitude distribution function

range statistical measure describing the dispersion of the data; determined by subtracting the two most extreme points from each other

Rapid Alternating Speech Perception (RASP) test central auditory test of brainstem integration consisting of sentence stimuli that are presented to each ear simultaneously with only a small portion going to each ear at any given time; presentation of the stimulus is alternated rapidly between the two ears

rapid speech transmission index (RASTI) a number between 0 and 1 that quantifies speech intelligibility; derived from the measurement of the modulation transfer function of two octave bands of pink-noise modulations that mimic the long-term speech spectrum; see also **articulation index (AI), modulation transfer function (MTF)**

Rapp-Hodgkin syndrome autosomal dominant disorder characterized by ectodermal dysplasia, cleft lip and palate, sparse hair, hypoplastic or absent nails, missing and abnormal teeth, maxillary deficiency; associated with conductive hearing loss caused by chronic otitis media secondary to clefting

rare stimulus a target signal that occurs with a lesser probability than a second signal; the subject is usually asked to make some response when the signal occurs; also referred to as the **infrequent signal**

rarefaction (1) the portion of the signal in which there is a reduction in the density of air molecules corresponding to the negative component of a sine wave; (2) form of a click stimulus produced by a negative-polarity electric pulse to an earphone; see also **condensation**

rarefaction polarity the initial displacement of the stimulus is negative polarity produced by a negative voltage electrical signal and inward movement of an acoustic transducer diaphragm; see also **rarefaction**

RASP Rapidly Alternating Speech Perception test; central auditory test of brainstem integration consisting of sentence stimuli that are presented to each ear simultaneously with only a small portion going to each ear at any given time; presentation of the stimulus is alternated rapidly between the two ears

RASTI rapid speech transmission index; a number between 0 and 1 that quantifies speech intelligibility; derived from the measurement of the modulation transfer function of two octave bands of pink-noise modulations that mimic the long-term speech spectrum; see also **articulation index (AI), modulation transfer function (MTF)**

rate the number of stimulus repetitions per unit time, usually in 1 second

rate-pitch the perception of pitch using the rate theory, which suggests that frequency perception is determined by the response of the nerve replicating the spectral envelope of the signal; most effective for low-frequency stimuli

ratio, compression (CR) ratio of the change in output level of a hearing aid that results from a given change in the input level in a compression amplifier

ratio, consonant-vowel relationship between the intensity of a consonant and its adjacent vowel(s)

ratio, critical based on indirectly derived measures of bandwidth; the ratio of the intensity of the tone to the intensity per cycle of the noise or the dB difference between the masked threshold and level-per-cycle of noise; critical ratios underestimate critical bands by about 2.5 times; see also **critical band**

ratio, message-to-competition relationship between the level of the desired signal (message) and the noise (competing signal) at the listener's ear; commonly reported as the difference in decibels between the intensity of the signal and the intensity of the background noise; also known as **signal-to-noise ratio (S/N, SNR)**

ratio, signal-to-noise (SNR, S/N) relationship between the sound levels of the signal and the noise at the listener's ear; commonly reported as the difference in decibels between the intensity of the signal and the intensity of the background noise (e.g., if the speech signal is meas-

ured at 70 dB and the noise is 64 dB, the signal-to-noise ratio is +6 dB)

ratio, speech-to-competition the signal-to-noise ratio or difference in decibels between the intensity of a speech signal and the intensity of a competing noise

ratio scale quantitative scale of measurement that has a true zero and ratios are valid; highest level of measurement

RCT rotary chair testing; a test of vestibular assessment that uses a computer-driven sinusoidal rotational chair that moves at different velocities and in different directions; electronystagmographic recordings are made during rotary chair testing for the assessment of bilateral vestibular loss

REA right ear advantage; a cerebral dominance phenomenon in which normal right-handed listeners have scores for the right ear that are consistently higher than scores for the left ear for dichotically presented signals

reactance (X) the opposition to alternating electrical current caused by capacitors and inductors in a circuit; the opposition to the flow of energy due to storage; see also **immittance**

reaction time the time between the presentation of the stimulus and the initiation of the response

readiness potential slow negative potential that occurs prior to the onset of movement

REAG real-ear aided gain; the value in decibels of the real-ear aided response at a specific frequency; the sound pressure level, as a function of frequency, at a specified measurement point in the ear canal for a specified sound field with the hearing aid in place and turned on; expressed as gain in decibels relative to the stimulus level

real ear refers to measurements of hearing aid performance conducted in the ear canal with probe-tube microphone instrumentation

real-ear aided gain (REAG) the value in decibels of the real-ear aided response at a specific frequency; the sound pressure level, as a function of frequency, at a specified measurement point in the ear canal for a specified sound field with the hearing aid in place and turned on; expressed as gain in decibels relative to the stimulus level

real-ear aided response (REAR) the sound pressure level, as a function of frequency, at a specified measurement point in the ear canal for a specified sound field with the hearing aid in place and turned on; expressed as gain in decibels relative to the stimulus level

real-ear attenuation at threshold (REAT) the reduction characteristics of hearing protection devices using probe microphone measurements; determined as the difference between the **real-ear unaided response (REUR)** and the **real-ear occluded response (REOR)**

real-ear gain gain of a hearing aid at the tympanic membrane measured with a probe microphone; the difference between the sound pressure level (SPL) in the external ear canal and the SPL at the field reference point for a specified sound field; see also **real-ear aided response (REAR), real-ear insertion response (REIR)**

real-ear insertion gain (REIG) the value in decibels of the real-ear insertion response at a specific frequency; see also **real-ear insertion response (REIR)**

real-ear insertion response (REIR) the difference in decibels as a function of frequency between the real-ear unaided response and the real-ear aided response measurements taken at the same measurement point in the same sound field; the amount of gain delivered to the patient wearing a hearing aid that he or she did not have before the hearing aid fitting; it is the electroacoustic equivalent of functional gain; see also **real-ear aided response (REAR), real-ear unaided response (REUR)**

real-ear measurement measurement of amplified sound in an ear canal through the use of a probe microphone; see also **probe microphone measurement**

real-ear occluded gain (REOG) the value in decibels of the real-ear occluded response at a specific frequency

real-ear occluded response (REOR) the sound pressure level, as a function of frequency, at a specified measurement point in the ear canal for a specified sound field with the hearing aid in place and turned off; the loss of gain from occluding the ear; insertion loss

real-ear probe microphone a tiny microphone often attached to a soft, small tube placed within the external ear canal to measure sound intensity level near the eardrum; used for real ear measurements for hearing aid fitting and verification; also known as **probe tube microphone**; see also **probe microphone measurement**

real-ear saturation response (RESR) the sound pressure level as a function of frequency at a specified measurement point in the ear canal with the hearing aid in place and turned on; the measurement is made with the stimulus level sufficiently intense to operate the hearing aid at its maximum output level

real-ear to coupler difference (RECD) the difference in decibels as a function of frequency between the outputs of a hearing aid measured in a real ear versus a 2-cc coupler; useful calculation when fitting amplification on young children to avoid overamplification in their smaller ear canals

real-ear unaided response (REUR) the sound pressure level as a function of frequency at a specified point in the unoccluded ear canal for a specified sound field; used as a reference value for calculation of insertion gain

real-time displaying information or results almost instantaneously

real-time captioning providing a typed dialog of a person's speech in real-time on a computer screen; can be used with a notebook computer or can be displayed on a large screen; see also **closed captioning (CC), open captioning**

real-time intraoperative monitoring monitoring the cochlear nerve action potential during surgery to prevent damage to cochlear function; also used to monitor the function of other nerves during surgery; see also **intraoperative monitoring**

real-time processing the instantaneous processing of information using a computer; the procedure is so rapid that the signal processing time is imperceptible

real-time speech the transitory, ephemeral nature of an ongoing speech signal; when speech is presented in a real-time manner, listeners must quickly recognize phonemes, syllables, and words based on preceding linguistic-contextual cues and ongoing acoustic-phonetic information

REAR real-ear aided response; the sound pressure level, as a function of frequency, at a specified measurement point in the ear canal for a specified sound field with the hearing aid in place and turned on; expressed as gain in decibels relative to the stimulus level

REAT real-ear attenuation at threshold; the reduction characteristics of hearing protection devices using probe microphone measurements;

determined as the difference between the real-ear unaided response and the real-ear occluded response

RECD real-ear to coupler difference; the difference in decibels as a function of frequency between the outputs of a hearing aid measured in a real ear versus a 2-cc coupler; useful calculation when fitting amplification on young children to avoid overamplification in their smaller ear canals

receiver component of a hearing aid that converts electrical amplified sound to acoustic energy; type of output transducer

receiver operating characteristic (ROC) graphic summary of the performance of a detector; detection probability is plotted on the ordinate, and false alarm probability is plotted on the abscissa

receiver tubing tubing that extends from the hearing aid receiver to the medial tip of a custom hearing aid; known for its propensity to become plugged with cerumen

receiver-stimulator a cochlear implant electronics package that decodes the transmitted signal into electrical stimuli to be presented to the electrode array

receptive language a patient's ability to receive and process verbal auditory information

receptor potential graded electrical potential that is always stimulus dependent; e.g., **cochlear microphonic (CM)** or **summating potential (SP)**

recessive pertaining to the transmission of a gene of which the effect is often masked or hidden

recessive hereditary sensorineural hearing loss common form of congenital hearing loss; caused by a 25% chance of autosomal recessive transmission of the gene to offspring; can be present on its own or as part of a syndrome

reconstructive middle ear surgery treatment techniques used to reconstruct the middle ear (e.g., tympanoplasty, myringoplasty, use of prosthetic ossicles, etc.) after ear disease has damaged the original structures; see also **tympanoplasty**

recovery time the time period immediately after a neural unit is depolarized (fires) during which it is unable to be activated

recruitment an abnormally rapid growth of loudness; for individuals with cochlear impairment, as the intensity of the sound increases, the perception of loudness increases very rapidly; also known as **loudness recruitment**

recruitment, complete a high-intensity tone is perceived as being equally loud in both ears although the thresholds are sustained differently; possible result of the alternate binaural loudness balancing test; see also **alternate binaural loudness balancing (ABLB), loudness recruitment, recruitment**

recruitment, loudness an abnormally rapid growth of loudness; for individuals with cochlear impairment, as the intensity of the sound increases, the perception of loudness increases very rapidly; considered a return to normal loudness

recruitment, partial possible result from loudness balance testing; abnormal growth of loudness in which the loudness of a high-intensity sound presented to the impaired ear comes close to but remains less than the perceived loudness in the normal ear

rectification the process whereby alternating electrical current is converted into direct current

rectilinear motion motion that travels in a straight line, back and forth manner

recurrent otitis media inflammation of the middle ear that reoccurs 3 to 6 times in a 6-month period

redundancy (1) the part of a message that can be eliminated without loss of information; (2) refers to stimulus items that have more information in them than is needed to understand the message (e.g., sentences are more redundant than nonsense syllables); see also **extrinsic redundancy, intrinsic redundancy**

reference electrode the relationship of one electrode to a second electrode; usually referred to as the common electrode

reference equivalent threshold force levels the vibratory force levels transmitted to the mechanical coupler when the vibrator is excited electrically at the level corresponding to the normal-hearing threshold

reference equivalent threshold sound pressure levels (RET-SPL) sound pressure levels produced in the acoustic coupler that correspond to the average normal threshold of hearing

reference microphone an electret microphone used in the comparison method of signal calibration in probe microphone measurement; acts as a standard against which the probe signal is compared

reference sound pressure level the amount of pressure against the eardrum that vibrates the eardrum and can be just detected by a normal hearing ear; (i.e., 0.0002 dyne/cm^2)

reference test gain (RTG) the acoustic gain of a hearing aid as measured in a hearing aid test box; the gain control of the aid is set to amplify a 60 dB SPL signal to a level 17 dB below the SSPL 90 value; the average values at 1000, 1600, and 2500 Hz determine reference test gain

reflected sound propagated sound after it has struck one or more objects or surfaces in a room

reflex a return flow of energy; an involuntary reflected action

reflex, acoustic (AR) response of the middle ear muscles (primarily the stapedius) and the ossicles to intense sound; also known as **acoustic stapedial reflex**

reflex, auropalpebral eye blink reflex associated with stimulation or startle from loud sounds

reflex, Babinski flexion of the foot and fanning of the toes in response to stimulation of the sole of the foot; normal reflex found in newborns and in children and adults having a lesion in the pyramidal tract

reflex, cochleopalpebral eye blink reflex associated with stimulation or startle from loud sounds

reflex, conditioned orientation (COR) a method for establishing auditory thresholds in young children; requires conditioning the child to make a response to a sound (e.g., head turn) that is reinforced

reflex, intra-aural contraction of the middle ear muscles (intra-aural muscles) in response to loud acoustic stimulation; the stapedius muscle provides the dominating response

reflex, light triangular-shaped light reflex seen when a light is shone down the external auditory canal toward the tympanic membrane with an otoscope; also known as **cone of light**

reflex, Moro response of infants (birth to 3 months of life) to acoustic stimuli characterized by extension and abduction of arms, hands, and fingers

reflex, stapedial a brainstem mediated reflex that causes the stapedial muscle in the middle ear to contract (via cranial nerve VII innervation) in response to a high-intensity stimulus

reflex, vestibulo-ocular (VOR) (1) a central vestibular-ocular pathway whose function is assessed during caloric electronystagmography; a response to angular acceleration (head turn); (2) when the head is turned to the right, there is excitation of the left lateral rectus and right medial rectus eye muscles so that the eyes are turned to the left

reflex decay reduction in the amplitude of the stapedial reflex in response to constant stimulation; 50% reduction in the first 5 seconds of the response suggests abnormal auditory adaptation; a component of the immittance battery that assesses the viability of cranial nerve VIII; a measure of auditory adaptation; also known as **stapedial reflex decay**; see also **auditory adaptation**

refraction a bending of the sound wave or a change in the direction of sound-wave propagation due to a change in the speed of propagation

refractory period the time following the excitation of a nerve or muscle fiber during which the fiber is either absolutely or relatively inexcitable; see also **absolute refractory period, relative refractory period**

Refsum syndrome autosomal recessive disorder characterized by retinitis pigmentosa, peripheral sensory and motor neuropathy, ichthyosis; associated with sensorineural hearing loss with onset in teen or early adult years, often beginning as asymmetric and progressing to severe in the high frequencies

rehabilitation instructional activities designed for the reteaching of particular skills (e.g., auditory, speech, language); see also **auditory rehabilitation (AR), habilitation**

REIG real-ear insertion gain; the value in decibels of the real-ear insertion response at a specific frequency; see also **real-ear insertion response (REIR)**

REIR real-ear insertion response; the difference in decibels as a function of frequency between the real-ear unaided response and the real-ear aided response measurements taken at the same measurement point in the same sound field; the amount of gain delivered to the patient wearing a hearing aid that he or she did not have before the hearing aid fitting; it is the electroacoustic equivalent of functional gain; see also **real-ear aided response (REAR), real-ear unaided response (REUR)**

Reissner's membrane membrane separating the scala media and the scala vestibuli; attached at one end to the inner part of the spiral limbus and at the other to the spiral ligament

relative refractory period the time following the excitation of a nerve or muscle fiber during which a new nerve discharge can occur only with increased stimulation; see also **absolute refractory period, refractory period**

relay system system used by persons with significant hearing loss to use the telephone; the individual contacts a relay operator who serves to transmit messages between the caller and the person called by means of text telephone or the use of voice

release from masking a measure of the improvement in the detectability of a signal that can occur under dichotic binaural listening conditions

release time (RT) the time required for nonlinear processing to reach the steady state value in a compression hearing aid; the time it takes for compression to be completely deactivated; see also **attack time (AT)**

reliability repeatability; reproducibility; the amount of agreement between multiple sequential averaged waveforms; high reliability implies confidence that the measurement has little error

remote control component of some programmable hearing aids (digitally controlled analog aids) that is used to program the electroacoustic characteristics of the aid as well as provide user controls such as volume control, directional microphones, and telecoil

remote masking downward spread of masking; situation in which low-frequency signals are masked by high-level high-frequency signals

renal disease pertaining to kidney dysfunction; can be associated with hearing loss

REOG real-ear occluded gain; the value in decibels of the real-ear occluded response at a specific frequency

REOR real-ear occluded response; the sound pressure level, as a function of frequency, at a specified measurement point in the ear canal for a specified sound field with the hearing aid in place and turned off; the loss of gain from occluding the ear; insertion loss

repair strategy tactic implemented by a participant in a conversation to rectify breakdowns in communication

repetition rate the rate chosen at which to present a stimulus; typically determined as the number of stimuli presented per second

reserve gain the residual gain in a hearing aid; the difference between the point at which feedback occurs and use gain; see also **headroom**

residential school state-supported schools for the deaf with dormitory accommodations; both academic learning and social enculturation of deaf children occurs in this environment

residual hearing hearing remaining after hearing loss from ear damage

residual inhibition the temporary reduction or elimination of tinnitus experienced by some patients after the masking signal has been discontinued; also known as the postmasking effect

resistance (R) a component of impedance that opposes or impedes the flow of energy by way of dissipation of that energy; see also **acoustic resistance**

resistor a device that introduces resistance into a circuit; controls the flow of energy that passes through the circuit

resonance the property of a mechanical or electrical system of oscil-

lating at a particular frequency with minimum dissipation of energy

resonant frequency the frequency at which a mass or a system vibrates with the least amount of external force (i.e., the natural frequency of vibration of a system); see also **natural resonant frequency**

resonator a device experiencing forced vibration; a device that increases sound energy through resonance

resource room a school room where students from regular classes go to receive tutoring or small group instruction; useful educational technique for children with hearing loss who are mainstreamed

respiration audiometry a technique used to predict hearing sensitivity by monitoring changes in respiration that occur in response to auditory stimuli

response (1) an observable behavior in behavioral audiometry that indicates that an individual heard a sound; (2) the output of a hearing aid as a function of frequency (i.e., frequency response)

response bias an individual's response criterion that influences his or her responses and test results

response time the amount of time it takes for an individual to respond to a stimulus

RESR real-ear saturation response; the sound pressure level as a function of frequency at a specified measurement point in the ear canal with the hearing aid in place and turned on; the measurement is made with the stimulus level sufficiently intense to operate the hearing aid at its maximum output level

resting potential (1) each cell in the body pumps ions across cell membranes to keep an electrical potential difference across the membrane: ions travel in and out of a cell through channels in the membrane; passive channels allow free movement; chemically gated channels are selective; (2) voltage potential differences that can be measured from the cochlea at rest; see also **endocochlear potential**

restoring force the force of gravity or elasticity that overcomes the force of inertia; the ability of an object to assume its original position once the force has been removed (i.e., the ability to return to the starting position); see also **elasticity**

reticular formation a complex, multisynaptic pathway in the central nervous system that is involved in consciousness and awakeness

reticular lamina a stiff membrane formed by a process of the supporting cells in which are incorporated the cuticular plates of the hair cells; the tectorial membrane within the scala media is superior to the reticular lamina

retinitis pigmentosa a group of diseases, usually genetic, marked by a progressive blindness due to retinal atrophy, attenuation of the retinal vessels, and contraction of the field

of vision; can be associated with hearing loss

retrocochlear the portion of the auditory system that is "behind or beyond the cochlea" (i.e., the auditory nerve or central auditory system); refers to dysfunction involving the auditory nerve

retrocochlear hearing loss a hearing loss in the portion of the auditory system that is "behind or beyond the cochlea" (i.e., cranial nerve VIII or central auditory system); refers to dysfunction involving cranial nerve VIII

retrocochlear lesion damage to the portion of the auditory system that is "behind or beyond the cochlea" (i.e., cranial nerve VIII or central auditory system); refers to dysfunction involving cranial nerve VIII

RETSPL reference equivalent threshold sound pressure level; sound pressure levels produced in the acoustic coupler that correspond to the average normal threshold of hearing

REUR real-ear unaided response; the sound pressure level as a function of frequency at a specified point in the unoccluded ear canal for a specified sound field; used as a reference value for calculation of insertion gain

reverberant sound sound that reaches a given location in a room only after being reflected from one or more barriers or partitions within a room

reverberant sound field an enclosed space with essentially no acoustic absorption in which the time average of the mean square sound pressure is the same everywhere and the flow of energy is equally probable in all directions; see also **sound field**

reverberation the persistence of sound in an enclosed space as a result of multiple reflections after the sound source has stopped; the amount of echo in a room; the more reverberant the room, the poorer the speech-to-noise ratio and the less intelligible the speech

reverberation chamber an enclosed space with essentially no acoustic absorption in which a reverberant sound field can be produced

reverberation measurement the careful use of a formula to measure the reverberation in a particular space such as a classroom (RT = .05 V/A where RT = reverberation time in seconds, V = volume of the room, and A = total absorption of the room surfaces)

reverberation time the time required for the mean-square sound pressure level of the sound to decrease 60 decibels after the source has stopped

Revised Hearing Performance Inventory (R-HPI) an assessment of self-perceived handicap imposed by hearing loss

Rh incompatibility the condition in which a baby may be born with jaundice if the baby's blood is Rh-positive and the mother's blood is Rh-negative; the blood of the fetus crosses the placenta and antibodies are formed which attack the fetus and poison its blood supply

rhinology branch of medicine specializing in the diagnosis and treatment of disorders involving the nose

rhombencephalon embryonic division of the brain from which the pons, cerebellum, and medulla oblongata ultimately arise

rhyme test a test of phonemic differentiation using rhyming monosyllabic words presented in a closed-set format

rhyming minimal contrasts a test designed to identify phoneme confusions in responses made for rhyming monosyllabic words presented in a closed-set format

rhythm timing and intensity information that aids in the comprehension of auditory signals; see also **prosody, suprasegmental**

RI rollover index; a decrease in performance (percent correct) scores for a speech audiometry procedure at a high stimulus intensity level versus maximum scores obtained at a lower intensity level

Richards-Rundle syndrome autosomal recessive disorder characterized by cognitive deficiency, ataxia, hypogonadism, nystagmus, deficiency of subcutaneous fat, joint contractures; when onset is early (in early childhood), sensorineural hearing loss progresses to severe; when late onset (teen years), progression is less severe

right ear advantage (REA) a cerebral dominance phenomenon in which normal right-handed listeners have scores for the right ear that are consistently higher than scores for the left ear for dichotically presented signals

right-beating nystagmus type of horizontal nystagmus in which the fast phase angles to the right

Rinne test a tuning fork test that compares a patient's hearing by air conduction with his and her hearing by bone conduction for a single frequency; see also **Weber test**

rise time the initial portion of a stimulus from its beginning at baseline to maximum or close-to-maximum amplitude; the amount of time it takes a gated signal to reach its maximum; see also **decay time**

rise-decay time the time it takes to initiate and terminate a signal's amplitude; also known as **rise-fall time**; see also **rise time, decay time**

rise-fall time the time it takes to initiate and terminate a signal's amplitude; also known as **rise-decay time**

risk criteria for infants/neonates a list of factors produced by the Joint Committee on Infant Hearing that place a child at risk for hearing loss; also known as **high-risk register (HRR)**

RMS root mean square; the long-term overall effective level of a signal; the square root of the mean of

the squared instantaneous values of a signal integrated over a time period long enough so that the result is not sensitive to small changes in the integration period

RMS amplitude a measure of amplitude that uses root mean square to calculate the long-term overall effective level of a signal; the square root of the mean of the squared instantaneous amplitude values of a signal integrated over a time period long enough so that the result is not sensitive to small changes in the integration period

Robinow syndrome autosomal dominant disorder characterized by frontal bossing, hypertelorism, wide palpebral fissures, short nose, macrocephaly, cleft palate and lip, progressive osteosclerosis of skull, shortening of the arms, brachydactyly, vertebral anomalies, skeletal anomalies, small penis, minor female genital anomalies; associated with conductive hearing loss in cases with clefts

ROC receiver operator characteristic; graphic summary of the performance of a detector; detection probability is plotted on the ordinate, and false alarm probability is plotted on the abscissa; also known as ROC curve

Rochester method an aural rehabilitation method that supplements oral communication with fingerspelling; see also **fingerspelling, manual alphabet**

rods of Corti two rows of stiff rodlike structures (inner and outer rods) supported by the basilar membrane; the heads of the rods are in contact with the reticular lamina and enclose the tunnel of Corti along with the basilar membrane; see also **outer pillars of Corti, pillars of Corti**

roll-off rate the rate at which the response of the system attenuates (rolls off) on either side of the center frequency; characteristic of a filter; expressed in dB per octave; see also **filter skirt**

rollover a decrease in performance (percent correct) scores for a speech audiometry procedure at a high stimulus intensity level versus maximum scores obtained at a lower intensity level

rollover index (RI) a test of retrocochlear dysfunction analyzing performance on high-intensity word identification tests compared to performance on lower-intensity word-identification tests; formula is (PB max − PB min)/PB max where PB max is the highest score obtained and PB min is the minimum score obtained; a rollover index of greater than 0.45 is indicative of a retrocochlear lesion; also known as **P-PB function**

Romberg test a test of vestibular assessment evaluating the maintenance of an erect stance while standing with the feet together and the head straight, first with eyes open and then with eyes closed; see also **Romberg's sign**

Romberg's sign an abnormal sway or falling during the Romberg test; see also **Romberg test**

root mean square (RMS) the long-term overall effective level of a signal; the square root of the mean of the squared instantaneous values of a signal integrated over a time period long enough so that the result is not sensitive to small changes in the integration period

Rosenthal's canal a channel that lies in the bony core of the cochlea that coils from the base to the apex in parallel with the cochlear spiral; the spiral ganglia lie in this canal

rostral (1) anatomical term referring to the head; (2) beak-shaped; toward the beak

rotary chair testing (RCT) a test of vestibular assessment that uses a computer-driven sinusoidal rotational chair that moves at different velocities and in different directions; electro-oculography recordings are made during rotary chair testing for the assessment of bilateral vestibular loss

rotary nystagmus type of nystagmus characterized by rotation of the eyes in a clockwise or counter-clockwise direction

round window an opening through the bone that separates the middle ear from the scala tympani of the cochlea; located behind and below the oval window and is closed by the round window membrane

round window electrode placement placement of cochlear implant electrodes outside the cochlea on the round window membrane

round window membrane thin membrane covering the round window; separates the fluid of the scala tympani from the air of the middle ear space

round window niche small indentation in the middle ear cavity (medial wall) that houses the round window

round window rupture a hole or tear in the round window that causes a perilymphatic leak

RT release time; the time required for nonlinear processing to reach the steady-state value in a compression hearing aid; the time it takes for compression to be completely deactivated; see also **attack time (AT)**

RTG reference test gain; the acoustic gain of a hearing aid as measured in a hearing aid test box; the gain control of the aid is set to amplify a 60 dB SPL signal to a level 17 dB below the SSPL90 value; the average values at 1000, 1600, and 2500 Hz determine reference test gain

rubella the German measles virus; viral infection that can cause multiple developmental anomalies of the fetus if contracted during the first trimester of pregnancy; can result in central nervous system damage, hearing loss, cardiac problems; associated with a cookie bite audiogram configuration resulting from degeneration of the membranous labyrinth

Runge test when the external ear is filled with water, low-frequency bone-conducted sound is normally lateralized to that side; no lateralization is a sign of a conductive hearing disorder

Rupp Feasibility Scale for Predicting Hearing Aid Use a prediction of the ability to use amplification successfully based on factors such as motivation, initial impression, age, self-assessment, manual dexterity, functional gain for speech, etc.

Rush-Hughes recordings distorted recordings of the PB-50 word lists used to assess speech perception

Rx prescription

S

S/N signal-to-noise ratio; relationship between the sound levels of the signal and the noise at the listener's ear; commonly reported as the difference in decibels between the intensity of the signal and the intensity of the background noise (e.g., if the speech signal is measured at 70 dB and the noise is 64 dB, the signal-to-noise ratio is +6 dB)

SAC Self Assessment of Communication; inventory that provides an estimate of the frequency with which a particular communication difficulty is experienced

saccade rapid, accurate change in the direction of eye movement by ocular muscles in following a target; the saccade test is one of the ocular-motor subtests of the electronystagmography test battery used to assess accuracy of eye movement and to calibrate the system

saccular macula vestibular sensory epithelia on the anterior wall of the saccule

saccular nerve portion of the vestibular branch of cranial nerve VIII that innervates the hair cells of the saccular macula

saccule the smaller of the vestibular sensory mechanisms housed within the vestibule of the inner ear; contains sensory epithelia called macula and is responsible for providing information about the static system of balance; see also **utricle**

sacculotomy surgical procedure used to treat a dilated saccule as a result of Ménière's disease; a needle is placed through the stapes footplate to perforate the saccule inside the membranous labyrinth

SADL Satisfaction with Amplification in Daily Life; self-assessment scale used with hearing aid wearers that determines their opinions about their hearing aids

saggital plane the midline division of the body that divides it into right and left halves

SAI Social Adequacy Index; a measure of the degree of hearing handicap that takes into account speech audiometry findings

SAL sensory acuity level; an audiometric procedure for assessing bone-conduction hearing in patients with serious conductive hearing loss; air-conduction thresholds are determined without masking and then with masking presented by bone conduction to the forehead; the size of the masked shift in hearing thresholds corresponds to the degree of the conductive hearing loss component

salicylates group of drugs used in the treatment of arthritis, rheumatic fever, and connective tissue disorders; including aspirin; can be ototoxic if taken in high doses

salicylic acid a component of aspirin used to temporarily deaden cochlear outer hair cells; results in a reversible mild to moderate sensorineural hearing loss

sampling the process of making a series of measurements from a continuous (analog) signal

sampling rate the rate at which a signal or process is sampled; in digital processing of speech, the sampling rate specifies the intervals at which the analog waveform is converted to digital form

SAT speech awareness threshold; the lowest intensity level at which a person can detect the presence of a speech signal; it approximates the best hearing level in the 250 to 8000 Hz audiometric frequency region; used clinically with children or others who have such poor speech understanding that a speech recognition threshold (SRT) cannot be obtained; also known as **speech detection threshold (SDT)**; see also **speech reception threshold (SRT)**

Satisfaction with Amplification in Daily Life (SADL) self-assessment scale used with hearing aid wearers

that determines their opinions about their hearing aids

saturation (1) when a neural unit, such as an auditory nerve fiber, reaches maximum firing rate; (2) may also be seen as a decrease in the output at high-stimulus inputs for hearing aids

saturation sound pressure level (SSPL) a hearing aid's maximum output expressed as a frequency response curve; the highest output produced by a hearing aid regardless of the level of input; see also **output sound pressure level (OSPL), maximum power output (MPO)**

saturation sound pressure level 90 (SSPL90) electroacoustic assessment of a hearing aid's maximum level of output signal expressed as a frequency response curve to a 90-dB signal with the hearing aid volume control set to full-on; see also **output sound pressure level (OSPL), maximum power output (MPO)**

SAV select-a-vent; venting option available in in-the-ear hearing instruments and earmolds providing the ability to alter the size of a vent; see also **vent, venting**

sawtooth noise a type of noise sometimes used in hearing science but now generally irrelevant for audiologists; made up of a fundamental frequency of 120 Hz with equal amplitude at all the harmonic frequencies

SBMPL simultaneous binaural median plane localization; outdated behavioral site-of-lesion test that requires the patient to adjust the intensity of identical tones delivered simultaneously to both ears until there is the sensation of a fused tone in the cranial midline; patient must have normal pure-tone configurations in both ears; if the patient cannot perceive the fused experience, or if the fused experience is perceived only with considerable interaural intensity differences, it is probably the result of some brainstem dysfunction

scala/scalae each of three cavities in the cochlea that coil around the modiolus: **scala media, scala tympani, scala vestibuli**

scala media the middle duct or passageway in the cochlea that is bordered on the outer (lateral wall) by the stria vascularis, medially by the spiral limbus, and inferiorly by the basilar membrane and organ of Corti; separated from the scala vestibuli by Reissner's membrane; filled with endolymph and has a closed end at the helicotrema; see also **scala tympani, scala vestibuli**

scala tympani the perilymph-filled passage of the cochlear canal that extends from the round window at the base to the helicotrema at the apex; it is separated from the scala media by the basilar membrane and the cellular structures attached to it; see also **scala media, scala vestibuli**

scala vestibuli the perilymph-filled passage of the cochlear canal that extends from the oval window at the base to the helicotrema at the

apex; it is separated from the scala media by Reissner's membrane; see also **scala media, scala tympani**

SCAN a screening test for central auditory processing disorders in children consisting of three subtests (filtered words, competing words, and auditory figure-ground); see also **SCAN-A**

SCAN-A a screening test for central auditory processing disorders in adolescents and adults consisting of four subtests (filtered words, competing words, auditory figure-ground, and competing sentences); see also **SCAN**

scaphoid fossa the region between the helix and the antihelix of the auricle

Scarpa's ganglion vestibular ganglion located medial to the vestibular end organ within the internal auditory canal of the petrous portion of the temporal bone

Scarpa's membrane round window membrane

SCCs semicircular canals; three canals of the vestibular system (lateral, superior, and posterior) responsible for sensation of movement (angular motion) of the head in space; the membranous semicircular canals are housed within the bony semicircular canals; also known as **semicircular ducts**

Scheibe dysplasia most common aplasia of the inner ear involving only the membranous labyrinth; patients may show a normal radiologic result with profound and total deafness; see also **Michel dysplasia, Mondini dysplasia**

Schwabach test a tuning fork test that compares a patient's hearing by bone conduction with the hearing of a presumably normal-hearing examiner

Schwann cell cell that produces the myelin sheath surrounding the axon of neurons in the peripheral nervous system

schwannoma encapsulated neoplasm arising from Schwann cells of the vestibular portion of cranial nerve VIII; also known as **vestibular schwannoma**

Schwartze's sign a pinkish blush detected by otoscopy through the tympanic membrane in some patients with early stages of otosclerosis that reflects vascularity or hyperemia (collection of blood) at the promontory; usually seen when there is active bone growth in the middle ear

scientific notation a system of denoting numbers as the product of some simple number and the base of 10 raised to some power (e.g., $2000 = 2 \times 10^3$)

SCIPS Screening Inventory of Perceptual Skills; battery of tests that assess the discrimination abilities of children having profound hearing impairments using single-word stimuli

sclerectomy the surgical removal of adhesions that form on middle ear

structures as a result of chronic or adhesive otitis media; see also **adhesive otitis media, chronic otitis media**

sclerosis a condition often caused by inflammation that results in hardening of body tissues

sclerosteosis autosomal recessive disorder characterized by progressive osteosclerosis with excessive bony overgrowth of craniofacial structures, clavicles, and pelvis; prognathism; associated with sensory hearing loss secondary to bony overgrowth of cranial foramina and damage to the auditory nerve

screening the use of tests that are quick and easy to administer to a large group for the purpose of identifying individuals who require further diagnostic testing

screening audiometer an electronic instrument that delivers calibrated pure-tone stimuli through air conduction only for the purpose of performing pure-tone air-conduction screenings; has limited capabilities for performing extensive clinical assessments of hearing sensitivity

Screening Instrument for Targeting Educational Risk (SIFTER) a checklist used by teachers to assess the educational effects of hearing loss on preschool and school-aged children

Screening Inventory of Perceptual Skills (SCIPS) battery of tests that assess the discrimination abilities of children having profound hearing impairments using single-word stimuli

Screening Test for Auditory Perception evaluation procedure focusing on auditory perception abilities and auditory memory and sequencing abilities

screw-set method used to adjust the gain of a hearing aid when the volume control wheel is not present

SDS speech discrimination score; percent correct score reflecting the number of word stimuli perceived correctly in speech perception testing; also known as **word-identification score (WIS)** and **word-recognition score (WRS)**

SDT speech detection threshold; the lowest intensity level at which a person can detect the presence of a speech signal; it approximates the best hearing level in the 250 to 8000 Hz audiometric frequency region; used clinically with children or others who have such poor speech understanding that a speech recognition threshold (SRT) cannot be obtained; also known as **speech awareness threshold (SAT)**; see also **speech reception threshold (SRT)**

sebaceous glands glands found in the lateral one third of the external auditory canal; secrete cerumen along with the ceruminous and apocrine glands

secretion (1) the release of a substance; (2) the release of a chemical substance produced by glandular organs

secretory otitis media inflammation of the middle ear with effusion that is sterile, pale yellow transudate of low viscosity; usually follows short-term illness (e.g., serous or mucoid otitis media); see also **serous otitis media (SOM)**

SEE1 Seeing Essential English; a manual communication system that incorporates some signs of American Sign Language and some English syntax; see also **Signing Exact English (SEE2)**

SEE2 Signing Exact English; a simplified version of Seeing Essential English; a manual communication system

Seeing Essential English (SEE1) a manual communication system that incorporates some signs of American Sign Language and some English syntax; see also **Signing Exact English (SEE2)**

segmental individual segment in spoken language; can be sentences, words, or syllables with their constituent phonetic units; see also **suprasegmental**

Seitelberger syndrome autosomal recessive disorder characterized by neuroaxonal degeneration, dementia, spastic quadriplegia, optic atrophy; associated with late onset sensorineural hearing loss

seizure fierce, involuntary muscle contractions caused by hyperexcitation of neurons in the brain

select-a-vent (SAV) venting option available in in-the-ear hearing instruments and earmolds providing the ability to alter the size of a vent; see also **vent, venting**

selective attention the observer is asked to attend specifically to a given condition and make a response; it may be a motor response (e.g., button press) or some mental counting task of the target stimulus; see also **selective listening**

selective listening (1) ability to attend to the primary message in one ear while relegating the background noise to the opposite ear and suppressing it; (2) how many spouses describe the listening of their mates; see also **selective attention**

Self Assessment of Communication (SAC) inventory that provides an estimate of the frequency with which a particular communication difficulty is experienced

self-contained FM receiver an FM receiver and a hearing aid contained in one wearable console

Self-Help for Hard-of-Hearing People (SHHH) non-profit self-help support organization for adults who have hearing loss and their relatives and friends; established in 1979

semantic(s) related to the meaning of words or groups of words in a language system

semi-aural device type of hearing protection consisting of flexible tips attached to a lightweight headband that provides a compromise between earmuffs and earplugs; see also **hearing protection device (HPD)**

semicanal of the tensor tympani location in the anterior wall of the

middle ear that houses the body of the tensor tympani muscle; see also **tensor tympani**

semicircular canal, horizontal the more horizontally placed semicircular canal, sensing movement in the transverse plane of the body; part of the vestibular labyrinth; also known as **lateral semicircular canal**

semicircular canal, lateral the more horizontally placed semicircular canal, sensing movement in the transverse plane of the body; part of the vestibular labyrinth; also known as **horizontal semicircular canal**

semicircular canal, posterior one of the three canals of the vestibular system that contains the sense organs (crista ampularis) for responding to angular motion; also know as the vertical-inferior canal

semicircular canal, superior the uppermost of the three canals of the vestibular system that contains the sense organs (crista ampularis) for responding to angular motion; also known as the **vertical semicircular canal**

semicircular canals (SCCs) three canals of the vestibular system (lateral, superior, and posterior) responsible for sensation of movement (angular motion) of the head in space; the membranous semicircular canals are housed within the bony semicircular canals; also known as **semicircular ducts**

semicircular ducts three canals or ducts of the vestibular system (lateral, superior, and posterior) responsible for sensation of movement (angular motion) of the head in space; the membranous semicircular canals are housed within the bony semicircular canals; also known as **semicircular canals (SCCs)**

Seminars in Hearing journal published quarterly by Thieme, each of which contains contributions about a particular issue related to hearing health care

sensation level (SL) the intensity of a sound above or below an individual's threshold; used as a reference point for presentation levels of speech perception testing

sensitivity (1) an amplifier setting that is defined by the positive and negative voltage limits for incoming electrical activity; greater sensitivity means more stringent voltage limits; expressed in terms of microvolts; (2) an individual's acuity or tolerance to sounds; (3) the ability of a test to identify individuals showing a particular abnormality

sensitivity control the dial on top of a cochlear implant speech processor that sets the responsiveness of the microphone to the sound source; with a low sensitivity setting, the sound source must be very close to the microphone; with a high sensitivity setting, the sound source can be further from the microphone

sensitivity prediction of the acoustic reflex (SPAR) a hearing loss prediction technique based on the normal difference expected in acoustic reflex thresholds for noise versus pure-tone signals

sensitization the enhanced perception to a sensory stimulus due to the presence of a preceding similar stimulus

sensorineural (SN) pertaining to the structures of the cochlea and the adjacent parts of the auditory nerve

sensorineural hearing loss (SNHL) type of hearing loss stemming from a lesion in the cochlea and in adjacent parts of the auditory nerve

sensory (1) the portion of a sensorineural hearing loss having to do with inner ear hair cell damage; (2) refers to afferent information coming from the extremities of the body to the central nervous system

sensory acuity level (SAL) an audiometric procedure for assessing bone-conduction hearing in patients with serious conductive hearing loss; air-conduction thresholds are determined without masking and then with masking presented by bone conduction to the forehead; the size of the masked shift in hearing thresholds corresponds to the degree of the conductive hearing loss component

sensory deprivation lack of sensory input caused by a hearing impairment that can cause delayed and/or deviant behaviors

sensory epithelia in the ear, the sense organs responsible for the process of hearing and balance; includes the cristae ampularis, saccular and utricular macula, and the sensory cells of the organ of Corti (e.g., inner and outer hair cells)

sensory gating the phenomenon whereby, given a paired stimulus, the second stimulus in the pair will produce a response of a smaller amplitude

sensory input input consisting of different sensory modalities (e.g., auditory, visual, tactile) that is provided to a listener

sensory organization test (SOT) a platform posturography procedure for assessment of balance (i.e., the integration of vestibular, visual, and somatosensory information); see also **posturography**

sensory presbycusis type of hearing loss due to aging resulting from a loss of sensory and supporting cells mostly at the base of the cochlea; see also **presbycusis**

sentence tests speech perception tests that allow an individual's performance in everyday listening situations to be measured because they are most similar to realistic listening situations

Senter syndrome autosomal recessive disorder characterized by growth deficiency, ichthyosis, dystrophic nails, anomalous teeth, corneal anomalies; associated with sensorineural hearing loss of varying severity

SEP somatosensory evoked potential; an evoked potential created by stimulation of the somatosensory system usually by electrical stimulation over a peripheral nerve or the spinal cord;

cortical and subcortical response to repetitive stimulation of sensory fibers of the peripheral nerves that are averaged by a computer

septum a divider, partition, or wall

sequence multiple anomalies resulting from a single defect or mechanical event; term for a constellation of developmental/health anomalies in which each is derived sequentially from another anomaly or structural disorder; a single malformation, deformation, or disruption can secondarily cause other anomalies

serial audiogram an audiogram that is part of a series; used in regular monitoring of hearing sensitivity as part of a hearing conservation program

serous a thin, watery fluid passed through a membrane that is uninfected; see also **serous otitis media, transudate**

serous otitis media (SOM) middle ear inflammation with effusion (uninfected fluid); see also **secretory otitis media (SOM)**

SERT Sound Effects Recognition Test; an auditory test for nonverbal children utilizing familiar environmental sounds

severe hearing loss hearing loss ranging between 71 and 90 dB HL

severe-to-profound hearing loss hearing loss ranging between 71 and 90 dB HL to poorer than 90 dB HL

sex-linked inheritance inherited form of genes located on the X chromosome; X-linked traits pass on only from mother to son; also known as **X-linked inheritance**

SF sound field; a space where sound is propagated; usually refers to audiometric testing conducted in a sound-treated suite through loudspeakers

SFOAE stimulus frequency otoacoustic emission; evoked otoacoustic emission generated in response to an ongoing pure-tone signal; not used clinically because the responses are difficult to interpret because they appear as ripples in the recording

SHA slow harmonic acceleration; a rotatory vestibular assessment technique utilizing a computer controlled rotary chair; see also **rotary chair testing**

shadow curve audiogram obtained without contralateral masking, usually in a patient with a "dead ear," that reflects the responses to sounds that have crossed over from the test ear to the nontest ear; see also **interaural attenuation (IA), masking**

shearing action the "bending" action of the hair cells arising from the relative movement of the basilar membrane and the tectorial membrane during auditory stimulation; causes excitation of the hair cells and their corresponding auditory nerve fibers

shell earmold type of earmold that completely fills the concha; can be made of silicone or lucite; see also **earmold**

SHHH Self-Help for Hard-of-Hearing People; non-profit self-help support organization for adults who have hearing loss and their relatives and friends; established in 1979

shielding material that protects a signal-carrying conductor of a cable from electrostatic or electromagnetic noise

SHM simple harmonic motion; a periodic motion whose displacement varies as a sinusoidal function of time

short increment sensitivity index (SISI) a clinical procedure based on a patient's ability to detect small changes (1 dB) in intensity of a pure tone presented at 20 dB SL; high SISI scores for low-intensity pure-tone stimuli are characteristic of cochlear (sensory) hearing impairment; at high stimulus intensity levels, normal hearers also yield high SISI scores; see also **high-level short increment sensitivity index, low-level short increment sensitivity index**

Short Isophonemic Word Lists speech perception test consisting of 15 different lists each with the same 30 phonemes arranged to form 10 CVC words; designed to solve some of the problems inherent in tests that measure speech understanding

short latency response (SLR) a term used to refer to early evoked potentials that occur within the first 12 to 15 ms following the stimulus onset (e.g., electrocochleography and auditory brainstem response)

short process (1) a slight extension from a bony structure; (2) portion of the incus extending medially from its body that is responsible for the rocking motion of the ossicular chain

short-term memory temporary storage of information capable of holding about seven units of information

Shrapnell's membrane superior anterior thin portion of the tympanic membrane (near the epitympanum); also known as **pars flaccida**; does not contain the fibrous layer making it more slack than the pars tensa portion; see also **pars flaccida**

sibilant consonants consonants produced by air flowing through a very narrow passageway between the top of the front part of the tongue, the hard palate, and the upper teeth (e.g., /s, z, ʃ, ʒ, tʃ, and dʒ/)

sideband one of the frequency bands on either side of a carrier frequency of a modulated radio wave

side-branching vent type of vent that runs up to the sound bore and branches into it (i.e., intersects the sound bore); results in a decrease in high-frequency gain of as much as 10 dB more than a parallel vent; the effect increases as vent diameter increases; also known as **diagonal vent**

SIFTER Screening Instrument for Targeting Educational Risk; a checklist used by teachers to assess the educational effects of hearing loss on preschool and school-aged children

sign language a system of hand, arm, and body positions and movements that are arbitrarily given meaning as words and thoughts, as in Signed English or American Sign Language; see also **Signed English, American Sign Language (ASL)**

signal (1) a term used interchangeably with stimulus indicating that it can be light, sound, or tactile energy; (2) an event that is being measured (i.e., evoked response) in contrast to extraneous activity (i.e., background electrical noise)

signal averaging a technique of averaging successive samples of encephalographic activity time-locked to a stimulus in order to reduce unrelated signals and thus enhance the measurement of the desired response by improving the signal-to-noise ratio

signal coding term used to describe different signal processing strategies used in cochlear implants

signal detection a process for determining the presence of an event (a signal) that usually is embedded within background activity (noise); it is a function of the size of the signal and the size of the noise

signal duration perceptual correlate of signal length; time

signal generator means by which a signal is created and presented

signal length the duration of a signal is determined by a physical measurement of the span of time occupied by the signal

signal processing manipulation of various parameters of a signal

signal processor a device or circuit that provides nonlinear modification of an audio signal; used in cochlear implants

signal-to-noise ratio (S/N, SNR) relationship between the sound levels of the signal and the noise at the listener's ear; commonly reported as the difference in decibels between the intensity of the signal and the intensity of the background noise (e.g., if the speech signal is measured at 70 dB and the noise is 64 dB, the signal-to-noise ratio is +6 dB)

Signed English manual communication system that utilizes English word order and syntax; the refinement, modification, and sequencing of American Sign Language to conform closely to the detail and syntax of the English spoken language; a sign system; see **Seeing Essential English (SEE1), Signing Exact English (SEE2)**

Significant Others Assessment of Communication (SOAC) a self-assessment inventory completed by the significant others of a patient who is hearing impaired to estimate the frequency with which a particular communication difficulty is experienced

Signing Exact English (SEE2) a simplified version of Seeing Essential English; a manual communication system; see also **Seeing Essential English (SEE1)**

SII speech intelligibility index; (1) the distribution of speech energy at normal conversational levels superimposed on an audiogram to provide a graphic representation of loudness as a function of frequency for conversational speech; (2) a number between 0 and 1 that expresses the degree of audibility of a speech signal that is highly correlated with traditional speech intelligibility scores (number of speech items repeated correctly); also known as **articulation index (AI)**

SIL speech interference level; the adverse effects of noise on the intelligibility of speech communication; used originally with the articulation index when evaluating communication systems

silhouette inductor a thin plate containing a coil that is worn between a behind-the-ear hearing aid and the head and transmits electromagnetic energy; a coupling option for assistive listening devices

simple harmonic motion (SHM) a periodic motion whose displacement varies as a sinusoidal function of time

simplex procedure an adaptive procedure designed to estimate the electroacoustic settings on more than one dimension of a hearing aid to maximize speech recognition scores

simultaneous binaural bithermal caloric test variation of the open-loop caloric irrigation as part of the electronystagmography test battery; both ears are irrigated simultaneously using cool water and then warm water

simultaneous binaural median plane localization (SBMPL) outdated behavioral site-of-lesion test that requires the patient to adjust the intensity of identical tones delivered simultaneously to both ears until there is the sensation of a fused tone in the cranial midline; patient must have normal pure-tone configurations in both ears; if the patient cannot perceive the fused experience, or if the fused experience is perceived only with considerable interaural intensity differences, it is probably the result of some brainstem dysfunction

simultaneous communication educational approach used with individuals with severe and profound hearing loss that integrates aural/oral communication and manual communication; also known as **total communication (TC)**

SIN speech in noise test; a speech perception test used to test a patient's ability to listen in noise in the sound field; often used for comparison with understanding speech in quiet

sine wave a waveform whose pressure variation as a function of time is a sine function; this is the function relating the sine of an angle to the size of the angle; also known as a **sinusoid**

sine wave generator an apparatus that generates pure tones at various frequencies

single-channel cochlear implant early type of cochlear implant that used an active ball electrode placed either at the round window or in the first turn of the scala tympani; a second ground electrode completed the path and was placed in the middle ear or muscle tissue; the coding strategy was limited to the single active electrode and its ground and relied mainly on rate-pitch discrimination

sintered filters materials placed in the tone-hook and/or tubing of a hearing instrument to control its maximum output; can provide an effective form of quasi-compression limiting

sinusoid a waveform whose pressure variation as a function of time is a sine function; this is the function relating the sine of an angle to the size of the angle; also known as **sine wave**

sinusoidal motion the representation of a sine wave called a waveform that is projected uniform circular motion

sinusoidal rotary chair test vestibular assessment tool for possible bilateral vestibular loss using electro-oculography techniques; performed in a dark room; nystagmus results in normal vestibular function; see also **rotary chair testing**

SIR speech intelligibility rating; a tool that documents the intelligibility of emerging speech and voice skills

SISI short increment sensitivity index; a clinical procedure based on a patient's ability to detect small changes (1 dB) in intensity of a pure tone presented at 20 dB SL; high SISI scores for low-intensity pure-tone stimuli are characteristic of cochlear (sensory) hearing impairment; at high stimulus intensity levels, normal hearers also yield high SISI scores; see also **high-level short increment sensitivity index, low-level short increment sensitivity index**

site of lesion (SOL) the location in the auditory system where disease or damage causing hearing impairment occurs; see also **site of lesion test battery**

site of lesion test battery battery of behavioral and physiologic tests designed to determine the location of pathology causing a particular auditory or hearing disorder; battery used to determine if the site of lesion is cochlear or retrocochlear; interpretation is based on the results from several tests, not just one or two

6-cc coupler a device for acoustic loading of earphones during calibration of audio equipment; designed to represent the volume of the human pinna and ear canal; measures the sound pressure level of the stimulus at the earphone under test; device meeting ANSI S3.6-1989 specifications for coupling an earphone to a sound level meter for audiometer calibration

60-cycle noise 60-Hz hum; electrical noise generated from the 60-Hz energy produced by appliances and lights; can interfere with recording electrical potentials; also referred to as 60-cycle hum

skeleton earmold type of earmold that fits around the outer portion of the concha but does not completely fill it; see also **earmold**

SKI*HI Language Development Scale a language test for children who are hearing impaired aged birth to 5 years

ski-slope audiogram an audiogram configuration characterized by progressively increasing high-frequency hearing loss that appears to "drop off" at or after some mid-frequency

skirt as in filter skirt; reflecting the degree to which a filter rolls off into adjoining frequencies above or below certain cut-off frequencies; usually measured in dB per octave roll-off

SL sensation level; the intensity of a sound above or below an individual's threshold; used as a reference point for presentation levels for audiometric and speech perception testing

slapback a discrete reflection of sound from a nearby surface

SLM sound level meter; an electronic instrument for measuring the rms level of sound in accordance with an accepted national or international standard

sloping a term used to describe the configuration of a pure-tone audiogram showing a progressively greater hearing loss for higher test frequencies

slow harmonic acceleration (SHA) a rotatory vestibular assessment technique utilizing a computer controlled rotary chair; see also **rotary chair testing**

slow negative response a relatively large, gradual negative voltage wave occurring in the 10-ms region in an auditory brainstem response recording; an analysis period of about 13 ms or more and a high-pass frequency filter setting of less than about 100 Hz is required to record this component; it is believed that the inferior colliculus is the generator site for this potential

slow phase the slower component of nystagmus induced by vestibular disease or caloric stimulation

slow phase velocity (SPV) the slower component of nystagmus induced by vestibular disease or caloric stimulation

slow potential refers to long latency or late auditory evoked potentials

slow pursuit component of the electronystagmography test battery that assesses the ability of the smooth pursuit eye movement system; its purpose is to match the angular velocity of the eye with a slowly moving object; the object moves sinusoidally and the patient is to track the object visually in the horizontal

and vertical plane; also known as **pendular tracking, smooth pursuit**

slow vertex response response that occurs between 50 and 250 ms after a sound is delivered to the ear for cortical evoked response audiometry

SLP speech-language pathologist; a professional who studies, diagnoses, and treats speech and language disorders

SLR short latency response; a term used to refer to early evoked potentials that occur within the first 12 to 15 ms following the stimulus onset (e.g., electrocochleography and auditory brainstem response)

Sly syndrome autosomal recessive disorder characterized by mucopolysaccharidosis VII with short stature, enlarged liver and spleen, facial coarseness, macrencephaly, skeletal and spine anomalies, inguinal hernia, mild cognitive deficiency with onset at approximately 2 years of age, all in childhood onset form, in congenital form there is early death; associated with conductive hearing loss secondary to chronic middle ear disease

smooth pursuit component of the electronystagmography test battery that assesses the ability of the smooth pursuit eye movement system; its purpose is to match the angular velocity of the eye with a slowly moving object; the object moves sinusoidally and the patient is to track the object visually in the horizontal and vertical plane; also known as **pendular tracking, slow pursuit**

SMSP spectral maxima speech processor; cochlear implant signal-processing strategy that uses amplitudes in each of its 16 bands ranging from 200 to 5400 Hz and uses rectifiers and low-pass filters; the best information found in the 16 bands is used as the output

SN sensorineural; pertaining to the structures of the cochlea and the adjacent parts of the auditory nerve

SNHL sensorineural hearing loss; type of hearing loss stemming from a lesion in the cochlea and in adjacent parts of the auditory nerve

SNR signal-to-noise ratio; relationship between the sound levels of the signal and the noise at the listener's ear; commonly reported as the difference in decibels between the intensity of the signal and the intensity of the background noise (e.g., if the speech signal is measured at 70 dB and the noise is 64 dB, the signal-to-noise ratio is +6 dB)

SN_{10} response slow negative auditory evoked response occurring approximately 10 ms after signal onset, usually acquired using low- frequency tone-burst stimuli

SOAC Significant Others Assessment of Communication; a self-assessment inventory completed by the significant others of a patient who is hearing impaired to estimate the frequency with which a particular communication difficulty is experienced

SOAE spontaneous otoacoustic emission; an otoacoustic emission recorded in some normal ears without acoustic stimulation; see also **otoacoustic emission (OAE)**

SOC superior olivary complex; a major collection of nuclei in the lower portion of the brainstem in the central auditory system; the first place where there is a neural interaction to stimulation of each ear (binaural stimulation)

Social Adequacy Index (SAI) a measure of the degree of hearing handicap that takes into account speech audiometry findings

Social Hearing Handicap Index self-assessment inventory designed to allow patients to rate psychological, social, vocational, and emotional handicaps imposed by their hearing loss

sociocusis hearing loss that occurs as a result of the process of aging and exposure to noise and environmental factors

sodium-potassium pump refers to an active neurological mechanism that occurs when a cell is stimulated; sodium (Na^+) ions are pumped out of the cell and potassium (K^+) ions that have left the cell are allowed to re-enter the cell

soft peak clipping form of output limiting used in linear hearing aids; the peaks of the waveform are removed in a gradual manner when the amplifier is saturated; results in a reduction of signal distortion compared to traditional peak clipping

SOL site of lesion; the location in the auditory system where disease or damage causing hearing impairment occurs; see also **site of lesion test battery**

solitary tract nucleus one of the cranial sensory nuclei of the brainstem that receives sensory input from the oral, pharyngeal, and laryngeal regions; some of the sensory input is involved with taste; interneurons within discrete subdivisions of the nucleus serve multiple functions including controlling blood pressure, respiratory regularity, swallowing, and taste

SOM serous otitis media; middle ear inflammation with effusion (uninfected fluid); see also **secretory otitis media (SOM)**

somatosensory evoked potential (SEP) an evoked potential created by stimulation of the somatosensory system usually by electrical stimulation over a peripheral nerve or the spinal cord; cortical and subcortical response to repetitive stimulation of sensory fibers of the peripheral nerves that are averaged by a computer

sone a linear unit of loudness; the ratio of the loudness of a sound to that of a 1000-Hz tone 40 dB above the threshold of hearing; a measure used to quantify the magnitude of the perception of loudness; e.g., a doubling in the perception of loudness is quantified as a doubling in the number of sones

SOT sensory organization test; a platform posturography procedure for assessment of balance (i.e., the integration of vestibular, visual, and somatosensory information); see also **posturography**

sound energy that is transmitted by pressure waves in air or other materials and is the objective cause of the sensation of hearing; commonly called noise if unwanted

sound absorption the attenuation of sound by porous materials in a sound field

sound absorption coefficient a number between 0 and 1 that expresses the sound-absorbing efficiency of a surface material at a specific frequency

sound bore the portion of the earmold through which amplified sound is directed into the external auditory canal; modifications to the shape and length of this hole can affect the acoustic nature of the sounds going through the sound bore

sound discrimination the ability to distinguish sounds in the environment including timing and intensity cues that make up the syllabic and prosodic patterns of speech

Sound Effects Recognition Test (SERT) an auditory test for nonverbal children utilizing familiar environmental sounds

sound field (SF) a space where sound is propagated; usually refers to audiometric testing conducted in a sound-treated suite through loudspeakers

sound field amplification system electronic equipment that amplifies an entire (class)room through the careful positioning of two to four loudspeakers; the teacher wears an FM microphone/transmitter

sound field equalization method used to create a balanced frequency response in a sound field

sound field testing calibrated auditory signals are presented through loudspeakers into a sound-isolated room rather than through headphones to test hearing; represented by the symbol "S" on an audiogram; often used when testing children who will not tolerate headphones and in evaluating hearing performance

sound level the level of sound measured with a sound level meter and one of its weighting networks

sound level meter (SLM) an electronic instrument for measuring the RMS level of sound in accordance with an accepted national or international standard

sound pressure level (SPL) an absolute value measured in dB representing the physical intensity of a sound; 20 times the log of the pressure output over the pressure reference (0.0002 dyne/cm^2 or 20 micropascals)

sound pressure level, peak equivalent (peSPL) a measure of sound intensity in which the maximum voltage of a transient stimulus (e.g., a click) is equated on an oscilloscope with the voltage of a tone stimulus

of known intensity level in dB sound pressure level (SPL); click intensity level is defined in terms of dB peSPL

sound pressure level, reference equivalent threshold (RETSPL) sound pressure level produced in the acoustic coupler that corresponds to the average normal threshold of hearing

sound pressure level, saturation (SSPL) a hearing aid's maximum output expressed as a frequency response curve; the highest output produced by a hearing aid regardless of the level of input; see also **output sound pressure level (OSPL), maximum power output (MPO)**

sound proof impenetrable by acoustic energy

sound quality the perceptual characteristics of a sound

sound reflection condition of sound propagation that is produced in addition to direct waves when the sound waves bounce off of objects lying in their path; results in reverberation and an increase in sound level

sound shadow a region in which a sound field is reduced in magnitude relative to the free-field value as a result of its incidence on an obstacle

sound source a body with mass and elasticity that produces sound waves

sound spectrum the distribution in frequency of the magnitudes of the components of sound waves; represented by plotting power, amplitude, or level as a function of frequency

sound transmission class a single number rating of transmission loss performance for a construction element tested over a standard frequency range

sound transmission loss logarithmic ratio of the sound intensity in decibels on one side of a partition to the sound intensity in decibels on the other side

sound treated room an acoustically treated room where hearing tests should be performed to obtain accurate results

sound velocity the rate which sound travels in a definite direction

sound wave the acoustical manifestation of physical disturbance in a medium

sound wave propagation movement of sound waves through an elastic medium

SP summating potential; a sustained direct current shift in the endocochlear potential that occurs when the organ of Corti is stimulated by sound; a direct-current electrical potential of cochlear origin that can be measured using **electrocochleography (ECochG)**

SP/AP summating potential/action potential ratio; ratio of the amplitudes of the summating potential and the action potential in electrocochleography measurement; used as a potential diagnostic indicator for Ménière's disease

SPAC Speech Pattern Contrast test; battery of tests designed to provide analytic data on speech perception at the sensory/phonetic level through a mostly closed-set format with one open-set task of word recognition

space of Nuel space between the outer rods of Corti and the outer hairs cells in the organ of Corti

space-occupying lesion pathologic condition that exists in a space as opposed to within a mass (e.g., neoplasm, tumor, cholesteatoma); a neoplasm that exerts its influence by impinging on neural tissues

SPAR sensitivity prediction of the acoustic reflex; a hearing loss prediction technique based on the normal difference expected in acoustic reflex thresholds for noise versus pure-tone signals

spatial localization the ability to use localization cues to determine a sound source in a spatial relationship; see also **localization**

SPEAK a cochlear implant signal processing strategy used in the spectra speech processor of the Nucleus-22 cochlear implant; it identifies the six most prominent peaks of the incoming signal and presents the information to electrodes that correspond to the frequency content of the signal

speaker an electroacoustic transducer that changes electrical energy to acoustical energy at the output stage of a sound system allowing amplified sound to be heard by many persons simultaneously

speaker-to-ear distance the physical distance between the auditory speaker and the listener's ear

specificity the ability of a test to categorize normal individuals as being normal

spectacle hearing aid a hearing aid that is built into the earpiece of eyeglasses; also known as **eyeglass hearing aid**

Spectra-22 speech processor the signal processing component of the Nucleus-22 cochlear implant system that provides ear-level speech processing

spectral analysis analysis of an acoustic signal to determine the relative contribution of individual frequency components

spectral content the frequency composition of an electrical or acoustic signal

spectral cues that portion of sound discrimination that focuses on selecting differences in vowel and consonant information within the same syllabic pattern

spectral maxima speech processor (SMSP) cochlear implant signal-processing strategy that uses amplitudes in each of its 16 bands ranging from 200 to 5400 Hz and uses rectifiers and low-pass filters; the best information found in the 16 bands is used as the output

spectrogram a process of characterizing a speech signal in the dimensions of time, intensity, and frequency; the horizontal axis shows time, the vertical axis represents frequency, and the intensity of the signal is shown by the darkness of the tracing

spectrum the distribution in frequency of the magnitudes of the components of the wave; represented by plotting power, amplitude, or level as a function of frequency

spectrum analyzer a sound-level measuring device that uses band-pass filters to determine the level of each frequency band in a complex sound

spectrum envelope the connection of the peaks of vertical lines representing frequency in a graph as a function of amplitude; see also **waveform envelope**

spectrum level the level of the part of the signal contained within a band unit width centered at a particular frequency; has most significance only for a signal having a continuous distribution of components within the frequency range under consideration

speculum instrument placed at the end of an otoscope that is used to examine orifices and canals; see also **otoscope**

speech coordination of respiration, phonation, articulation, and resonation for the purpose of producing spoken language

speech, compressed speech that has had segments removed and then compressed and yet maintains intact frequency composition

speech, cued a system for making all the sounds of speech visible; utilizes eight hand shapes, placed in four different locations around the face, to remove any ambiguity about what is seen and heard by a person with a hearing loss

speech, digitized storage of a person's actual words and sentences in the form of "digitized" sounds, which are recorded by a peripheral device that converts sound input from a stereo system, an instrument, or a microphone into a form that a computer can process, store, and play back as speech synthesis

speech, expanded recorded speech altered by duplicating small segments of the signal so that the speech sounds as if it were produced with a slow speaking rate; no additional spectral information is introduced

speech, filtered speech that has been passed through filter banks for the purpose of removing, alternating, or amplifying frequency bands in the signal

speech, fluent speech characterized by the continuity or blending of words within phrases and a rapid rate that in adults is about 15 sounds per second

speech, low-pass filtered speech that has been passed through filter banks, leaving the lower, but not the higher frequencies

speech, real-time the transitory, ephemeral nature of an ongoing speech signal; when speech is presented in a real-time manner, listeners must quickly recognize phonemes, syllables, and words based on preceding linguistic-contextual cues and ongoing acoustic-phonetic information

speech audiometry measurement of speech perception skills including speech awareness, speech recognition, and word recognition; one component of an audiometric test battery; (e.g., speech recognition threshold and word-identification testing)

speech awareness threshold (SAT) the lowest intensity level at which a person can detect the presence of a speech signal; it approximates the best hearing level in the 250 to 8000 Hz audiometric frequency region; used clinically with children or others who have such poor speech understanding that a speech recognition threshold (SRT) cannot be obtained; also known as **speech detection threshold (SDT)**; see also **speech reception threshold (SRT)**

speech coding term used to describe different signal processing strategies used in cochlear implants

speech conservation active intervention as part of auditory rehabilitation to preserve the speech production skills of an individual who is hard-of-hearing

speech contour an outline of the distribution of speech energy in all directions

speech detection threshold (SDT) the lowest intensity level at which a person can detect the presence of a speech signal; it approximates the best hearing level in the 250 to 8000

Hz audiometric frequency region; used clinically with children or others who have such poor speech understanding that a speech recognition threshold (SRT) cannot be obtained; also known as **speech awareness threshold (SAT)**; see also **speech reception threshold (SRT)**

speech discrimination outdated term used to describe an individual's ability to understand and identify speech

speech discrimination score (SDS) percent correct score reflecting the number of word stimuli perceived correctly in speech perception testing; preferred terms are **word-identification score (WIS), word-recognition score (WRS)**

speech discrimination testing procedures that measure a patient's ability to repeat phonetically balanced single-syllable word lists presented at a suprathreshold level or at a comfortable listening level; more commonly referred to as **word recognition**

speech frequencies frequencies within the 500 to 2000 or 3000 Hz region that are most important for the perception of speech

Speech in Noise (SIN) test a speech perception test used to test a patient's ability to listen in noise in the sound field; often used for comparison with understanding speech in quiet

speech intelligibility the percentage of the speech of a talker that is understood by a listener

speech intelligibility index (SII) (1) the distribution of speech energy at normal conversational levels superimposed on an audiogram to provide a graphic representation of loudness as a function of frequency for conversational speech; (2) a number between 0 and 1 that expresses the degree of audibility of a speech signal that is highly correlated with traditional speech intelligibility scores (number of speech items repeated correctly); also known as **articulation index (AI)**

speech intelligibility rating (SIR) a tool that documents the intelligibility of emerging speech and voice skills

speech interference level (SIL) the adverse effects of noise on the intelligibility of speech communication; used originally with the articulation index when evaluating communication systems

speech noise type of stimulus consisting of filtered white noise with a frequency spectrum containing the typical spectrum of speech

Speech Pattern Contrast (SPAC) test a battery of tests designed to provide analytic data on speech perception at the sensory/phonetic level through a mostly closed-set format with one open-set task of word recognition

speech perception the ability to understand speech through listening

Speech Perception in Noise (SPIN) sentence test presented in a background of multitalker babble used to measure listeners' utilization of linguistic-situational aspects of speech in comparison to their utilization of acoustic-phonetic information

speech processor component of a cochlear implant that transmits the signal across the skull from the external transmitter to the internal receiver

speech reception threshold (SRT) old term for a test that determines the softest level at which a person can just barely understand speech 50% of the time; same as **speech recognition threshold (SRT)**

speech reception threshold testing using sentence stimuli a measure of the speech recognition threshold (SRT) using open-set sentence stimuli; designed to improve the reliability of the SRT

speech recognition threshold (SRT) a test that determines the softest level at which a person can just barely understand speech 50% of the time; also referred to as **speech reception threshold (SRT)**

speech spectrogram a process of characterizing a speech signal in the dimensions of time, intensity, and frequency; the horizontal axis shows time, the vertical axis represents frequency, and the intensity of the signal is shown by the darkness of the tracing

speech Stenger modified Stenger test that uses spondees instead of pure tones; also known as the **modified Stenger test**; see also **Stenger test**

speech stimulus a type of stimulus composed of speech characteristics

speech threshold (ST) the lowest level at which a patient can repeat bisyllabic words; measured using speech recognition threshold procedures; used to be called speech reception threshold; see also **speech recognition threshold (SRT), speech reception threshold (SRT)**

speech tracking a speechreading technique that requires the individual to repeat verbatim a paragraph that is being read; scored according to the number of words perceived per minute; also known as **continuous discourse tracking (CDT)**

speech transmission index (STI) a number between 0 and 1 that quantifies speech intelligibility on the basis of seven modulation transfer function curves; see also **modified speech transmission index (MSTI), rapid speech transmission index (RASTI)**

speech viewer device that compares the speaker's attempt to a standard and provides a proximity metric (i.e., a graphic display based on the score)

speech visualization therapeutic system primarily used for speech training and communication aids

speech waveform the shape of a wave comprised of speech stimuli plotted with amplitude as a function of time

speech with alternating masking index (SWAMI) a test of the ability of a person to understand a speech signal while a white noise masker is alternated between the ears at an intensity level that is 20 dB higher than the speech

speech-language pathologist (SLP) a professional who studies, diagnoses, and treats speech and language disorders

speech-language pathology professional discipline related to the study, diagnosis, and treatment of speech and language disorders

speech-to-competition ratio the signal-to-noise ratio or difference in decibels between the intensity of a speech signal and the intensity of a competing noise; see also **message-to-competition ratio (MCR)**, **signal-to-noise ratio (S/N, SNR)**

speech-weighted composite signal a broadband, complex sound that has the same crest factor as speech (12 dB); used for electroacoustic analysis of hearing aids

speechreading speech recognition using auditory and visual cues; see **lipreading**

spherical wave a waveform caused by alternate regions of compression and rarefaction in an air mass caused by vibration of a point source of sound

spike a very sharp increase in electrical or acoustic energy; electrical potential recording from single neurons may appear as spikes

SPIN Speech Perception in Noise test; sentence test presented in a background of multitalker babble used to measure listeners' utilization of linguistic-situational aspects of speech in comparison to their utilization of acoustic-phonetic information

spiral ganglia the collection of cell bodies of afferent auditory nerve fibers found within the modiolus of the cochlea; located after the fibers leave the hair cells of the cochlea but before they form the auditory nerve

spiral lamina thin shelf of bone arising from the medial end of the cochlea near the modiolus; auditory nerve fibers travel through the spiral lamina to and from the hair cells; see also **osseous spiral lamina**

spiral ligament the periosteumlike outer wall of the scala media; it is attached to the outer border of the basilar membrane at the basilar crest and is covered by the stria vascularis within the cochlear duct

spiral limbus an extension of the osseous spiral lamina toward the scala vestibuli; near its inner edge it is attached to Reissner's membrane and on its outer edge it forms the inner spiral sulcus, which is attached to the tectorial membrane

SPL sound pressure level; an absolute value measured in dB representing the physical intensity of a sound; 20 times the log of the pressure output over the pressure reference (0.0002 dyne/cm^2 or 20 micropascals)

SPL-O-GRAM a plot used in the desired sensation level approach to hearing aid fitting that compares aided and unaided performance; the plot includes the minimal audibility level, the patient's thresholds, the long-term average speech spectrum, levels for amplified speech, and hearing aid saturation levels

spondaic word two-syllable word with equal stress on each syllable; (e.g., baseball); used in obtaining the speech recognition threshold; also referred to as **spondee**

spondee two-syllable word with equal stress on each syllable; (e.g., baseball); used in obtaining the speech recognition threshold; also referred to as **spondaic word**

spondee threshold (ST) the lowest level at which a patient can repeat bisyllabic words; measured using speech recognition threshold procedures; used to be called **speech reception threshold (SRT)** and is now called **speech recognition threshold (SRT)**

spondyloepiphyseal dysplasia autosomal dominant disorder characterized by short stature, skeletal anomalies, cleft palate, Robin sequence; possible conductive hearing loss caused by middle ear disease secondary to clefting, occasional high-frequency sensorineural hearing loss

spontaneous neural discharge the firing of neurons without an evoking stimulus

spontaneous nystagmus the presence of nystagmus without an evoking stimulus

spontaneous otoacoustic emission (SOAE) an otoacoustic emission recorded in some normal ears without acoustic stimulation; see also **otoacoustic emission**

spontaneous recovery the return of hearing sensitivity to its original state that occurs without treatment or intervention after exposure to loud noise; occurs in **temporary threshold shift (TTS)**

sporadic inheritance a trait that appears in a single individual in a family with no evident genetic basis

spring-mass system a system in which there is always a restoring force to return the mass to its position of equilibrium; the magnitude of the restoring force is proportional to the change in the length of the spring whether it is compressed or stretched

SPV slow phase velocity; the slower component of nystagmus induced by vestibular disease or caloric stimulation

squamous cell carcinoma a cancerous lesion of the squamous cells that tends to grow slowly and may initially appear as an ulcer, polyp, or subcutaneous mass; can be found on the skin of the external ear

square wave a complex periodic wave with energy only at odd integral multiples of the fundamental frequency

squelch effect (1) improved speech perception in noise as a result of binaural listening; (2) prevention of a radio receiver output unless the incoming signal has predetermined characteristics

SRT speech reception threshold; speech recognition threshold; a test that determines the softest level at which a person can just barely understand speech 50% of the time; used as a comparison to the **pure-tone average (PTA)**

SSEP steady-state evoked potential; an auditory evoked potential in which the response waveform approximates the rate of stimulation; also referred to as steady state evoked response

SSI Synthetic Sentence Identification test; a measure of central auditory function that involves identification of syntactically incomplete sentences (a closed-set of 10 sentences) presented simultaneously with a competing message (an ongoing story about Davy Crockett)

SSI-CCM Synthetic Sentence Identification-Contralateral Competing Message; central auditory processing test in which the stimuli resemble nonsense sentences presented in the target ear while a competing message consisting of continuous discourse is presented to the contralateral ear; the listener must choose which sentence was presented among a list of 10 sentences; see also **Synthetic Sentence Identification (SSI)**

SSI-ICM Synthetic Sentence Identification-Ipsilateral Competing Message; central auditory processing test in which the stimuli resemble nonsense sentences presented in the target ear while a competing message consisting of continuous dis-

course is presented to the ipsilateral ear; the listener must choose which sentence was presented among a list of 10 sentences; see also **Synthetic Sentence Identification (SSI)**

SSPL saturation sound pressure level; a hearing aid's maximum output expressed as a frequency response curve; the highest output produced by a hearing aid regardless of the level of input

SSPL90 saturation sound pressure level 90; electroacoustic assessment of a hearing aid's maximum level of output signal expressed as a frequency response curve to a 90-dB signal with the hearing aid volume control set to full-on; see also **output sound pressure level (OSPL), maximum power output (MPO)**

SSW Staggered Spondaic Word test; a measure of central auditory function that utilizes spondees presented dichotically so that the second syllable of the first spondee overlaps with the presentation of the first syllable of the second spondee; the remaining syllables are presented in isolation

ST speech threshold; spondee threshold; the lowest level at which a patient can repeat bisyllabic words; measured using speech recognition threshold procedures; used to be called speech reception threshold; used as a comparison for the **pure-tone average (PTA)**; see also **speech reception threshold (SRT), speech recognition threshold (SRT)**

Staggered Spondaic Word (SSW) test a measure of central auditory function that utilizes spondees presented dichotically so that the second syllable of the first spondee overlaps with the presentation of the first syllable of the second spondee; the remaining syllables are presented in isolation

standard deviation a statistical measure of dispersion; equal to the square root of the mean of the squares of the deviations from the mean of the distribution

standard threshold shift (STS) a change in hearing from the baseline hearing test of more than an average of 10 dB for the test frequencies of 2000, 3000, and 4000 Hz for either ear

standing wave standing waves occur when two progressive waves, the incident wave and the reflected wave of the same frequency and amplitude, travel through the same medium in opposite directions; they are called standing waves because they appear to be "standing still" rather than moving, although both the incident wave and reflected wave are moving—in opposite directions; it is the resultant wave, the sum of the incident and reflected waves, that is stationary

stapedectomy surgical removal and replacement of the stapes due to fixation of the footplate; the stapes is replaced with a prosthesis that reconnects the ossicular chain to the oval window; a treatment used to manage otosclerosis; see also **otosclerosis**

stapedial ankylosis fixation of the stapes due to a growth of new bone from otosclerosis; see also **otosclerosis, ankylosis**

stapedial reflex a brainstem-mediated reflex that causes the stapedial muscle in the middle ear to contract (via VIIth nerve innervation) in response to a high-intensity stimulus; see also **acoustic reflex, stapedius**

stapedial reflex decay reduction in the amplitude of the stapedial reflex in response to constant stimulation; 50% reduction in the first 5 seconds of the response suggests abnormal auditory adaptation; a component of the immittance battery that assesses the viability of cranial nerve VIII; a measure of auditory adaptation; also known as **reflex decay**

stapedial tendon tendon (branch of cranial nerve VII) from the stapedius muscle that attaches to the neck of the stapes

stapedius muscle the smallest muscle in the human body attached to the posterior portion of the neck of the stapes and innervated by cranial nerve VII; it contracts in response to high-intensity sound; the combined action of the stapedius and tensor tympani muscles limits the motion of the auditory ossicles and thereby protects the inner ear from damage from intense sound; see also **acoustic reflex, tensor tympani**

stapedius reflex threshold the lowest level at which the stapedius

s

muscle contracts to high-intensity sound

stapedotomy a hole placed in the footplate of the stapes as a treatment for otosclerosis; the hole is used for insertion of a piston-type prosthesis that is used to reestablish the function of the middle ear system; see also **otosclerosis**

stapes the innermost and smallest of the three auditory ossicles located in the middle ear; the head of the stapes is attached to the lenticular process of the incus and the footplate nearly fills the oval window; the stapes footplate is attached to the oval window by way of the annular ligament

stapes fixation inability of the stapes footplate to move in and out of the oval window; usually due to otosclerosis; see also **otosclerosis**

stapes footplate flat oval-shaped part of the stapes bone that is connected to the oval window by way of the annular ligament; average length is 1.08 to 1.66 mm; average area is 2.65 to 3.75 mm²; also known as **footplate**

stapes mobilization surgical procedure in which spongy bone is chipped away from the stapes footplate to allow its movement in and out of the oval window; a treatment used to manage **otosclerosis**

startle response noticeable, surprise behavioral reaction to a loud sound; used to verify hearing ability in very young children

STAT Suprathreshold Adaptation Test; a test of tone decay that is presented at high stimulus intensities; if the patient hears the tone for a full 60 seconds for pure-tone signals of 500, 1000, and 2000 Hz, the test result is interpreted as negative for retrocochlear auditory dysfunction

static acoustic admittance component of the immittance test battery that reflects the amplitude of the peak of a tympanogram; indication of the amount of compliance (mobility) in the eardrum; see also **static compliance**

static compliance a measure of the flexibility (or stiffness) of the middle ear system at rest (i.e., at atmospheric pressure and without contraction of the stapedius muscle); see also **immittance, static acoustic admittance**

statoconia very small crystals of calcium carbonate embedded in a gelatinous material of the otolithic membrane; also known as **otoconia, otolith**

steady state the response level in a circuit with a response that changes over time after which no additional changes occur

steady-state evoked potential (SSEP) an auditory evoked potential in which the response waveform approximates the rate of stimulation; also referred to as steady-state evoked response

Stenger principle the psychoacoustic phenomenon that states that when two tones of the same frequency are introduced simultaneously into both ears, only the louder tone will be perceived; the basis for the Stenger test; see also **Stenger test**

Stenger test an pseudohypacusic evaluation technique used with unilateral hearing loss; the Stenger threshold test is used to estimate threshold while the Stenger screening test determines if the patient is malingering; based on the Stenger principle; see also **Stenger principle**

stenosis (1) an abnormally small and narrow ear canal; (2) narrowing of an anatomical area; laryngeal or tracheal stenosis may occur from injuries related to airway management procedures

stereocilia hairlike protein rods located on top of the inner and outer hair cells of the cochlea; arranged in an orderly fashion on top of each hair cell and contain actin filaments; shearing of the stereocilia excites the hair cell and causes ion exchange; see also **sodium-potassium pump**

Stewart-Bergstrom syndrome autosomal dominant disorder characterized by hand anomalies including curved digits with contractures; sensorineural hearing loss, nonprogressive, ranging from mild to severe, unilateral or bilateral

STI speech transmission index; a number between 0 and 1 that quantifies speech intelligibility on the basis of seven modulation transfer function curves; see also **modified speech transmission index (MSTI), rapid speech transmission index (RASTI)**

Stickler syndrome autosomal dominant disorder characterized by round face, micrognathia, maxillary deficiency, cleft palate, Robin sequence, myopia, joint laxity, associated with occasional high-frequency sensorineural hearing loss or conductive hearing loss caused by middle ear effusion secondary to clefting

stiffness ratio of the change in force to the corresponding change in displacement of an elastic element

stigmata the evidence of a disease or condition; symptoms

stimulation, bipolar (BP) the stimulation mode often used in some cochlear implants in which the active and indifferent electrodes that are stimulated are beside each other; two-electrode array

stimulation, caloric irrigation of warm or cool water into the external auditory canal during caloric testing as part of the electronystagmography test battery

stimulation, monopolar refers to the stimulation mode in which one electrode of a pair is detecting the response and the second electrode is inactive; usually located distant from the response generator and not detecting the response

stimulation, promontory a test used to measure the degree of neuron survival by placing an electrode on the promontory of the cochlea and evaluating psychophysical capabilities; used in cochlear implant evaluations

stimulation mode the determination of how much of the electrode array in a cochlear implant is stimulated each time; when more current is required to obtain threshold and comfort levels, an increase in the area of stimulation will occur by changing the stimulation mode

stimulation rate (1) the number of times electrodes transmit a pulse during 1 second; also referred to as pulses per second; (2) the number of stimuli presented per second; also known as **rate**

stimulus a form of sound, light, tactile, or electrical energy that is presented to an organism

stimulus artifact a form of electrical interference, usually observed during electrophysiologic measurements that is a result of changes in the stimulus or the response that are not a result of the original stimulus or generator site

stimulus complexity refers to the intricacy of the components in a complex sound and their relationships

stimulus duration the length of time a stimulus is on (presented)

stimulus ear refers to the ear that receives the stimulus signal; also known as the **test ear**

stimulus familiarity knowledge of specific stimuli in a given test; an

important consideration in administering individual speech perception tests

stimulus frequency otoacoustic emission (SFOAE) evoked otoacoustic emission generated in response to an ongoing pure-tone signal; not used clinically because the responses are difficult to interpret because they appear as ripples in the recording

stirrup outdated term for the last bone in the middle ear ossicular chain known as the stapes; see also **stapes**

streptomycin an aminoglycoside antibiotic used in the treatment of certain severe infections that are resistant to other antibiotics; known to be ototoxic; vestibular and permanent bilateral auditory ototoxicity can occur in patients with preexisting renal damage

stria vascularis vascularized tissue arising from the spiral ligament of the scala media; thought to be the source of the endolymph and the electrical polarization within the cochlea

strial atrophy disease resulting in hearing loss and the following clinical features: bilaterally symmetric hearing loss, similar degree of threshold elevation across frequencies, good speech recognition ability, and very slow progression

strial presbycusis type of hearing loss due to aging that is characterized by a slow, progressive, flat, bilaterally symmetrical sensorineural hearing loss starting in the third through sixth decades of life; results from atrophy of the stria vascularis and a general reduction in sensitivity of all hair cells due to the metabolic changes in the endolymph

STS standard threshold shift; a change in hearing from the baseline hearing test of more than an average of 10 dB for the test frequencies of 2000, 3000, and 4000 Hz for either ear

stylomastoid foramen an opening near the mastoid bone, behind and below the ear, from which the facial nerve exits before it courses toward the face; site of stimulation for electroneuronography

subdural hematoma an accumulation of blood in the subdural space; often a result of some injury or trauma to the head

subharmonic a frequency obtained by dividing a fundamental frequency by an integer greater than zero

subjective based on one's perceptions; not physically measurable

subjective tinnitus type of tinnitus that others cannot hear; most common type of tinnitus; see also **objective tinnitus, tinnitus**

subjective vertigo the sensation that one is spinning; see also **vertigo**

substitution method method of calibration in which the output of a device is measured and correction factors are used to compare the measured outputs to standard output levels

sudden deafness deafness that occurs with a quick onset time, not gradual; due to factors such as viral infections, vascular disease, autoimmune disturbances, or perilymphatic fistula

sudden hearing loss hearing loss with an acute and rapid onset

summating potential (SP) a sustained direct current shift in the endocochlear potential that occurs when the organ of Corti is stimulated by sound; a direct-current electrical potential of cochlear origin that can be measured using electrocochleography

summating potential/action potential ratio (SP/AP) ratio of the amplitudes of the summating potential and the action potential in electrocochleography measurement; used as a potential diagnostic indicator for **Ménière's disease**

summation, binaural the advantage in dB of binaural over monaural listening; the binaural threshold is approximately 3 dB better than the monaural threshold

summation, loudness an increase in loudness when the bandwidth of a complex sound is increased so that it exceeds a critical bandwidth even when the sound pressure level of the complex sound is kept constant

summation, temporal the integration of timing information in a tone that occurs as the duration of the tone is increased up to a critical length of time (i.e., 200 ms)

summation tone a combination tone with a frequency equal to the sum of the frequencies to two primary tones or of their harmonics

superficial (1) pertaining to the skin or another surface; (2) anatomical direction referring to structures that are away from the center of the body

superior the upper point; nearer the head

superior colliculus central nucleus in the midbrain of the visual system; located superior to the inferior colliculus of the central auditory system

superior malleolar ligament one of the ligaments of the middle ear responsible for suspension of the ossicular chain; connects from the head of the malleus to the roof of the tympanic cavity

superior olivary complex (SOC) a major collection of nuclei in the lower portion of the brainstem in the central auditory system; the first place where there is a neural interaction to stimulation of each ear (binaural stimulation)

superior olive, lateral (LSO) nuclear aggregate of the superior olivary complex involved in processing interaural intensity differences

superior olive, medial (MSO) nuclear aggregate of the superior olivary complex involved in processing interaural time (phase) differences

superior semicircular canal the uppermost of the three canals of the vestibular system that contains the sense organ (crista ampularis) for responding to angular motion; also known as the **vertical canal**; see also **semicircular canals (SCCs)**

superior temporal gyrus a rounded elevation on the temporal lobe of either side of the brain

superior vestibular nerve superior portion of the vestibular branch of cranial nerve VIII that innervates the superior and horizontal semicircular canal crista ampularis, the utricular macula, and the anterior superior part of saccular macula

supine position of the body when an individual is lying flat on his or her back facing upward

supporting cells a group of cells extending from the basilar membrane that support the organ of Corti; the free ends of these cells form the reticular lamina; consist of the inner rods of Corti, outer rods of Corti, inner phalangeal cells, outer phalangeal cells (Deiter's cells), border cells, Claudius cells, and Hensen cells

suppression (1) a reduction in the audibility of tinnitus; (2) a reduction in the amplitude of otoacoustic emissions with the introduction of an external stimulus presented simultaneously during the recording of the response

suppuration the discharge of pus; see also **purulence**

suppurative labyrinthitis an acute inflammatory response in the scala tympani and scala vestibuli portions of the inner ear membranous labyrinth; results in a proteinaceous exudate within the scalae

suppurative otitis media acute and/ or chronic otitis media with infected fluid (suppuration); inflammation of the middle ear with infected fluid (effusion); also known as **tubotympanic disease**

supra-aural on or over the outer ear

supra-aural cushions the portion of the earphones that couples the transducer to the ear so that it lies on top of the pinna

supra-aural earphones a device for presenting a sound stimulus to the ear that consists of an acoustic transducer for converting an electrical signal into an acoustic one and a cushion that couples the transducer on top of the ear

suprasegmental information above the level of individual sounds; prosodic aspects of speech including variations in pitch, rate, intensity, rhythm, intonation, and stress patterns

suprathreshold the number of decibels above (on top of) a reference point (e.g., patient's threshold); referred to as a suprathreshold intensity

Suprathreshold Adaptation Test (STAT) a test of tone decay that is presented at high stimulus intensities; if the patient hears the tone for a full 60 seconds for pure-tone signals

of 500, 1000, and 2000 Hz, the test result is interpreted as negative for retrocochlear auditory dysfunction

surface electrode an electrode placed on the skin's surface for audiometric testing

surface wave a wave that moves along a surface; the vertical-phase difference observed on the vocal fold during vibration

susceptance (B) a component of impedance that is the reciprocal of reactance; energy flow is associated with reactance

SWAMI speech with alternating masking index; a test of the ability of a person to understand a speech signal while a white noise masker is alternated between the ears at an intensity level that is 20 dB higher than the speech

sweep-frequency audiometry a method of presenting pure-tone audiometric testing in which the stimulus frequency sweeps steadily from one end of the range to the other at a rate of 1 octave per minute

swimmer's ear informal term for external otitis resulting from infection transmitted in the water of a swimming pool; characterized by edema, erythema, desquamation, and pus; see also **external otitis, otitis externa**

Swinging Story test test of pseudohypacusis used in unilateral feigned deafness; the story phrases are presented at changing thresholds in the "good ear" and the "bad ear" singularly or simultaneously

syllabic compression type of hearing aid compression system that is characterized by short time constants (attack and release times) and a low compression threshold; results in compression of virtually all signals presented to the listener; also known as **wide-dynamic range compression (WDRC)**

symmetric condition of being the same on both sides

symmetric hearing loss hearing loss that is essentially the same in both ears

symmetric peak clipping form of output limiting seen in linear class B amplifiers in hearing aids; the peaks of the positive portion of the waveform are eliminated when the amplifier is saturated; results in significant signal distortion; see also **peak clipping (PC), asymmetric peak clipping**

sympathetic nervous system thoracolumbar autonomic nervous system portion, with effects including heart rate increase, bronchiole and pupil dilation, skin, viscera, and skeletal muscle vasodilation, peristalsis moderation, liver conversion of glycogen to glucose, and secretion of epinephrine and norepinephrine by the adrenal medulla; tends to prepare the body to deal with stress

synapse the junction between two communicating neurons; the axon of one neuron approaches the cell body or dendrite of another neuron; neural transmission depends on biochemical communication between two nerves occurring at synapses

synaptic cleft the region between two communicating neurons into which a neurotransmitter is released

synaptic transmitter the chemical messenger released by the presynaptic terminal of a neuron on arrival of an action potential; released as a packet that moves across the synaptic cleft to link with receptors on the postsynaptic membrane; more than one type of transmitter can be released from one neuron and more than one type of postsynaptic receptor can combine with the transmitter

synaptic vesicles the saccules within the end bouton of an axon that contain the neurotransmitter substance for neural transmission

syndactyly the joining of two or more digits by soft tissue; webbing

syndrome a collection of anomalies that co-occur; hearing impairment often accompanies other disabilities or abnormalities, such as skeletal malformations or endocrine disorders

syndromology the study of the diagnosis and delineation of multiple anomaly syndromes

syntax word order in a given language

Synthetic Sentence Identification (SSI) test a measure of central auditory function that involves identification of syntactically incomplete sentences (a closed-set of 10 sentences) presented simultaneously with a competing message (an ongoing story about Davy Crockett)

Synthetic Sentence Identification Test with Contralateral Competing Message (SSI-CCM) central auditory processing test in which the stimuli resemble nonsense sentences presented in the target ear while a competing message consisting of continuous discourse is presented to the contralateral ear; the listener must choose which sentence was presented among a list of 10 sentences; see also **Synthetic Sentence Identification (SSI)**

Synthetic Sentence Identification Test with Ipsilateral Competing Message (SSI-ICM) central auditory processing test in which the stimuli resemble nonsense sentences presented in the target ear while a competing message consisting of continuous discourse is presented to the ipsilateral ear; the listener must choose which sentence was presented among a list of 10 sentences; see also **Synthetic Sentence Identification (SSI)**

synthetic speech speech generated by a computer

syphilis (1) an in utero infection whose presence is part of the high-risk hearing register warranting a newborn infant screening to identify a possible hearing loss due to infection; (2) a sexually transmitted disease

syringe (1) a device used to inject or withdrawal fluids; (2) used in cerumen management to inject water for the purpose of flushing out cerumen; (3) used in making ear mold impressions

T

t-coil telecoil; an induction coil built into nearly all behind-the-ear hearing aids and some in-the-ear hearing aids that picks up electromagnetic signals and converts them into an electrical voltage which is then amplified when the hearing aid is switched to the "T" setting; useful for coupling to the telephone and assistive listening devices; see also **induction loop**

t-switch telecoil switch; control on some hearing aids that allows the user to activate the telecoil on the hearing aid for use with the telephone or an assistive listening device

TAC Test of Auditory Comprehension; a battery of three subtests developed to examine a child's ability to discriminate suprasegmentals using speech and nonspeech stimuli

TACL Test of Auditory Comprehension of Language; picture-pointing task designed to assess auditory comprehension in children ages 3 to 9; see also **Test of Auditory Comprehension of Language–Revised (TACL-R)**

TACL-R Test of Auditory Comprehension of Language–Revised; revised version of the Test of Auditory Comprehension of Language (TACL); see also **Test of Auditory Comprehension of Language (TACL)**

Tactaid a commercially available single-channel vibrotactile device that receives sound through a microphone, divides the sound into bands of information based on acoustic frequency, and uses the information in each band to drive a stimulator worn on the skin that reacts proportionally to the energy in its corresponding band

Tactaid II a two-channel vibrotactile aid with improved performance over the original Tactaid; see also **Tactaid, Tactaid VII**

Tactaid VII a seven-channel vibrotactile aid with improved performance over the Tactaid and Tactaid II; see also **Tactaid, Tactaid II**

tactile communication device refers to a generic communication device that uses tactile input to assist the user in speechreading; see also **Tactaid**

tactile stimulation (1) referring to the sense of touch; (2) using the sense of touch as the modality for signal presentation

tangible reinforcement operant conditioned audiometry (TROCA) a

304

pediatric behavioral audiometry technique that reinforces a response to auditory signals with food; the patient is conditioned to manipulate the reinforcer; used mainly with individuals who are mentally handicapped or developmentally delayed

TAPS Test of Auditory Perception Skills; a test designed to measure auditory perceptual skills in areas such as digit span, sentence memory, dictation, and word recognition for children ages 4 through 11

target gain the desired amount of hearing aid gain at each frequency for a particular patient, based on the audiogram, the prescriptive fitting method, and the patient's ear canal resonance measurement; see also **prescriptive gain targets**

TBI traumatic brain injury; severe head injury that causes damage to various areas of function in the brain

TC total communication; a communication philosophy that suggests that all forms of communication (e.g., speech, manual communication, auditory, and speechreading) are available for both receptive and expressive communication

TD threshold of discomfort; the minimum effective sound pressure level of a signal that stimulates the ear to a point that is uncomfortable

TDD telecommunication device for the deaf; assistive device for individuals with severe and/or profound hearing impairment capable of sending or receiving messages that are typed by the sender, transmitted via telephone lines, and read by the receiver; used to be known as a **teletypewriter (TTY)**

TDH-39/TDH-49 earphones specialized types of headphones acceptable for clinical use in audiology; use MX-41/AR supra-aural cushions

tectorial membrane a cellular fibrous structure in the scala media that is attached on its inner edge to the spiral limbus and connected to the reticular lamina on its undersurface; consists of three regions: limbal, middle, and marginal zones and is superior to the organ of Corti

tegmen tympani the superior wall of the middle ear space; the roof of the tympanic cavity; also known as **tegmental wall**

tegmental wall the superior wall of the middle ear space; the roof of the tympanic cavity; also known as **tegmen tympani**

telecoil t-coil; a series of interconnected wire loops in a hearing aid that respond electrically to a magnetic signal to enhance telephone use

telecoil switch t-switch; an external control (switch) on a hearing aid that turns off the microphone and activates a telecoil in the device that picks up magnetic leakage from a telephone or the loop of an assistive listening device

telecommunication device for the deaf (TDD) assistive device for individuals with severe and/or profound hearing impairment capable of sending or receiving messages that are typed by the sender, transmitted via telephone lines, and read by the receiver; used to be known as a **teletypewriter (TTY)**

telephone amplifier an amplification device that can be integrated with a telephone to boost the signal coming through the receiver portion of the handset; can be an in-line amplifier or an amplified handset

telephone induction coil a telecoil that specifically picks up the electromagnetic signal from telephones; assists the hearing aid listener with telephone communication

teletypewriter (TTY) a communication device used by individuals with severe or profound hearing loss for communicating via the telephone channel; see also **telecommunication device for the deaf (TDD)**

television captioning printed text or printed dialog that corresponds to the auditory speech signal from a television program or movie; also referred to as **closed captioning (CC)**

Television Decoder Circuitry Act Public Law 101-431 requiring all televisions manufactured in the United States with a 13-inch diagonal or larger screen to contain circuitry necessary for closed captioning; see also **closed captioning (CC)**

temporal (1) having to do with time or timing; (2) referring to the anatomical region of the head just above the outer ear

temporal acuity the differential sensitivity to changes in the timing of a signal

temporal bone one of the seven bones of the skull, a very dense bone that houses the structures of the ear including the enclosure for the external auditory canal, the middle and inner ears, and cranial nerve VIII housed within the internal auditory canal; has four portions: the squamous, mastoid, tympanic, and petrous

temporal bone fracture fracture of the temporal bone resulting in possible hearing loss; can be a **longitudinal fracture** that spares the inner ear or a **transverse fracture** that directly affects the inner ear structures; see also **temporal bone**

temporal coding coding or processing sound based on the temporal (timing) patterns in the firing of auditory nerve fibers

temporal discrimination the ability to detect short timing/interval changes in sound that deteriorates with age

temporal distortion subjective or physiological reduction in loudness sensation caused by auditory adaptation

temporal information timing cues detected by auditory nerves firing at particular points in the cycle of a periodic tone; this information is used along with interaural timing and intensity differences to localize sound

temporal integration a time versus intensity relationship in which the intensity of a tone must be increased to reach threshold when the duration of the tone is decreased below a critical minimum (less than 200 ms); see also **temporal summation**

temporal lobe the area of the brain responsible for auditory perception, smell, memory, and learning

temporal masking obscuring the perception of a sound by pre- or poststimulatory presentation of a masker; see also **backward masking, forward masking**

temporal ordering detection of a sequence of sounds over time

temporal patterning changes in acoustic signal contours that provide important information for sound perception

temporal processing auditory mechanisms and processes responsible for temporal patterning (e.g., phase locking, synchronization) of neural discharges and the following behavioral phenomena: temporal resolution, temporal ordering, temporal integration, and temporal masking

temporal resolution the detection of changes in the durations of auditory stimuli and in the time intervals between auditory stimuli over time

temporal summation the integration of timing information in a tone that occurs as the duration of the tone is increased up to a critical length of time (i.e., 200 ms); see also **temporal integration**

temporal theory of pitch perception theory of hearing developed by Rutherford in 1886, which states that every hair cell responds to every tone and that the perception of frequency is determined by the rate of firing of nerve impulses

temporary threshold shift (TTS) a change in threshold that returns to its pre-exposure level over time; temporary threshold shift is not permanent; usually seen after exposure to high-intensity noise; see also **permanent threshold shift (PTS)**

temporomandibular joint (TMJ) point of articulation between the temporal bone and the mandible; improper alignment or weakening in the temporomandibular joints of the mandible can cause TMJ dysfunction

10-20 International Electrode System a systematic standard for uniform electrode placement that is computed as a percentage of head circumference

tensor tympani muscle an intra-aural muscle of the middle ear whose tendon is attached to the manubrium of the malleus; its contraction increases tension on the tympanic membrane; the combined action of the tensor tympani and the stapedius muscles limits the motion of the auditory ossicles and thereby helps to protect the inner ear from damage from intense sound, especially low frequencies; see also **stapedius muscle**

tensor veli palatini muscle muscle in the region of the neck that contracts along with other muscles to open the eustachian tube; see also **levator veli palatini**

TEOAE transient evoked otoacoustic emission; otoacoustic emission measured in the external auditory canal in response to a transient evoking stimulus (e.g., a click with rapid onset and short duration); useful technique for determining cochlear function in infants; also known as **click evoked otoacoustic emission (CEOAE), transient otoacoustic emission (TOAE)**; see also **otoacoustic emission (OAE)**

teratogen any external agent causing congenital malformations and disease

teratogenic drugs a class of pharmacological agents that can harm a developing fetus if ingested by the mother during pregnancy; includes quinine, dilantin, and thalidomide; may result in malformation of the ear

test ear (TE) the ear to be evaluated in an audiometric procedure

Test for Auditory Comprehension of Language (TACL) picture-pointing task designed to assess auditory comprehension in children ages 3 to 9; see also **Test of Auditory Comprehension of Language–Revised (TACL-R)**

Test for Auditory Comprehension of Language–Revised (TACL-R) revised version of the Test of Auditory Comprehension of Language (TACL); see also **Test of Auditory Comprehension of Language (TACL)**

Test of Auditory Analysis Skills a central auditory test that assesses auditory perception skills

Test of Auditory Comprehension (TAC) a battery of three subtests developed to examine a child's ability to discriminate suprasegmentals using speech and nonspeech stimuli

Test of Auditory Perception Skills (TAPS) a test designed to measure auditory perceptual skills in areas such as digit span, sentence memory, dictation, and word recognition for children ages 4 through 11

Test of Language Development–Intermediate (TOLD-I) test of receptive and expressive language for older children (8 to 12 years) that assesses vocabulary, syntax, and phonology; see also **Test of Language Development–Primary (TOLD-P)**

Test of Language Development–Primary (TOLD-P) test of receptive and expressive language for younger children (4 to 6 years) that assesses vocabulary, syntax, and phonology; see also **Test of Language Development–Intermediate (TOLD-I)**

Test of Nonverbal Auditory Discrimination a central auditory processing assessment tool of auditory discrimination using nonverbal stimuli

Test of Receptive Language Competence a test for patients who are deaf or hearing in which subjects are required to judge whether simple sentences generated by correct and incorrect rules are "right" or "wrong"

Test of Word Finding (TWF) a test that assesses the accuracy and speech of word retrieval for a child's existing vocabulary; consists of six sections; designed for children aged 6 to 12 years

test-retest reliability the ability of a test to produce the same results when retested on the same subject; an indication of the repeatability of test findings indicating a low standard error of measurement

text telephone (TT) an assistive device for telephone use that consists of a keyboard and a display with a built-in modem that allows signals representing the characters on the keyboard to be sent along the telephone line; personal computers can be adapted for this use; see also **telecommunication device for the deaf (TDD)**

thalamus a subcortical oval-shaped structure on each side of the central nervous system that serves as a major relay station for sensory pathways (auditory, visual, and somatosensory) between the brainstem and the cortex; the medial geniculate body is an important central auditory structure that is located on the posterior portion of the thalamus; see also **medial geniculate body (MGB)**

THD total harmonic distortion; a measure of nonlinear distortion that assesses the relative strength of any new frequencies created by the nonlinearity of a hearing instrument when sine-wave signals of one or more frequencies are presented as the input to the device; electroacoustic measurement occurs as a percentage of distortion at 500, 800, and 1600 Hz

thickened tympanic membrane a tympanic membrane thickened by some type of dysfunction that interferes with immittance measurements due to changes in eardrum mobility

third-octave filter a filter whose upper-to-lower passband limits are one-third of an octave

third-order English sentence type of sentence material used with the Synthetic Sentence Identification (SSI) test; has normal phonology and syntax, but no semantic content

three-alternative forced-choice test (THRIFT) testing paradigm in which a listener must decide whether a signal is present during the first, second, or third observation period

three-dB rule (3-dB rule) in calculating temporary threshold shift with noise exposure, for each doubling of a sound's duration, the sound power must be decreased by 3 dB to maintain equal threshold shift; also known as the **equal energy rule of noise exposure**

3M/House cochlear implant a single-channel, single-electrode cochlear implant producing analog stimulation used in children and adults; one of the first cochlear implants available; created by Dr. W. F. House and colleagues at the House Ear Institute in Los Angeles, CA

3M/Vienna cochlear implant an early cochlear implant design that was a single-channel cochlear implant producing analog stimulation used in children and adults via extracochlear stimulation

threshold the intensity at which an individual can just barely hear a sound 50% of the time; all sounds louder than threshold can be heard, but sounds below threshold cannot be detected

threshold, absolute the minimum stimulus that evokes a response in a specified fraction of trials; the difference between audibility and inaudibility

threshold, acoustic reflex (ART) the lowest level of the acoustic activating signal that produces an observable, time-locked change in acoustic immittance

threshold, air-conduction the lowest level that one can hear a pure-tone signal delivered via insert or supra-aural earphones 50% of the time

threshold, bone-conduction absolute hearing threshold perceived from a bone-conducted pure-tone signal providing information about sensorineural function

threshold, compression (CT) the lowest input level at which the compression operates; the level that activates compression; also known as **compression kneepoint**

threshold, detection the lowest intensity level at which a person can detect the presence of a speech or nonspeech signal; it approximates the best hearing level in the 250 to 8000 Hz audiometric frequency region; also known as **speech awareness threshold (SAT), speech detection threshold (SDT)**

threshold, differential the minimal increment in a stimulus needed to produce a just-noticeable difference in sensation; the relative difference limen is the ratio of the difference limen to the value of the stimulus to which it is added

threshold, hearing level of intensity at which a sound is just audible to an individual

threshold, masked the threshold of audibility for a specified sound in the presence of another (masking) sound

threshold, pure-tone the lowest level that a patient can hear a pure sinusoid that provides a direct indication of the amount of hearing loss the individual has at each frequency for both air and bone conduction

threshold, speech (ST) the lowest level at which a patient can repeat bisyllabic words; measured using speech recognition threshold procedures; used clinically with children or others who have such poor speech understanding that a speech recognition threshold (SRT) cannot be obtained; used to be called **speech reception threshold**; see also **speech recognition threshold (SRT)**

threshold, speech awareness the lowest intensity level at which a person can detect the presence of a speech signal; it approximates the best hearing level in the 250 to 8000 Hz audiometric frequency region; used clinically with children or others who have such poor speech understanding that a speech recognition threshold (SRT) cannot be obtained; also known as **speech detection threshold (SDT)**; see also **speech reception threshold (SRT)**

threshold, speech detection the lowest intensity level at which a person can detect the presence of a speech signal; it approximates the best hearing level in the 250 to 8000 Hz audiometric frequency region; used clinically with children or others who have such poor speech understanding that a speech recognition threshold (SRT) cannot be obtained; also known as **speech awareness threshold (SAT)**; see also **speech reception threshold (SRT)**

threshold, speech reception the lowest intensity level at which a person can detect the presence of a speech signal; it approximates the best hearing level in the 250 to 8000 Hz audiometric frequency region; also known as **speech recognition threshold (SRT)**

threshold, speech recognition the lowest intensity level at which a

person can detect the presence of a speech signal; it approximates the best hearing level in the 250 to 8000 Hz audiometric frequency region; also known as **speech reception threshold (SRT)**

threshold, spondee the lowest level at which a patient can repeat bisyllabic words; measured using speech recognition threshold procedures; used to be called **speech reception threshold (SRT)**

threshold, unmasked pure-tone or speech threshold obtained with no masking presented to the nontest ear

threshold curve the configuration of threshold across frequencies on the audiogram

threshold estimation a clinical application of the auditory brainstem response to measure responses to low-level stimuli to estimate threshold; useful with infants and children whose hearing is difficult to evaluate

threshold measurement the procedure followed to obtain threshold levels for various stimuli; often uses a bracketing procedure

threshold of audibility the minimum effective sound pressure level of the signal that is capable of evoking an auditory sensation in a specified fraction of the trials; see also **minimal audible pressure (MAP), minimal audible field (MAF)**

threshold of discomfort (TD) the minimum effective sound pressure level of a signal that stimulates the ear to a point that is uncomfortable

threshold of pain the minimum effective sound pressure level of a signal that will stimulate the ear to a point at which the discomfort gives way to definite pain; distinct from a non-noxious feeling of discomfort

threshold shift an increase (worsening) in the threshold of audibility for an ear at a specified frequency; the amount of threshold shift is expressed in decibels; see also **temporary threshold shift (TTS), permanent threshold shift (PTS)**

threshold variability large differences measured in the thresholds obtained for one subject across the frequencies

THRIFT three-alternative forced-choice test; testing paradigm in which a listener must decide whether a signal is present during the first, second, or third observation period

TILL treble increase at low levels; type of automatic signal processing in hearing aids that increases gain for low-intensity signals and reduces gain for high-intensity stimuli; results in an overall increase in high-frequency amplification; circuitry used in the K-Amp; see also **bass increase at low levels (BILL), programmable increase at low levels (PILL)**

timbre the attribute of auditory sensation in which a listener can judge that two sounds having the same loudness and pitch are perceived as dissimilar; see also **quality**

time compression signal processing technique applied to speech and nonspeech stimuli that does not alter the frequency components of the signal; portions of the signals are removed and accelerated

time delay spectrography a method used by a time-energy-frequency (TEF) system for obtaining anechoic room results in echoic spaces

time domain waveform a graph that illustrates the nature of simple vibratory motion by plotting changes in the magnitude (amplitude) of displacements over time

time-compressed speech signal processing technique applied to speech stimuli that does not alter the frequency components of the signal; speech signals are accelerated to assess central auditory function

time-intensity tradeoff the relationship between the time of exposure and the level of the noise to which an individual is exposed; damage risk criteria set by the Occupational Safety and Health Administration (OSHA) recommending that for every 5 dB increase in noise level, the time of exposure should be cut in half

time-weighted average (TWA) amplitude measures in dB taken moment to moment to reflect a single decibel value that is considered to be equivalent in energy to the time-varying amplitudes experienced in the real world

tinnitus the perception of noise in the ear when the internally perceived sound is absent externally; any of a number of internal head noises that can accompany hearing impairment; also called "ringing in the ears"

tinnitus masker electronic hearing instrument designed to emit low-level noise to mask the presence of tinnitus

tinnitus matching test procedure that requires the patient to match his or her tinnitus for pitch and loudness using pure tones

tinnitus suppression the effect produced by a tinnitus masker that emits a low-level noise to mask the perception of tinnitus by the patient

TIPtrode a special electrode design with gold foil covering a foam insert contacting the wall of the external auditory canal that detects the evoked responses; useful in measuring electrocochleography and the auditory brainstem response

TM tympanic membrane; the membranous separation between the outer and middle ears; responsible for initiating the mechanical impedance-matching process of the middle ear; has three layers: cutaneous, fibrous, mucous

TM electrode an electrode that makes contact with the tympanic membrane

TMJ temporomandibular joint; point of articulation between the temporal bone and the mandible; improper alignment or weakening in the temporomandibular joints of the mandible can cause TMJ dysfunction

TOAE transient otoacoustic emission; otoacoustic emission measured in the external auditory canal in response to a transient evoking stimulus (e.g., a click with rapid onset and short duration); also known as **transient evoked otoacoustic emission (TEOAE)**

tobramycin an aminoglycoside antibiotic used in the treatment of certain severe infections that are resistant to other antibiotics; has the inherent potential for causing ototoxicity and nephrotoxicity

Token Test for Children a measure of receptive language that assesses a child's ability to understand verbal instructions of progressively increasing length and intensity; designed for children 3 to 12 years of age

TOLD-I Test of Language Development–Intermediate; test of receptive and expressive language for older children (8 to 12 years) that assesses vocabulary, syntax, and phonology; see also **Test of Language Development–Primary (TOLD-P)**

TOLD-P Test of Language Development–Primary; test of receptive and expressive language for younger children (4 to 6 years) that assesses vocabulary, syntax, and phonology; see also **Test of Language Development–Intermediate (TOLD-I)**

tolerance maximum decibel deviation permissible in the specification of frequency response; tolerance values are provided with manufacturer's electroacoustic characteristics and instrument calibrations

tomography sectional imaging; see also **computed tomography (CT)**

tone (1) a sound wave capable of exciting an auditory sensation that has a certain vibration or pitch; includes complex tones, pure tones, and overtones; (2) musical or vocal sound of a specific quality; see also **sine wave**

tone, combination produced when two tones act simultaneously on a nonlinear transducer; may have a frequency equal to the difference between the two tones or any of their harmonics (difference tones) or it may have a frequency equal to the sum of two tones or any of their harmonics (summation tones)

tone, complex (1) a sound wave containing simple sinusoidal components of different frequencies; (2) a sound sensation characterized by more than one pitch

tone, difference a combination tone with a frequency equal to the difference between the frequencies of two primary tones or of their harmonics

tone, frequency-modulated a tone that alters its frequency at a fixed rate; see also **FM**

tone, probe steady-state stimulus used in immittance audiometry that provides a known quantity of sound pressure; used indirectly to measure changes in the mobility of the middle ear system; low-frequency probe tone is typically 226 Hz

tone, pure (PT) sound produced by an instantaneous sound pressure that is a simple sinusoidal function of time; a single-frequency tonal sound (e.g., 1000 Hz); a sinusoid

tone, warble (WT) acoustic signal produced by modifying a pure tone with small and rapid changes in frequency; used in sound-field audiometry to minimize the likelihood of standing waves

tone burst a signal having a rise time, plateau time, and decay time of sufficient duration to be perceived as having tonal information; tone refers to a sinusoid or a combination of sinusoids; see also **tone pip**

tone control a potentiometer in a hearing aid used to alter its frequency response

tone decay a clinical measure of auditory adaptation in which a tone is presented continuously to a hearing-impaired ear until it becomes inaudible; excessive tone decay (>30 dB) is a sign of a retrocochlear site of lesion; see also **auditory adaptation**

tone pip a brief-tone stimulus sometimes defined as one complete cycle of the tone in the rise, plateau, and fall portions of the stimulus (e.g., a 1000-Hz tone pip has a rise, duration, and fall time of 1 ms each); see also **tone burst**

tonotopic organization the arrangement of auditory nerve fibers such that fibers innervating the apex of the cochlea process low-frequency information, while fibers in the basal region process high-frequency information; see also **tonotopicity**

tonotopicity organization of auditory neurons in a particular structure according to their responsiveness to specific frequencies; tonotopicity is present throughout the auditory system (e.g., cochlea, auditory nerve, central auditory system, and temporal lobe); see also **tonotopic organization**

top-down processing information processing that is knowledge—or concept—driven such that higher level constraints guide data processing leading to data interpretation consistent with these constraints; see also **bottom-up processing**

TORCH a group of perinatal medical problems often linked to hearing loss: t = toxoplasmosis; o = other (e.g., syphilis); r = rubella; c = cytomegalovirus; h = herpes; more current term is TORCH+S complex; see also **TORCH+S complex**

TORCH+S complex a group of perinatal medical problems often linked to hearing loss: t = toxoplasmosis; o = other (e.g., associated ophthalmologic disease); r = rubella; c = cytomegalovirus; h = herpes; s = syphilis; see also **TORCH**

TORP total ossicular replacement prosthesis; used during tympanoplasty to assist in reconstructing the ossicular chain; see also **PORP**

torsion swing test older, relatively simple clinical vestibular test in which the patient is seated in a chair equipped with a calibrated spring oscillated with decreasing amplitude; see also **rotary chair testing**

total communication (TC) a communication philosophy that suggests that all forms of communication (e.g., speech, manual communication, auditory, and speechreading) are available for both receptive and expressive communication

total harmonic distortion (THD) a measure of nonlinear distortion that assesses the relative strength of any new frequencies created by the nonlinearity of a hearing instrument when sine-wave signals of one or more frequencies are presented as the input to the device; electroacoustic measurement occurs as a percentage of distortion at 500, 800, and 1600 Hz

Townes (or Townes-Brocks) syndrome autosomal dominant disorder characterized by facial asymmetry, ear tags and pits, microtia, commissural cleft, digital anomalies, radial anomalies, anal anomalies, renal anomalies; associated with sensorineural hearing loss of variable severity

toxin a poison that is produced by a microorganism

toxoplasmosis an infection caused by an intracellular parasite; can be transmitted to humans via cat feces

Toynbee maneuver a method for forcing the eustachian tube open by swallowing with the nostrils and mouth closed; see also **Valsalva maneuver**

TPP tympanometric peak pressure; the pressure at which the peak of the tympanogram occurs; provides an estimate of the volume in the middle ear and the status of the tympanic membrane

tracking (1) continuous discourse tracking technique in which the listener attempts to repeat verbatim text that is presented by a speaker; (2) part of the electronystagmography battery of tests in which the patient's eye movements are recorded while he or she follows a visual target moving in the horizontal plane; see also **continuous discourse tracking (CDT), pursuit tracking test, speech tracking**

tragus small protrusion of tissue just anterior to the opening (meatus) of the external ear canal

transcranial CROS hearing aid unilateral hearing aid fitting using contralateral routing of signals (CROS); a power in-the-ear hearing aid is placed on the poorer ear for transmission of sound via bone conduction to the better ear's cochlea

transcranial transmission loss the amount of sound that is lost when crossing the skull

transcutaneous link in cochlear implants, a way of passing the stimulus from the speech processor to the electrode(s) in which a transmitter worn outside the skin is coupled to a receiver placed on the mastoid under the skin

transcutaneous signal transmission in cochlear implants, a way of passing the stimulus from the speech processor to the electrode(s) in which a transmitter worn outside the skin is coupled to a receiver placed on the mastoid under the skin

transcutaneous transducer a transducer for a bone-conduction implant that consists of an internal magnet and an external sound processor

transdermal stimulation in cochlear implants, a way of passing the stimulus from the speech processor to the electrode(s) in which a transmitter worn outside the skin is coupled to a receiver placed on the mastoid under the skin

transduce (1) to change; (2) to convert from one form of energy to another

transducer a device such as a microphone or loudspeaker that converts one form of energy to another (e.g., a microphone changes acoustic energy into electricity and a loudspeaker changes electricity into acoustic sound)

transduction the conversion of energy from one form to another

transection a surgical cut that runs through or across a structure

transfer function a filter curve that has the following parameters: natural frequency, center frequency, upper cuttoff frequency, lower cutoff frequency, bandwidth, and attenuation rate

transformer a two-coil induction device for increasing or decreasing the voltage of alternating current

transient (1) a very brief duration (e.g., 0.1 ms) sound with almost instantaneous onset that is effective in eliciting auditory evoked responses (e.g., click); (2) lasting only a brief time; (3) the response of a transducer to a short-duration signal such as a click

transient distortion the inaccurate reproduction of a signal as a result of sudden changes in voltage; distortion created by initiating and terminating a signal

transient evoked otoacoustic emission (TEOAE) otoacoustic emission measured in the external auditory canal in response to a transient evoking stimulus (e.g., a click with rapid onset and short duration); useful technique for determining cochlear function in infants; also known as **click evoked otoacoustic emission (CEOAE), transient otoacoustic emission (TOAE)**; see also **otoacoustic emission (OAE)**

transient otoacoustic emission (TOAE) otoacoustic emission measured in the external auditory canal in response to a transient evoking stimulus (e.g., a click with rapid onset and short duration); also known as **click evoked otoacoustic emission (CEOAE), transient evoked otoacoustic emission (TEOAE)**

transistor a type of amplifier currently used in hearing aids that provides higher reliability and lower noise than amplifiers used prior to 1952

transmissibility the ratio of the amplitude response of a system in steady-state vibration to the excitation amplitude

transmission gain hearing aid gain measured in an ear simulator or a 2-cc coupler in a test box

transmitter (1) an apparatus that sends out electromagnetic rays; (2) the component of an FM system that modulates the frequency of the radio signal in an audio frequency signal and sends the radio waves through the air to the antenna of the amplifier/receiver

transmitter coil component of a cochlear implant that delivers the processed signal from the speech processor to the internal receiver; attaches to the side of the head via transdermal magnetic connections or percutaneous plugs

transmitter cord the short cord that runs from the microphone to the transmitter coil

transpositional hearing aid hearing aid fitting in which high-frequency energy is converted into low-frequency signals to take advantage of residual hearing in the low frequencies

transtympanic ABR an auditory brainstem response obtained by placing a needle electrode through the tympanic membrane

transtympanic action potential action potential measurement through electrocochleography in which a needle electrode is placed through the tympanic membrane and rests on the promontory of the cochlea; also known as **transtympanic ECochG**

transtympanic ECochG electrocochleography measure obtained with a needle electrode that is placed through the tympanic membrane and rests on the promontory of the cochlea; also known as **transtympanic action potential**

transtympanic electrode a needle electrode that is inserted through the tympanic membrane and rests on the promontory at the medial end of the middle ear; used for electrophysiology measurements; see also **transtympanic action potential, transtympanic ECochG**

transtympanic SP/AP ratio measurement of the ratio of the amplitudes of the summating potential compared to the action potential in electrocochleography (ECochG) that is obtained when a transtympanic needle electrode is placed on the promontory; results in a smaller SP/AP ratio than an ECochG measured with an electrode placed farther away from the cochlea

transudate a thin, watery fluid passed through a membrane that is uninfected

transverse anatomic plane that crosses the long axis of the body; perpendicular to a given structure or phenomenon, such as a muscle fiber or airflow

transverse fracture fracture of the temporal bone resulting in possible hearing loss; directly affects the inner ear structures

transverse wave wave that moves in a medium perpendicular to the direction that the sound wave travels; motion is at right angles to wave movement

transverse wave motion "stretched rope" motion of a wave with the particles moving alternately up and down over time at right angles to the direction of wave motion from left to right

trapezoid body transverse fiber tract in the lower brainstem's ventral portion; auditory brainstem pathway crossing from one side of the brain to the other; the first (lowest) such decussation (crossing) in the auditory system is located in the pons

trauma physical injury due to a violent disruption to a system or any part of a system; can also be in the form of acoustic trauma that affects the auditory structures as a result of an extremely loud sound or vibration (e.g., explosion)

traumatic brain injury (TBI) severe head injury that causes damage to various areas of function in the brain

traveling wave the wavelike action of the basilar membrane arising from stimulation of the perilymph of the scala vestibuli and scala tympani; the traveling wave moves from the base of the cochlea to the apex, and the point of maximum displacement of the basilar membrane indicates the frequency location where the stimulus is perceived; also known as **Békésy traveling wave**

traveling wave theory frequency analysis in the cochlea that ascribes the ability of the ear to analyze sound strictly to the mechanical gradient of stiffness along the organ of Corti; Georg von Békésy's (1899–1972) Nobel Prize-winning work led to this theory; see also **traveling wave**

Treacher Collins syndrome autosomal dominant form of mandibulofacial dysostosis that may be associated with craniofacial anomalies, aural atresia, micrognathia, absent or hypoplastic zygomas, defects of lower eyelids, absent lashes of inner two-thirds of lower eyelids, malar clefts, cleft palate, Robin sequence, cleft lip (uncommon), microtia, ossicular malformation, airway obstruction, and choanal atresia; associated with conductive hearing loss of varying degree ranging from mild to maximum depending on the degree of microtia; fixation of the footplate of the stapes is also common; there is occasionally a sensorineural hearing loss; see also **mandibulofacial dysostosis**

treble increase at low levels (TILL) type of automatic signal processing in hearing aids that increases gain for low-intensity signals and reduces gain for high-intensity stimuli; results in an overall increase in high-frequency amplification; type of circuitry used in the K-Amp; see also **bass increase at low levels (BILL), programmable increase at low levels (PILL)**

triangular fossa depressed region between the crura of the antihelix of the pinna

triangular wave a complex periodic wave with energy at odd integral multiples of the fundamental frequency

trigeminal nerve cranial nerve V responsible for chewing, face sensitivity, and muscle innervation; innervates the tensor tympani middle ear muscle and muscles used to open and close the eustachian tube; see also **tensor tympani**

trimmer a control for adjustment with a screwdriver for the tone, gain, or maximum output of an amplifier; also known as **potentiometer**

trisomy the presence of an extra chromosome in an individual's genetic makeup

trisomy 18 disorder resulting from an extra chromosome 18 characterized by severe cognitive deficiency and brain anomalies, hypertonicity, micrognathia, heart anomalies, renal anomalies, esophageal atresia, limb anomalies, loose neck skin; also known as **Edwards syndrome**

trisomy 21 a chromosomal, congenital condition that results from the presence of an extra chromosome on chromosome 21; characterized by flat occiput, upslanting eyes, strabismus, small ears, large protruding tongue, short neck, micropenis, inguinal hernias, brachydactyly, short 5th finger, hyperextensible joints, obesity, cognitive impairment, small teeth, maxillary hypoplasia, heart anomalies, immune deficiency, blood disorders, occasional cleft lip and palate, airway obstruction, and hypertrophic lymphoid tissue; hearing is usually normal although conductive hearing loss secondary to chronic otitis media is common; also known as **Down syndrome**

TROCA tangible reinforcement operant conditioned audiometry; a pediatric behavioral audiometry technique that reinforces a response to auditory signals with food; the patient is conditioned to manipulate the reinforcer; used mainly with individuals who are mentally handicapped or developmentally delayed

trochaic a two-syllable word with the emphasis on the first syllable; (e.g., father); also known as a **trochee**

trochee a two-syllable word with the emphasis on the first syllable; (e.g., father); also known as a **trochaic word**

trochlear nerve cranial nerve IV responsible for efferent innervation for eye movement

trochleariform process bony outcropping of the middle ear from which the tendon for the tensor tympani arises

troubleshooting performing various visual and listening inspections to determine whether an amplification unit or piece of audiometric equipment is malfunctioning and, if so, evaluating the nature and severity of the malfunction

TT text telephone; an assistive device for telephone use that consists of a keyboard and a display with a built-in modem that allows signals representing the characters on the keyboard to be sent along the telephone line; personal computers can be adapted for this use; see also **telecommunication device for the deaf (TDD)**

TTS temporary threshold shift; a change in threshold that returns to its pre-exposure level over time; temporary threshold shift is not permanent; usually seen after exposure to high-intensity noise; see also **permanent threshold shift (PTS)**

TTY teletypewriter; a communication device used by individuals with severe or profound hearing loss for communicating via the telephone channel; see also **telecommunication device for the deaf (TDD)**

tubal insert earphones earphones that are inserted into the ear canal for a better seal than circumaural or supra-aural headphones; see also **insert earphones**

tuberculum auriculae the outer portion or rim around the pinna; also known as the **helix**

tubing flexible tube that is inserted in earmolds; serves to connect the earmold to a behind-the-ear hearing aid; diameter and length can be changed to affect the acoustic properties

tubing expander hand-held instrument used to enlarge the opening of earmold tubing for easy attachment to the earhook of a behind-the-ear hearing aid

tubotympanic disease disorder of the tubotympanum (middle ear space and/or eustachian tube) that is benign or safe mucosal disease; an example of an intrinsic eustachian tube disorder

tumor an abnormal growth of tissue resulting from an excessively rapid proliferation of cells

tuning curve a graph depicting the response of a neuron, plotted as a function of stimulus intensity versus frequency; the lowest sound level to which the neuron responds is represented by the tip of the tuning curve (i.e., characteristic frequency); see also **characteristic frequency (CF), psychophysical tuning curve**

tuning fork tests evaluation procedures that use tuning forks (two-pronged metal instruments) to estimate the type and degree of hearing loss

tunnel of Corti region of the organ of Corti produced by the articulation of the rods of Corti

tunnel radial fibers efferent fibers from cranial nerve VIII that connect directly to the base of the outer hair cells

Turner syndrome disorder resulting from the deletion of an entire X chromosome characterized by short stature, webbed neck, short neck, low posterior hairline, lack of sexual development, heart anomalies, renal anomalies, small nails, osteoporosis, occasional cleft palate, and occasional cognitive impairment; associated with conductive hearing loss

TWA time-weighted average; amplitude measures in dB taken moment to moment to reflect a single decibel value that is considered to be equivalent in energy to the time-varying amplitudes experienced in the real world

tweeter a loudspeaker for reproducing high-frequency sounds usually those higher than 6000 Hz

TWF Test of Word Finding; a test that assesses the accuracy and speech of word retrieval for a child's existing vocabulary; consists of six sections; designed for children aged 6 to 12 years

two-alternative forced-choice procedure testing paradigm in which a listener must decide whether a signal is present during the first or the second observation period

2-cc coupler a precisely bored tube in a metal block that represents the volume of air occupying the human ear canal for the use of checking hearing aid conformance to manufacturers' specifications

2-cc coupler gain the amount of acoustic gain measured in a 2-cc coupler; see also **acoustic gain**

two-channel ABR an auditory brainstem response recorded using two channels allowing for ipsilateral and contralateral recordings simultaneously

2k notch bone-conduction hearing loss measured at 2000 Hz often seen in patients with otosclerosis; see also **Carhart notch**

tympanic aditus posterior-superior region of the middle ear space containing the head of the malleus and greater part of the incus; communicates upward and backward to the mastoid antrum

tympanic annulus fibrous tissue and cartilage that forms the rim of the tympanic membrane

tympanic antrum posterior-superior region of the middle ear space containing the head of the malleus and greater part of the incus; communicates upward and backward to the mastoid antrum

tympanic cavity the air-filled middle ear space

tympanic membrane (TM) the membranous separation between the outer and middle ears; responsible for initiating the mechanical impedance-matching process of the middle ear; has three layers: cutaneous, fibrous, mucous

tympanic membrane displacement procedure of assessing the mobility of the tympanic membrane in order to determine indirectly the function of the eustachian tube

tympanic membrane perforation a hole or laceration in the tympanic membrane (eardrum); may be marginal or central

tympanic membrane retraction pocket negative pressure in a portion of the tympanic membrane that forms a pocket behind the eardrum; results from abnormal middle ear pressure; see also **attic retraction pocket**

tympanic sulcus groove in the osseous portion of the external auditory meatus in which the tympanic membrane is seated

tympanogram a measure of tympanic membrane mobility as a function of changes in air pressure within the ear canal; a plot of eardrum mobility (admittance) as a function of pressure; types include **Type A, Type As, Type Ad, Type B,** and **Type C**

tympanomastoiditis infection of the mastoid and tympanic portions of the ear

tympanometric peak pressure (TPP) the pressure at which the peak of the tympanogram occurs; provides an estimate of the volume in the middle ear

tympanometric width a measure used to evaluate the shape of a tympanogram; involves measurement across the peak of the tympanogram at a level that is halfway between the baseline and the peak of the tracing; value is reported in daPa to correspond to the horizontal scale on the tympanogram; see also **gradient**

tympanometry a routine clinical procedure that involves measures of acoustic immittance as air pressure in the ear canal is varied above and below the atmospheric level; results in a plot called a **tympanogram**

tympanoplasty surgical repair of damaged or removed middle ear structures; includes operations such as myringoplasty, stapedectomy, PORP, TORP

tympanosclerosis scarring on the tympanic membrane exhibited by whitish plaques on the eardrum itself; results from chronic otitis media or repeated healed perforations

tympanostomy tubes tiny ventilating tubes that are surgically inserted through the eardrum to compensate for a malfunctioning eustachian tube by allowing ventilation of the middle ear space; see also **pressure equalization (PE) tube**

tympanotomy the surgical incision into the tympanic membrane to remove middle ear effusion; also known as **myringotomy**

tympanum the tympanic cavity of the middle ear that connects not only the posterior parts of the nose by way of the eustachian tube, but also the air-filled spaces in the mastoid bone

Type A tympanogram a tympanogram type with normal static admittance, gradient, tympanometric peak pressure, and ear canal volume that indicates normal middle ear function; see also **tympanogram**

Type Ad tympanogram a tympanogram with abnormally high static admittance, normal gradient, ear canal volume, and tympanometric peak pressure; often results from a flaccid middle ear system such as ossicular disarticulation; see also **tympanogram**

Type As tympanogram a tympanogram type characterized by abnormally low static admittance and normal ear canal volume, tympanometric peak pressure, and gradient; often associated with a stiff middle ear system such as otosclerosis; see also **tympanogram**

Type B tympanogram a flat tympanogram that indicates the possibility of middle ear fluid or tympanometric perforation (with a large ear canal volume); characterized by no peak, low static admittance, wide gradient, and variable ear canal volume; see also **tympanogram**

Type C tympanogram a tympanogram type with normal static admittance, gradient, and ear canal volume but negative tympanometric peak pressure; the negative middle ear pressure is often from impending or resolving otitis media; see also **tympanogram**

Type I fibers radial afferent fibers of cranial nerve VIII innervating inner hair cells; many fibers connect to each inner hair cell; also known as **inner radial fibers**

Type I hair cells vestibular receptor hair cells characterized by a flask shape and innervation by very large afferent nerve fibers

Type 1 sound level meter a sound measuring device that meets the most rigorous specifications; capable of performing integrating sound level measurements; used most often in any litigation involving sound measurements; see also **sound level meter (SLM)**

Type II fibers outer spiral afferent fibers of cranial nerve VIII innervating outer hair cells; each nerve fiber connects to many outer hair cells; also known as **outer spiral fibers**

Type II hair cells vestibular receptor hair cells characterized by a cylindrical shape and innervation by multiple afferent nerve fiber terminals

Type 2 sound level meter a general purpose sound measuring device that is adequate for most industrial measurements; see also **sound level meter (SLM)**

type-token ratio (TRR) the ratio of the number of different words used (types) to the total number of words used (tokens)

U

UCL uncomfortable loudness level; an intensity level at which speech or a pure-tone signal is perceived as being so loud that it causes discomfort; also known as **loudness discomfort level (LDL)**; see also **upper limit of comfortable loudness (ULCL)**

UHF ultra-high frequency; refers to frequencies that are above the conventional audiometric frequencies (e.g., 10,000 to 20,000 Hz)

ULCL upper limit of comfortable loudness; the highest level of a suprathreshold measure of speech to be amplified by a hearing instrument without overamplifying and causing discomfort; see also **maximum comfort level, uncomfortable loudness level (UCL, ULL)**

ULL uncomfortable loudness level; an intensity level at which speech or a pure-tone signal is perceived as being so loud that it causes discomfort; also known as **loudness discomfort level (LDL)**; see also **upper limit of comfortable loudness (ULCL)**

ultra-high frequency refers to frequencies that are above the conventional audiometric frequencies (e.g., 10,000 to 20,000 Hz)

ultrasound (1) sound at frequencies above the audible range (i.e., above about 20,000 Hz); (2) medical procedure used to provide images of internal structures by the reflected signals that are produced when a high-frequency signal is projected throughout the body

umbo central depressed portion of the tympanic membrane where the malleus is attached on the medial surface; the point of most concavity of the tympanic membrane; see also **tympanic membrane (TM)**

unaided response a measurement of residual hearing that quantifies a patient's response to different stimuli without the use of an amplification device

uncomfortable loudness level (UCL, ULL) an intensity level at which speech or a pure-tone signal is perceived as being so loud that it causes discomfort; also known as **loudness discomfort level (LDL)**; see also **upper limit of comfortable loudness (ULCL)**

uncrossed acoustic reflex threshold the lowest level that can activate the acoustic reflex of the middle ear by using test signals that are presented to the same ear as the measuring device (i.e., probe)

underfitted condition in which the amount of gain provided by a hearing aid is insufficient for the user's hearing loss

undermasking condition in clinical masking in which the masking level is insufficient to prevent cross hearing and the test ear is still responding to the signal; occurs when the presentation level minus the masking level is greater than interaural attenuation

unidirectional microphone a microphone that is more sensitive to sound coming from one direction than from another direction; also known as **directional microphone**

unilateral one side; affecting one side or one ear; see also **bilateral**

unilateral deafness a patient with total deafness in one ear and normal hearing in the other

unilateral hearing loss a patient with some degree and type of hearing loss in one ear and better or normal hearing in the other; see also **bilateral hearing loss**

unilateral tinnitus the experience of tinnitus (ringing) in only one ear; see also **tinnitus**

unisensory unimodal; used to refer to an educational philosophy in which stimulation is presented primarily through the auditory modality; see also **auditory-verbal approach**

unity acoustic gain term used to describe the condition in which the hearing aid provides neither amplification nor attenuation of the incoming sound

universal newborn hearing screening a screening program adopted by many states since the 1993 National Institutes of Health (NIH) consensus statement recommending that all newborns (those who are healthy and at risk) have their hearing screened to promote early identification of hearing loss; see also **neonatal screening**

universal precautions exercising caution when handling hearing instruments, cerumen, earphones, etc., that may be contaminated with fresh blood or dried blood; precautions taken to prevent disease transmission including hand washing, use of protective barriers (e.g., gloves, eye protection, masks, etc.), disinfection, and sterilization

University of Oklahoma Closed-Response Speech Test (UOCRT) a closed-set monosyllabic word-identification test designed to minimize word frequency, familiarity, and contextual cue effects so that any errors are due to the acoustic characteristics of the phonemes

unmasked a response obtained with no masking presented to the nontest ear

unmasked threshold pure-tone or speech threshold obtained with no masking presented to the nontest ear

unoccluded not blocked; open; e.g., the normal external auditory meatus is unoccluded

UOCRT University of Oklahoma Closed-Response Speech Test; a closed-set monosyllabic word-identification test designed to minimize word frequency, familiarity, and contextual cue effects so that any errors are due to the acoustic characteristics of the phonemes

up-beating nystagmus type of vertical nystagmus in which the fast phase beats upward; can be pathological

upper cutoff frequency the frequency parameter of a filter that designates the 3-dB down point for which the amplitude of the response is 3 dB less than the amplitude at its highest frequency

upper limit of comfortable loudness (ULCL) the highest level of a suprathreshold measure of speech to be amplified by a hearing instrument without overamplifying and causing discomfort; see also **maximum comfort level, uncomfortable loudness level (UCL, ULL)**

upward spread of masking the effect of masking that spreads from low-frequency sounds to high-frequency sounds; often occurs in speech where weaker high-frequency consonants are masked by stronger low-frequency phonemes such as vowels

use gain amount of gain provided by a hearing aid when the volume control is set where it is commonly used by the wearer

user control component of a hearing instrument that influences its operation; can be changed by the patient or by the hearing health care professional

Usher syndrome autosomal recessive disorder characterized by retinitis pigmentosa with night blindness followed by visual deterioration in adult life with blindness in approximately half of cases, occasional ataxia and mental illness; associated with variable severity of sensorineural hearing loss, ranging from moderate to profound, usually sloping to most severe in the high frequencies

Utley lipreading test a diagnostic test of speechreading/lipreading ability the results of which can be used to measure the appropriateness of school placement and progress, to monitor the growth and development of the individual, and to compare the effectiveness of different methodologies and teaching techniques

utricular macula vestibular sensory epithelia on the lateral wall of the utricle

utricle one of two sacs within the membranous labyrinth of the inner ear that communicates with the semicircular canals; contains sensory epithelia called macula and is responsible for providing information about the static system of balance; see also **saccule**

utriculitis inflammation of the utricle

utriculofugal stimulation caused by endolymph movement away from the utricle of the horizontal semicircular canals; see also **utriculopetal**

utriculopetal stimulation caused by endolymph movement toward the utricle of the horizontal semicircular canals; see also **utriculofugal**

V

V volt; unit of force or electrical potential; pressure that causes the current of 1 ampere to flow through the resistance of 1 ohm

vacuum tube a sealed glass tube with little or no air; electrodes from the outside project from it; component of early hearing aids

vagus nerve cranial nerve X named for its wandering course that extends through the neck, thorax, and abdomen; provides neural innervation to the external ear and the speech mechanism including the larynx, tongue, and palate

validity how closely a test reflects what it is supposed to measure; when a measurement produces the desired results; types include **concurrent, construct, content, criterion-related, external, internal,** and **face**

validity, concurrent criterion-related validity index employed to predict real-life performance

validity, construct statistical term meaning the extent to which a test measures what it is supposed to measure, usually a trait or a skill; the extent to which a test measurement corresponds to theoretical concepts (as when a measure expected to vary over time does so)

validity, content statistical term referring to the extent to which a test adequately samples what it is supposed to measure (the domain studied); e.g., measurement for sentence perception would include sentence or phrase stimuli

validity, criterion-related test effectiveness of an individual's behavior or abilities in specific situations

validity, external generalizability of results; results can lead to unbiased inferences about the target population and not just the study subjects

validity, face how well test items represent what they claim to test

validity, internal variability between the control and comparison groups may, other than sampling error, be from the effect being studied

Valsalva maneuver inflation of the middle ear produced by closing the mouth and pinching the nose and then exhaling (forcing) air through the eustachian tube; see also **Toynbee maneuver**

Van Buchem syndrome autosomal recessive disorder characterized by osteosclerosis, compression of cranial nerves with sequella; associated with late onset hearing loss, mixed or sensorineural due to osteosclerosis

van der Hoeve disease autosomal dominant disorder characterized by bone fragility, blue sclerae, and dental anomalies; associated with conductive hearing loss related to fixation of the footplate of the stapes or fracture of the ossicles; sensorineural and mixed hearing loss are also common, all of late onset; also known as **osteogenesis imperfecta**

variable release time compression circuitry that provides changeable release times depending on the duration of the input signal; release time decreases as the duration of the signal decreases

variable venting valve (VVV) a device that can be inserted into the vent of an earmold or hearing aid to change its diameter

vascular presbycusis a type of hearing loss due to aging that is caused by vascular insufficiency (i.e., poor levels of oxygen or other blood-borne metabolites) to the cochlea; see also **presbycusis**

VC (1) volume control; the dial on hearing aids and cochlear implants that controls the loudness of the sound transmitted through the device; (2) vowel-consonant; a nonsense syllable or real word comprised of a vowel followed by a consonant (e.g., ab, ad, ag, at, it)

VCN ventral cochlear nucleus; one of the nuclei in the cochlear nucleus complex that is part of the auditory pathway and acoustic reflex arc; sound that leaves the cochlea by

way of cranial nerve VIII travels first to the ventral cochlear nucleus

VCV vowel-consonant-vowel; a nonsense syllable comprised of a vowel followed by a consonant followed by a vowel (e.g., aba, ada, aga)

vector tympanogram an immittance measure involving the use of one low-frequency probe tone (typically 226 Hz) and the measurement of one component, generally the acoustic admittance vector

velo-cardio-facial syndrome autosomal dominant disorder characterized by cleft palate, heart anomalies, facies characterized by a long nose with bulbous or dimpled tip and prominent root, puffy upper eyelids, small ears with attached lobules and overfolded helices, learning disabilities, attention deficit hyperactivity disorder (ADHD), eventual mental illness, scoliosis, immune deficiency, vascular anomalies, kidney anomalies, feeding difficulties, hypotonia; associated with conductive hearing loss caused by chronic middle ear disease, sensorineural hearing loss found in approximately 15% and may be unilateral or bilateral, usually mild although moderate to severe cases have been seen

velocity a vector quantity that specifies time rate of change of displacement

venous hum tinnitus the sensation of a "humming" sound (ringing in the ears) resulting from a venous disorder; see also **tinnitus**

vent an opening (e.g., 1 mm or 2 mm in diameter) traveling from the lateral face to the medial tip of an earmold or hearing aid; used for pressure equalization and sound transmission; see also **venting**

vent, diagonal type of vent that runs up to the sound bore and branches into it (i.e., intersects the sound bore); results in a decrease in high-frequency gain of as much as 10 dB more than a parallel vent; the effect increases as vent diameter increases; also known as **side-branching vent**

vent, parallel a bore made in an earmold or hearing aid that is parallel to the sound bore and runs from outside the mold to the external auditory meatus

vent, pressure a bore made in an earmold or hearing aid that is approximately 0.06 to 0.8 mm in diameter; has no measurable effect on the frequency response but provides pressure equalization in the external auditory meatus

vent, side-branching type of vent that runs up to the sound bore and branches into it (i.e., intersects the sound bore); results in a decrease in high-frequency gain of as much as 10 dB more than a parallel vent; the effect increases as vent diameter increases; also known as **diagonal vent**

ventilation tube a tube that is inserted in the eardrum of individuals suffering from otitis media; used to help ventilate and equalize pressure within and outside the middle ear; also known as a **grommet**; see also **pressure equalization (PE) tube**

venting a modification of an earmold in which an additional tube is bored next to or into the existing sound tube; it has a considerable effect on low-frequency responses depending on the size of the hole bored; see also **vent**

ventral toward the front; referring to a position toward the front of the body

ventral cochlear nucleus (VCN) one of the nuclei in the cochlear nucleus complex that is part of the auditory pathway and acoustic reflex arc; sound that leaves the cochlea by way of cranial nerve VIII travels first to the ventral cochlear nucleus; see also **cochlear nucleus (CN)**

VEP visual evoked potential; activity in visual organs (e.g., retina), pathways (e.g., optic nerve and tracts), and centers of the brain (e.g., calcarine fissure in the occipital lobe) that is elicited by photic (light) stimuli and recorded with electrodes

verbotonal method an aural rehabilitation method founded by Peter Guberina that involves auditory training of a person who is hearing impaired by maximizing input at those frequencies where the most residual hearing exists; often uses tactile stimulation

vertebrobasilar vascular insufficiency a reduction in the flow of blood to the vertebral and basilar arteries that supply nutrients to the inner ear; often results in vertiginous episodes

vertex (1) a location on top of the head, in the center, defined as the intersection of lines constructed from one external ear canal to the other and from front to back along the midline (nasion to inion); (2) a common electrode site in evoked potential measurement

vertex electrode the electrode placed on the top of the head in the center; the active (noninverting) electrode used in auditory brainstem response measurement

vertical semicircular canal the uppermost of the three canals of the vestibular system that contains the sense organs (crista ampularis) for responding to angular motion; also known as the **superior semicircular canal**; see also **semicircular canals (SCCs)**

vertigo a vestibular symptom in which the patient has a spinning sensation or senses that the environment is spinning around; may have many causes; types include **benign paroxysmal positioning, objective, paroxysmal, positional,** and **subjective**

vertigo, benign paroxysmal positioning (BPPV) a specific vestibular disorder that causes vertigo, lightheadedness, and rotatory nystagmus when provoked by head motion or changes in body position (e.g., Dix Hallpike maneuver); vertigo is sudden and brief and may be accompanied by nausea and vomiting; often seen in older persons

vertigo, objective the sensation that the room is spinning around the patient

vertigo, paroxysmal sudden, brief sensation of dizziness and spinning often accompanied by nausea and vomiting; see also **benign paroxysmal positioning vertigo (BPPV)**

vertigo, positional dizziness and the sensation of spinning with specific stationary head positions

vertigo, subjective the sensation that the patient is spinning

vestibular aqueduct a part of the bony labyrinth running from the labyrinth to the posterior surface of the petrous bone containing one or more small veins and the endolymphatic duct

vestibular dysfunction inappropriate functioning of the vestibular system

vestibular evaluation diagnostic techniques used to assess the function of the vestibular system that might include electronystagmography, rotary chair testing, posturography, and medical evaluation

vestibular hypofunction a diminished or inadequate level of activity in the vestibular system

vestibular labyrinth intricate passageways within the vestibular portion of the inner ear including the membranous semicircular canals, utricle, and saccule, and the bony semicircular canals and vestibule

vestibular labyrinthitis inflammation of the labyrinthine semicircular canals of the vestibular portion of the inner ear

vestibular membrane structure separating the cochlear duct from the vestibular canal

vestibular Ménière's disease form of Ménière's disease that has only vestibular symptoms; no hearing loss is present

vestibular nerve branch of cranial nerve VIII responsible for carrying balance sensations to the brain; runs alongside the auditory and facial nerves inside the internal auditory canal

vestibular neurectomy surgical procedure that involves cutting the vestibular nerve

vestibular neuronitis a sudden, severe attack of vertigo (dizziness) that is not associated with any hearing loss; results from inflammation of the vestibular nerve often caused by an upper respiratory infection

vestibular nuclei the first stop in the central vestibular system where the vestibular nerve fibers synapse; there are four vestibular nuclei: superior, inferior, lateral, and medial

vestibular rehabilitation procedures followed after an operation on the vestibular system in which patients learn what they can and cannot do as a result of the surgery; the limiting factors to a patient's activity are often disequilibrium, fatigue, or headache

vestibular schwannoma neoplasm typically arising on the vestibular

portion of the eighth nerve that often begins in the Schwann cells surrounding the nerve

vestibular system the portion of the inner ear, comprised of the saccule, utricle, and semicircular canals, that functions to regulate balance; it coordinates changes in head position, acceleration and deceleration, and gravitational effects

vestibular tinnitus a clinical type of tinnitus reflecting dysfunction of the vestibular labyrinth; see also **tinnitus**

vestibule bony cavity within the temporal bone connecting the vestibular semicircular canals and the cochlea; the oval window in the vestibule permits communication with the middle ear; contains the utricle and saccule

vestibulo-ocular reflex (VOR) (1) a central vestibular-ocular pathway whose function is assessed during caloric electronystagmography; a response to angular acceleration (head turn); (2) when the head is turned to the right, there is excitation of the left lateral rectus and right medial rectus eye muscles so that the eyes are turned to the left

vestibulo-spinal reflex a central vestibular-spinal pathway that plays a major role in vestibular reflex reactions initiated by head movements; helps maintain neck muscles to stabilize the position of the head

vestibulocochlear nerve cranial nerve VIII with its auditory and vestibular branches

vestibulocochlear neuritis an inflammatory disorder of cranial nerve VIII

vestibulotoxicity deterioration of the vestibular system due to ingestion of ototoxic drugs; the poisonous effect of toxic substances to the sense organs of the membranous labyrinth (e.g., cristae and maculae); see also **ototoxicity, cochleotoxicity**

vibration continuing or periodic motion; see also **forced vibration, free vibration, simple harmonic motion (SHM)**

vibrotactile pertaining to the detection of vibrations through the sense of touch

vibrotactile aid an assistive listening device that converts acoustic energy into vibratory patterns that are delivered to the skin; different systems are available that can be single or multichannel and that have different processing strategies; see also **Tactaid**

vibrotactile response the sensation of feeling a stimulus rather than hearing the signal when high intensities at low frequencies of 250 and 500 Hz are presented

video otoscope a simple, compact unit that incorporates a rod system, fiberoptic illumination, and a high-resolution color video camera capable of recording images of patients' ear canals and tympanic membranes

VIIIth nerve cranial nerve VIII, known as the vestibulocochlear nerve consisting of vestibular and cochlear branches

VIOLA visual input/output locator algorithm; tool used as part of the Independent Hearing Aid Fitting Forum (IHAFF) protocol to determine the electroacoustic characteristics of a hearing aid to allow soft sounds to be judged as soft and audible, average speech to be judged as comfortable, and loud speech to be judged as loud, but okay; see also **Independent Hearing Aid Fitting Forum (IHAFF)**

viral labyrinthitis inflammation of the labyrinthine systems as a result of a pathogenic virus; potential etiologies include **rubella, mumps, measles, herpes zoster oticus**

virus a group of microscopic organisms that, with few exceptions, can pass through filters that retain bacteria; they are incapable of growth or reproduction outside living cells

viseme a speech sound that sounds different but appears identical on the lips (e.g., p, b, m); see also **homophene**

Visipitch computer-based device that displays speech spectrograms, spectral displays, or F2 versus F1 formant displays; often requires articulatory interpretation to the displayed acoustic pattern

visual alerting systems assistive devices that include alarm clocks, doorbells, and smoke detectors in which the altering mechanism is a flashing light; useful for individuals with profound deafness

visual coding the process of visually associating the place of the oral mechanism with words or letters

visual evoked potential (VEP) activity in visual organs (e.g., retina), pathways (e.g., optic nerve and tracts), and centers of the brain (e.g., calcarine fissure in the occipital lobe) that is elicited by photic (light) stimuli and recorded with electrodes

visual input/output locator algorithm (VIOLA) tool used as part of the Independent Hearing Aid Fitting Forum (IHAFF) protocol to determine the electroacoustic characteristics of a hearing aid to allow soft sounds to be judged as soft and audible, average speech to be judged as comfortable, and loud speech to be judged as loud, but okay; see also **Independent Hearing Aid Fitting Forum (IHAFF)**

visual reinforcement audiometry (VRA) a pediatric behavioral audiometry procedure that reinforces localization responses to acoustic signals with a visual event (e.g., an animal playing an instrument); see also **visual reinforcement operant conditioning audiometry (VROCA), tangible reinforcement operant conditioning audiometry (TROCA)**

visual reinforcement operant conditioning audiometry (VROCA) a behavioral procedure used in pediatric audiometry that reinforces localization responses to acoustic signals with a visual event (e.g., an animal playing a musical instrument); it differs from visual reinforcement audiometry in that the child can manipulate the reinforcer; see also **visual reinforcement audiometry (VRA), tangible reinforcement operant conditioning audiometry (TROCA)**

visual-analog scale a type of graphical rating scale used to obtain subjective estimates of values of perceptual stimuli on a relevant psychological dimension by having a subject make marks at points along undifferentiated straight lines

vocal folds muscles and connective tissue located within the larynx used to produce voice (through vocal fold vibration); the two vocal folds are attached anteriorly to the thyroid cartilage and posteriorly to the arytenoid cartilages

vocoder a device that transposes the frequencies of speech into some equivalent signal such as vibratory stimulation

voice-onset time (VOT) the amount of time it takes for the voicing of a sound to begin; measure used to distinguish voiced and voiceless consonants

voiced speech produced using the vibrating vocal folds; all vowels are voiced and some consonants are voiced (e.g., /b, g, d, n, m/); see also **voiceless, voicing**

voiceless phonemes produced without the use of the vocal folds; some consonants are voiceless (e.g., /p, k, t, s, ʃ/); see also **voiced, voicing**

voicing classification of a speech sound according to whether it is produced with or without voice (e.g., /b/ versus /p/)

volley principle one of the theories of hearing that postulates that when the frequency limits of a nerve fiber are reached, additional and adjacent nerve fibers become activated; these nerves fire as a volley of activity allowing the brain to perceive the combined input

volt (V) unit of force or electrical potential; pressure that causes the current of 1 ampere to flow through the resistance of 1 ohm

voltmeter an instrument that measures the number of volts between any two points in an electric circuit; used to test batteries when troubleshooting amplification devices

volume (1) the aspect of auditory sensation in which sounds may be ordered on a scale running from "small" to "large;" the volume of a tone increases with increased intensity, but decreases with increased frequency; (2) intensity adjustment via gain control or volume control

volume conduction instantaneous transmission or conduction of electrical activity from a neural generator through a medium to a relatively distant point

volume control (VC) the dial on hearing aids and cochlear implants that controls the loudness of the sound transmitted through the device

volume unit (VU) meter a device that records the exact output level produced in order to permit precise presentation of auditory signals in decibels

von Recklinghausen's disease (NF-1) neurofibromatosis; a neuropathologic disease that is characterized by tumors within the central nervous system that may involve one or both auditory nerves and may cause auditory evoked potential abnormalities; also known as **neurofibromatosis;** see also **NF-2**

VOR vestibulo-ocular reflex; (1) a central vestibular-ocular pathway whose function is assessed during caloric electronystagmography; a response to angular acceleration (head turn); (2) when the head is turned to the right, there is excitation of the left lateral rectus and right medial rectus eye muscles so that the eyes are turned to the left

VOT voice onset time; the amount of time it takes for the voicing of a sound to begin; measure used to distinguish voiced and voiceless consonants

vowel a speech sound identified by its unrestricted voice flow

vowel discrimination the ability to determine whether vowels are the same or different; see also **vowel recognition**

vowel recognition the identification of vowels based on cues in the speech signal (e.g., vowel duration, loudness, and spectral composition); see also **vowel discrimination**

vowel spectra the frequency composition of vowel sounds based on hearing level in dB HL as a function of frequency in Hz

vowel-consonant (VC) a nonsense syllable or a real word comprised of a vowel followed by a consonant (e.g., ab, ad, ag, at, it)

vowel-consonant-vowel (VCV) a nonsense syllable comprised of a vowel followed by a consonant followed by a vowel (e.g., aba, ada, aga)

VRA visual reinforcement audiometry; a pediatric behavioral audiometry procedure that reinforces localization responses to acoustic signals with a visual event (e.g., an animal playing an instrument); see also **visual reinforcement operant conditioning audiometry (VROCA), tangible reinforcement operant conditioning audiometry (TROCA)**

VROCA visual reinforcement operant conditioning audiometry; a behavioral procedure used in pediatric audiometry that reinforces localization responses to acoustic signals with a visual event (e.g., an animal playing a musical instrument); it differs from visual reinforcement audiometry in that the child can manipulate the reinforcer; see also **visual reinforcement audiometry (VRA), tangible reinforcement operant conditioning audiometry (TROCA)**

VU volume unit; a device that records the exact output level produced in order to permit precise presentation of auditory signals in decibels; also known as **VU meter**

VU meter a device that records the exact output level produced in order to permit precise presentation of auditory signals in decibels

VVV variable venting valve; a device that can be inserted into the vent of an earmold or hearing aid to change its diameter

W

W watt; a unit of electrical power equal to a flow of 1 ampere under the force of 1 volt in an electric circuit

W-1 CID W-1 test; early test of speech perception measuring threshold of intelligibility; developed at the Central Institute for the Deaf (CID)

W-2 CID W-2 test; open-set test for rapid estimation of the intelligibility threshold by sweeping intensity; developed at the Central Institute for the Deaf (CID)

W-22 CID W-22 test; monosyllabic word-recognition test with multiple randomized lists; developed at the Central Institute for the Deaf (CID)

Waardenburg syndrome autosomal dominant integumentary disorder characterized by pigmentary anomalies of hair and skin (depigmentation), a broad nasal root, widely spaced medial canthai, confluent eyebrows, a white forelock in the hair, a characteristically shaped mouth, heterochromia iridium (two different colored eyes), and occasional cleft lip and palate; associated with a variable degree of sensorineural hearing loss, ranging from mild to severe, usually flat or U-shaped audiograms

Walsh-Healey noise standard basis of Department of Labor regulations established in 1969 for setting allowable levels and durations of noise exposure

warble tone (WT) acoustic signal produced by modifying a pure tone with small and rapid changes in frequency; used in sound-field audiometry to minimize the likelihood of standing waves

watt (W) a unit of electrical power equal to a flow of 1 ampere under the force of 1 volt in an electric circuit

wave a disturbance that is propagated in a medium as a function of time; the amount of disturbance is reflected in the displacement at any point

wave, longitudinal a pressure wave that moves in a medium in the direction that the sound wave travels; motion is parallel to wave movement

wave, mucosal undulation along the vocal fold surface traveling in the direction of the airflow

wave, sound the acoustical manifestation of physical disturbance in a medium

wave, surface a wave that moves along a surface; the vertical-phase difference observed on the vocal fold during vibration

wave, transverse wave that moves in a medium perpendicular to the direction that the sound wave travels; motion is at right angles to wave movement

wave, traveling the wavelike action of the basilar membrane arising from stimulation of the perilymph of the scala vestibuli and scala tympani; the traveling wave moves from the base of the cochlea to the apex, and the point of maximum displacement of the basilar membrane indicates the frequency location where the stimulus is perceived; also known as **Békésy traveling wave**

wave I the first component or bump of the auditory brainstem response recording, normally occurring at about 1.5 ms and generated in the distal region of cranial nerve VIII

wave II an auditory brainstem response component normally occurring at about 2.5 ms and generated within the lower portion of the auditory brainstem, possibly in the cochlear nucleus

wave III an auditory brainstem response component normally occurring at about 3.5 ms and generated within the lower (pons) portion of the auditory brainstem

wave IV an auditory brainstem response component normally occurring at about 4.5 ms and generated within the upper (pons or midbrain) portion of the auditory brainstem

wave propagation movement of a wave through an elastic medium such as air; the speed of sound in air is 1130 ft/sec

wave V an auditory brainstem response component normally occurring at about 5.5 ms and thought to be generated within the upper (pons or midbrain) portion of the auditory brainstem; the most robust wave in the auditory brainstem response

waveform may be acoustic or electrophysiologic; (1) a disturbance that is propagated in a medium as a function of time; the amount of disturbance is reflected in the displacement at any point; (2) for evoked potentials, it is a series of waves or fluctuations in voltage with a characteristic normal waveform

waveform acceleration the quality of a wave that changes velocity, either positive or negative; the time-rate change in velocity

waveform analysis the process of decomposing any complex waveform to determine the amplitudes, frequencies, and phases of the sine waves that make up the complex wave; also known as **Fourier analysis**

waveform envelope in acoustics, the shape of the overall waveform of an acoustic stimulus that follows the rise, plateau, and fall portions of the stimulus; also known as **envelope**

waveform morphology the qualitative features of an evoked potential; considers the "noisiness," the "smoothness," and the replicability of the recording, and how the recording compares to an ideal recording

wavelength (λ) the distance between the same point (determined in degrees) on two successive cycles of a tone (i.e., from the beginning of one wave to the beginning of the next); calculated by the speed of sound in air (1130 ft/sec)/f, where f = frequency

wax a substance secreted from the combination of the sebaceous and ceruminous glands in the outer ear canal; helps lubricate, protect, and cleanse the ear canal; also known as **cerumen, ear wax**

WDRC wide-dynamic range compression; a type of compression circuitry that can provide much greater amplification for low-intensity signals than for medium-intensity signals while providing less or no gain for high-intensity signals; useful for individuals with a very narrow dynamic range; has a low compression threshold; see also **syllabic compression**

wearable speech processor component of a cochlear implant that helps with signal processing, especially in frequencies used for speech perception

Weber fraction the expression of a difference threshold in terms of the proportional or relative change in the stimulus that is detectable; provides information about whether there is regularity in the size of difference limen across the stimulus range, i.e., if there is a consistent relationship between the standard stimuli and the increment needed to judge a change in the stimuli; the Weber fraction is a ratio that is calculated as the absolute difference limen divided by the standard level of the stimulus

Weber test a tuning fork test in which bone-conducted signals are presented to a midline site on the frontal bone; the sound lateralizes to the ear with the conductive hearing loss (middle ear dysfunction); see also **tuning fork tests**

Wechsler Intelligence Scale for Children (WISC) an assessment of verbal language and speech that uses four verbal subtests

weighting the filter circuitry setting of a sound level meter that can be adjusted to meet different sound measurement conditions; see also **weighting scale**

weighting scale sound level meter filtering network in which the measurement of one band of frequencies is emphasized over another; see also **dBA, dBB, dBC, weighting**

Wernicke's aphasia fluent, mostly receptive language disorder caused by cerebral cortex dysfunction in the posterior temporal lobe of the dominant hemisphere for language which may include deficits in comprehension, jargon speech, and word-finding problems

whisper test an unstandardized method of providing a rough estimate of an individual's hearing; single words or short sentences are whispered to the patient

white noise (WN) a broadband noise with approximately equal energy per cycle; the bandwidth is limited by the characteristics of the transducer

whole nerve action potential (1) gross neural potential; summed or averaged activity of action potentials of cranial nerve VIII in response to acoustic stimulation; (2) in auditory evoked potential measurements, it is the whole-nerve response of cranial nerve VIII; (3) the main component of the electrocochleogram and wave I of the auditory brainstem response; also known as **action potential (AP)**

wide-band noise a band of noise covering a wide range of frequencies; e.g., **white noise**; also known as **broad-band noise (BBN)**

wide-dynamic range compression (WDRC) a type of compression circuitry that can provide much greater amplification for low-intensity signals than for medium-intensity signals while providing less or no gain for high-intensity signals; useful for individuals with a very narrow dynamic range; has a low compression threshold; see also **syllabic compression**

Wildervanck syndrome characterized by facial asymmetry, Klippel-Feil anomaly (cervical vertebrae fusion), Duane syndrome (eye motility disorder), occasional cognitive impairment, occasional cleft palate; associated with mixed or sensorineural hearing loss, occasionally purely conductive, occasionally unilateral, ranges from mild to severe

Williams syndrome disorder characterized by cognitive impairment, short stature, heart anomalies, hypercalcemia, microcephaly, large mouth, thick lips, microdontia, enamel hypoplasia, limited joint movement, scoliosis strabismus, hypertension, hyperopia; associated with hyperacusis

windscreen a covering placed over the microphone inlet of an amplification device to keep wind noise, breath, and low-frequency energy out of the sound system

WIPI Word Intelligibility by Picture Identification; a picture pointing pediatric speech audiometry procedure consisting of six color pictures depicting words that are phonetically similar

wireless microphone the microphone component of a wireless transmitter; see also **wireless system**

wireless system consists of an FM transmitter and an FM receiver; the speaker and listener are connected by radio waves not wires

wireless transmitter a battery-powered FM transmitter; part of a wireless system; see also **wireless system**

WIS word-identification score; percent correct score reflecting the number of word stimuli perceived correctly in speech perception testing; also known as **word-recognition score (WRS)**

WISC Wechsler Intelligence Scale for Children; an assessment of verbal language and speech that uses four verbal subtests

WNL within normal limits

WN white noise; a broadband noise with approximately equal energy per cycle; the bandwidth is limited by the characteristics of the transducer

woofer a loudspeaker for producing sounds below the treble register, or usually below 500 Hz and always below 1500 Hz

word deafness term used to describe a characteristic of receptive aphasia; the inability to understand the words of spoken language; not considered to be a peripheral hearing problem

word discrimination outdated term referring to the percentage of monosyllabic words correctly repeated when presented at an intensity well above the speech recognition threshold; more appropriate term is **word recognition**

Word Intelligibility by Picture Identification (WIPI) a picture pointing pediatric speech audiometry procedure consisting of six color pictures depicting words that are phonetically similar

Word List, CID W-22 monosyllabic word-recognition test with multiple randomized lists; developed at the Central Institute for the Deaf (CID)

Word List, Kindergarten Phonetically Balanced (PB-K) phonetically balanced (PB) lists of monosyllabic words used to test speech recognition by young children

Word List, NU-6 commonly used test of phonetically balanced monosyllabic word lists; a word-recognition test

Word Lists, Gardner High-Frequency an open-set monosyllabic word-identification test designed to provide an accurate measure of the effects from earmold modifications for those with high-frequency sensorineural hearing loss

Word Lists, Harvard PB-50 word-identification lists that were developed in 1948 that are highly sensitive to differences in hearing loss among patients

Word Lists, Short Isophonemic speech perception test consisting of 15 different lists each with the same 30 phonemes arranged to form 10 consonant-vowel-consonant (CVC) words; designed to solve some of the problems inherent in tests that measure speech understanding

word recognition a patient's ability to perceive and correctly identify a set of words usually presented at suprathreshold intensities

word-identification score (WIS) percent correct score reflecting the number of word stimuli perceived correctly in speech perception testing; also known as **word-recognition score (WRS)**

word-recognition score (WRS) percent correct score reflecting the number of word stimuli perceived correctly in speech perception testing

word-recognition test a speech audiometry measure that typically uses monosyllabic words presented at a suprathreshold level in an open-set format; provides an assessment of a patient's speech understanding as a percent correct score

WRS word-recognition score; percent correct score reflecting the number of word stimuli perceived correctly in speech perception testing; also known as **word-identification score (WIS)**

WT warble tone; acoustic signal produced by modifying a pure tone with small and rapid changes in frequency; used in sound-field audiometry to minimize the likelihood of standing waves

X (1) symbol used to reflect an unmasked, left ear, air-conduction threshold on an audiogram; (2) acoustic reactance; the opposition to alternating current or motion

X-linked inheritance inherited form of genes located on the X chromosome; X-linked traits pass on only from mother to son; also known as **sex-linked inheritance**

X-linked mixed hearing loss a mixed type hearing loss resulting from a morphogenetic defect of the inner ear and a widening of the internal auditory meatus through which the auditory nerve leaves the inner ear

X-linked nonsyndromic hearing loss congenital hearing loss due to hereditary factors that is not associated with any other syndromal attributes

X-linked sensorineural hearing loss a sensorineural hearing loss due to a genetic defect

X-ray electromagnetic radiation that can penetrate most substances used to determine the integrity of certain structures of interest

x-y recorder a device that displays the relationship between two variables on the x and y axes; used in Békésy audiometry

xeroderma pigmentosa autosomal recessive disorder characterized by skin hypersensitivity to sunlight, skin lesions and possible malignancy, occasional short stature, cognitive impairment, neuropathy, small genitals; associated with progressive sensorineural hearing loss

Y

Y admittance; the reciprocal of impedance; the amount of energy flow through the middle ear system

y-cord used with body-style hearing aids to transmit electrical signals to two ear-level receivers; bilateral, not truly binaural

yes-no test a test used to determine auditory thresholds in children who are malingering; patients are instructed to say "yes" when they hear a tone and "no" when they do not; see also **pseudohypacusis**

Z

Z impedance; opposition to the flow of energy; the reciprocal of admittance; expressed in ohms

z check a check of the interelectrode impedance for auditory evoked potential testing

zero reference curves minimal audible pressure and minimal audible field sound pressure levels curves developed by Sivian and White; see also **minimal audible field, minimal audible pressure**

zero-crossing an algorithm used by computer systems to identify the fundamental frequency of a complex (speech) signal

zeta noise blocker early form of digital signal processing applied to hearing instruments to reduce noise; based on temporal characteristics of the noise

zinc-air battery a hearing aid battery with an adhesive tab to cover tiny air holes; once the tab is removed, the battery is activated by exposure to the air and is ready for use; has a long shelf life until the tab is removed; see also **mercury battery**

zona arcuata medial portion of the basilar membrane supporting the structures from the outer rods of Corti medially to the inner hair cells; see also **basilar membrane**

zona pectinata portion of the basilar membrane supporting the structures from the outer rods of Corti laterally to the spiral ligament; see also **basilar membrane**

Zwislocki coupler a 1.5-cc device for coupling a hearing aid for measurements of hearing aid performance developed in 1970; more closely resembles the real ear than the commonly used 2-cc coupler; see also **1.5-cc coupler**

zygomatic arch prominent portion of the zygomatic bone that is attached to the lateral surface of the squamous portion of the temporal bone

zygomatic bone portion of the facial bone that is inferior to the eye socket and adjacent with the temporal and frontal bones of the skull; the zygomatic process is attached to the lateral surface of the squamous portion of the temporal bone

APPENDIX

A

Acronyms

AAA American Academy of Audiology, p. 1

AAO-HNS American Academy of Otolaryngology-Head and Neck Surgery, p. 1

AABER aided auditory brainstem evoked response, p. 1

AABR automated auditory brainstem response audiometry, p. 1

AAS American Auditory Society, p. 1

ABG air-bone gap, p. 1

ABI auditory behavior index; auditory brainstem implant, p. 1

ABLB alternate binaural loudness balancing, p. 2

ABONSO automated brain operated noise suppressor option, p. 2

ABR auditory brainstem response, p. 2

AC air conduction; alternating current, p. 2

ACE Award for Continuing Education, p. 3

Ach acetylcholine, p. 3

AD auris dextra (right ear), p. 7

ADA Academy of Dispensing Audiologists; Americans with Disabilities Act, p. 7

ADC analog-to-digital converter, p. 7

ADD attention deficit disorder, p. 7

ADHD attention deficit and hyperactivity disorder, p. 8

AEP auditory evoked potential, p. 8

AER auditory evoked response, p. 8

AFR adaptive frequency response, p. 8

AG Bell Alexander Graham Bell Association for the Deaf, p. 9

AGC automatic gain control, p. 9

AGC-I automatic gain control-input, p. 9

AGC-O automatic gain control-output, p. 9

AI articulation index; audibility index, p. 9

AIDS acquired immunodeficiency syndrome, p. 10

AIT auditory integration therapy, p. 27

AJA American Journal of Audiology, p. 10

ALD assistive listening device, p. 10

ALR auditory late response, p. 11

ALS adrenoleukodystrophy, p. 11

AM amplitude modulation, p. 12

AMA American Medical Association, p. 12

AMLB alternate monaural loudness balancing, p. 13

AMLR auditory middle latency response, p. 13

amp ampere, p. 13

AN acoustic neuroma; auditory nerve, p. 15

ANOVA analysis of variance, p. 16

ANS autonomic nervous system, p. 16

ANSI American National Standards Institute, p. 16

ANT Auditory Numbers Test, p. 28

AP action potential, p. 17

APHAB Abbreviated Profile of Hearing Aid Benefit, p. 17

APR auropalpebral reflex, p. 18

AR acoustic reflex; auditory rehabilitation, p. 18

ARA Academy of Rehabilitative Audiology, p. 18

ARC auditory response cradle, p. 18

ARO Association for Research in Otolaryngology, p. 18

ART acoustic reflex threshold, p. 19

AS auris sinistra (left ear), p. 19

ASA American Standards Association, p. 19

ASHA American Speech-Language-Hearing Association, p. 19

ASL American Sign Language, p. 19

ASP adaptive signal processing; automatic signal processing, p. 20

ASR automatic speech recognition, p. 20

AT attack time; auditory trainer, p. 20

ATA American Tinnitus Association, p. 20

AU aures unitas (both ears), p. 21

AuD doctor of audiology, p. 21

AVC automatic volume control, p. 32

AVCN anterior ventral cochlear nucleus, p. 32

B susceptance, p. 34

BAEP brainstem auditory evoked potential, p. 34

BAER brainstem auditory evoked response, p. 34

BBN broad-band noise, p. 36

BC bone conduction, p. 36

BEAM brain electrical activity mapping, p. 36

BHI Better Hearing Institute, p. 38

BI-CROS bilateral contralateral routing of signals, p. 38

BILL bass increase at low levels, p. 39

BMLD binaural masking level difference, p. 40

BOA behavioral observation audiometry, p. 42

BP bipolar stimulation, p. 44

BP+1 bipolar plus one, p. 44

BP+2 bipolar plus two, p. 44

BP+3 bipolar plus three, p. 44

BPPN benign paroxysmal positional nystagmus, p. 44

BPPV benign paroxysmal positional vertigo, p. 44

BSER brainstem evoked response, p. 46

BTE behind-the-ear, p. 46

CA chronologic age, p. 47

CANS central auditory nervous system, p. 48

CAOHC Council for Accreditation in Occupational Hearing Conservation, p. 48

CAP central auditory processing; compound action potential, p. 48

CAPD central auditory processing disorder, p. 48

CAST computer-aided speechreading training, p. 50

CBA cost-benefit analysis, p. 73

cc cubic centimeter, p. 50

CC closed captioning, p. 50

CCB clinical certification board, p. 50

CCC certificate of clinical competence, p. 50

CCM contralateral competing message, p. 51

CCT California Consonant Test, p. 51

CD communication disorder; compact disc, p. 51

CDP computerized dynamic posturography, p. 51

CDT continuous discourse tracking, p. 51

CEA cost-effective analysis, p. 73

CF center frequency; characteristic frequency; clinical fellowship, p. 54

CHIP Children's Implant Profile, p. 55

CI cochlear implant, p. 56

CIC completely-in-the-canal, p. 57

CICI Cochlear Implant Club International, p. 57

CID Central Institute for the Deaf, p. 57

CIS continuous interleaved sampling, p. 58

CM cochlear microphonic, p. 60

CMR common mode rejection, p. 60

CMRR common mode rejection ratio, p. 60

CMV cytomegalovirus, p. 60

CN cochlear nucleus; cranial nerves, p. 60

CNC consonant-nucleus-consonant, p. 60

CNS central nervous system, p. 60

CNT could not test, p. 61

CNV contingent negative variation, p. 61

COR conditioned orientation reflex, p. 72

CORFIG coupler response for flat insertion gain, p. 72

COSI Client Oriented Scale of Improvement, p. 73

CPA cerebellopontine angle, p. 75

cps cycles per second, p. 75

CPT current procedural terminology, p. 75

CPU central processing unit, p. 75

CR compression range; compression ratio, p. 75

CR-NST Closed-Response Nonsense Syllable Test, p. 75

CROS contralateral routing of signals, p. 77

CSF cerebrospinal fluid, p. 78

CST Connected Speech Test, p. 78

CT compression threshold; computed tomography, p. 79

CTS compound threshold shift, p. 79

CV consonant-vowel, p. 80

CVA cerebrovascular accident, p. 80

CVC consonant-vowel-consonant, p. 80

DAC digital-to-analog converter, p. 81

DAF delayed auditory feedback, p. 81

DAI direct audio input, p. 81

daPa decaPascal, p. 81

DASL Developmental Approach to Successful Listening, p. 81

DAT digital audio tape, p. 82

dB decibel, p. 82

dB HL decibels hearing level, p. 82

dB HTL decibels hearing threshold level, p. 82

dB nHL decibels normal hearing, p. 82

dB peSPL decibels peak sound pressure level, p. 82

dB SL decibels sensation level, p. 82

dB SPL decibels sound pressure level, p. 82

dBA decibels, A-weighted, p. 82

dBB decibels, B-weighted, p. 82

dBC decibels, C-weighted, p. 82

DC direct current, p. 82

DCA digitally controlled analog, p. 82

DCN dorsal cochlear nucleus, p. 82

DFD Distinctive Feature Difference Test, p. 86

DI directivity index, p. 86

DIP Discrimination by the Identification of Pictures, p. 91

DL difference limen, p. 87

DLF difference limen for frequency, p. 88

DLI difference limen for intensity, p. 88

DLT difference limen for time , p. 88

DMic directional microphone, p. 93

DNE did not evaluate, p. 93

DNT did not test, p. 93

DP directional preponderance; distortion product, p. 94

DPOAE distortion product otoacoustic emission, p. 94

DR dynamic range, p. 94

DRC damage risk criteria, p. 94

DRF Deafness Research Foundation, p. 84

DRT Diagnostic Rhyme Test; Dichotic Rhyme Test, p. 94

DSI Dichotic Sentence Identification, p. 84

DSL desired sensation level, p. 94

DSL (I/O) desired sensation level (input/output), p. 95

DSP digital signal processing, p. 95

EAA Educational Audiology Association, p. 97

EAC ear canal; external auditory canal, p. 97

EAM external auditory meatus, p. 97

ECochG electrocochleography, p. 100

ECV ear canal volume, p. 100

ED-NST Edgerton-Danhauer Nonsense Syllable Test, p. 101

EEE external ear effects, p. 101

EEG electroencephalogram; electroencephalography, p. 101

EIN equivalent input noise level, p. 102

ELC equal loudness contours, p. 102

EM effective masking, p. 105

EMG electromyography, p. 105

ENG electronystagmography, p. 107

ENoG electroneuronography, p. 107

ENT ear, nose, & throat physician, p. 107

EOAE evoked otoacoustic emission, p. 107

EOG electro-oculography, p. 107

EP evoked potential, p. 107

ERA electric response audiometry, p. 109

ERP event related potential, p. 109

ESP Early Speech Perception Test, p. 109

EST Environmental Sounds Test, p. 109

ET eustachian tube, p. 109

f frequency, p. 113

F force, p. 113

F$_0$, f$_0$ fundamental frequency, p. 113

F1 first formant, p. 113

F2 second formant, p. 113

F3 third formant, p. 113

F4 fourth formant, p. 113

FAAA Fellow of the American Academy of Audiology, p. 113

FDA Food and Drug Administration, p. 115

FDC frequency dependent compression, p. 115

FDRC full dynamic range compression, p. 115

FET field effect transistor, p. 116

FFR fixed frequency response; frequency following response, p. 117

FFS failure of fixation suppression, p. 117

FFT fast Fourier transform, p. 117

FG functional gain, p. 117

FM frequency modulation, p. 120

FN false negative, p. 114

FP false positive, p. 114

FOG full-on gain, p. 120

FTC frequency tuning curve, p. 125

G conductance, p. 126

GASP Glendonald Auditory Screening Procedure, p. 126

HA hearing aid, p. 130

HAE hearing aid evaluation, p. 130

HAIC Hearing Aid Industry Conference, p. 131

HAO hearing aid orientation, p. 131

HAPI Hearing Aid Performance Inventory, p. 131

HC hair cell, p. 132

HCP hearing conservation program, p. 132

HEAR Hearing Education and Awareness for Rockers, p. 133

HFA high-frequency average, p. 142

HFE high-frequency emphasis, p. 142

HHIA Hearing Handicap Inventory for Adults, p. 143

HHIE Hearing Handicap Inventory for the Elderly, p. 143

HHIE-S Hearing Handicap Inventory for the Elderly–Screening version, p. 143

HHS Hearing Handicap Scale, p. 143

HIA Hearing Industries Association, p. 143

HICROS high-frequency contralateral routing of signals, p. 143

HINT Hearing in Noise Test, p. 144

HIV human immunodeficiency virus, p. 144

HL hearing level, p. 145

HOH hard-of-hearing, p. 145

HMO health maintenance organization, p. 145

HPD hearing protection device, p. 145

HPI Hearing Performance Inventory; Hearing Problem Inventory, p. 145

HRHR high-risk hearing register, p. 146

HRR high-risk register, p. 146

HTL hearing threshold level, p. 146

Hx history, p. 146

Hz Hertz, p. 147

I/O input/output function, p. 149

IA interaural attenuation, p. 149

IAC internal auditory canal, p. 149

IAM internal acoustic meatus; internal auditory meatus, p. 149

IC inferior colliculus; integrated circuit, p. 149

ICM ipsilateral competing message, p. 149

ICU intensive care unit, p. 150

IDEA Individuals with Disabilities Education Act, p. 150

IDL intensity difference limen, p. 150

IEP individualized educational plan, p. 150

IFSP individualized family service plan, p. 150

IHAFF Independent Hearing Aid Fitting Forum, p. 150

IHC inner hair cell, p.150

IHS International Hearing Society, p. 150

IID interaural intensity difference, p. 150

IL intensity level, p. 150

ILD interaural latency difference, p. 151

IPA International Phonetic Alphabet, p. 158

IPL interpeak latency, p. 159

IROS ipsilateral routing of signals, p. 161

ISI interstimulus interval, p. 161

ISO International Standards Organization, p. 161

ITC in-the-canal hearing aid, p. 162

ITD interaural timing difference, p. 162

ITE in-the-ear hearing aid, p. 162

J joule, p. 163

JAAA Journal of the American Academy of Audiology, p. 163

JASA Journal of the Acoustical Society of America, p. 163

JCAHO Joint Commission on Accreditation of Health Care Organizations, p. 163

JCIH Joint Committee on Infant Hearing, p. 163

jnd just-noticeable difference, p. 164

JSHD Journal of Speech and Hearing Disorders, p. 164

JSLHR Journal of Speech, Hearing, and Language Research, p. 164

k kilo, p. 166

K+ potassium, p. 166

kbyte kilobyte, p. 166

KEMAR Knowles Electronics Manikin for Acoustic Research, p. 167

kg kilogram, p. 167

kHz kiloHertz, p. 167

LD learning disability, p. 172

LDFR level dependent frequency response, p. 172

LDL loudness discomfort level, p. 172

LED light emitting diode, p. 172

Leq equivalent level, p. 172

LI latency-intensity function, p. 175

LL lateral lemniscus, p. 177

LNTB lateral nucleus of trapezoid body, p. 177

LPC linear predictive coding, p. 177

LPFS Low-Pass Filtered Speech Test, p. 180

LSHSS Language, Speech, and Hearing Services in the Schools, p. 180

LSO lateral superior olive, p. 180

LTASS long-term average speech spectrum, p. 180

MA mental age, p. 181

MAA minimal audible angle, p. 181

MAC Minimal Auditory Capabilities battery, p. 181

MAF minimal audible field; minimum auditory field, p. 181, 194

MAIS Meaningful Auditory Integration Scale, p. 181

MAP minimal audible pressure; minimum auditory pressure, p. 183, 194

MCL most comfortable level, p. 186

MCR message-to-competition ratio, p. 186

MCT minimal contact technology earmold, p. 187, 194

ME middle ear, p. 187, 192

mg milligram, p. 190

MGB medial geniculate body, p. 190

MHz megaHertz, p. 190

MLB monaural loudness balance test, p. 195

MLD masking level difference, p. 195

MLE microphone location effect, p. 195

MLR middle latency response, p. 195

MLS maximum length sequence, p. 195

MLU mean length of utterance, p. 195

MLV monitored live voice, p. 195, 197

mm millimeter, p. 196

mmho millimho, p. 196

MML minimum masking level, p. 196

MMN mismatched negativity, p. 196

MPO maximum power output, p. 199

MRHT Modified Rhyme Hearing Test, p. 199

MRI magnetic resonance imaging, p. 199

MRT Modified Rhyme Test, p. 199

ms millisecond, p. 199

MS multiple sclerosis, p. 201

MSO medial superior olive, p. 199

MSP multispeak speech processor, p. 199, 201

MSTI modified speech transmission index, p. 199

MTF modulation transfer function, p. 197, 199

MTS Monosyllable-Trochee-Spondee test, p. 198, 199

mV millivolt, p. 202

μPa microPascal, p. 190

μs microsecond, p. 192

μV microvolt, p. 192

N Newton, p. 203

N/m² Newton per square meter, p. 203

Na+ sodium, p. 203

NAD National Association of the Deaf, p. 203

NAL National Acoustics Laboratory, p. 203

NAL-R National Acoustic Laboratory–Revised, p. 204

NBN narrow-band noise, p. 204, 205

NCC noise criterion curve, p. 205

NECCI Network of Educators of Children with Cochlear Implants, p. 205

NESPA National Examination in Speech-Language Pathology and Audiology, p. 204, 207

NF1 neurofibromatosis I, p. 209

NF2 neurofibromatosis II, p. 209

NH normal hearing, p. 209

nHL normal hearing level, p. 210

NHAS National Hearing Aid Society, p. 210

NHCA National Hearing Conservation Association, p. 210

NICU neonatal intensive care unit, p. 210

NIDCD National Institute on Deafness and Other Communicative Disorders, p. 210

NIHIS National Institute for Hearing Instrument Sciences, p. 210

NIHL noise-induced hearing loss, p. 210

NIOSH National Institute for Occupational Safety and Health, p. 210

NIPTS noise-induced permanent threshold shift, p. 210

NITTS noise-induced temporary threshold shift, p. 210, 212

NR no response, p. 214

NRR noise reduction rating, p. 214

NSSLHA National Student Speech-Language-Hearing Association, p. 214

NST Nonsense Syllable Test, p. 214

NTE nontest ear, p. 214

NU-6 Northwestern University Auditory Test No. 6, p. 214

NU-CHIPS Northwestern University Children's Perception of Speech, p. 214

nV nanovolt, p. 215

OAE otoacoustic emission, p. 217

OCB olivocochlear bundle, p. 217, 220

OE occlusion effect, p. 219

OHC outer hair cell, p. 219

OHCP occupational hearing conservation program, p. 219

OKN optokinetic nystagmus, p. 220

OM otitis media, p. 220, 221

OME otitis media with effusion, p. 221

OSHA Occupational Safety and Health Administration, p. 223

OSPL output sound pressure level, p. 223

SOC superior olivary complex, p. 284

SOL site of lesion, p. 285

SOM serous otitis media, p. 285

SOT sensory organization test, p. 285

SP summating potential, p. 287

SP/AP summating potential/action potential ratio, p. 287

SPAC speech pattern contrasts, p. 287

SPAR sensitivity prediction of the acoustic reflex, p. 287

SPIN speech perception in noise, p. 292

SPL sound pressure level, p. 292

SPV slow phase velocity, p. 293

SRT speech recognition threshold, p. 294

SSEP steady-state evoked potential, p. 294

SSI Synthetic Sentence Identification test, p. 294

SSI-CCM Synthetic Sentence Identification Test with Contralateral Competing Message, p. 294

SSI-ICM Synthetic Sentence Identification test with Ipsilateral Competing Message, p. 294

SSPL saturation sound pressure level, p. 294

SSPL90 saturation sound pressure level 90, p. 294

SSW Staggered Spondaic Word test, p. 294

ST speech threshold; spondee threshold, p. 294

STAT Suprathreshold Adaptation Test, p. 296

STI speech transmission index, p. 297

STS standard threshold shift, p. 299

SWAMI speech with alternating masking index, p. 301

t-coil telecoil, p. 304

t-switch telecoil switch, p. 304

TAC Test of Auditory Comprehension, p. 304

TACL Test for Auditory Comprehension of Language, p. 304

TACL-R Test for Auditory Comprehension of Language–Revised, p. 304

TAPS Test of Auditory Perception Skills, p. 305

TBI traumatic brain injury, p. 305

TC total communication, p. 305

TD threshold of discomfort, p. 305

TDD telecommunication device for the deaf, p. 305

TE test ear, p. 308

TEOAE transient evoked otoacoustic emission, p. 308

THD total harmonic distortion, p. 309

THRIFT three-alternative forced-choice test, p. 312

TILL treble increase at low levels, p. 312

TM tympanic membrane, p. 313

TMJ temporomandibular joint, p. 313

TOAE transient otoacoustic emission, p. 313

TOLD-I Test of Language Development–Intermediate, p. 313

TOLD-P Test of Language Development–Primary, p. 313

TORP total ossicular replacement prosthesis, p. 315

TPP tympanometric peak pressure, p. 316

TROCA tangible reinforcement operant conditioned audiometry, p. 320

TTR type-token ratio, p. 324

TT text telephone, p. 320

TTS temporary threshold shift, p. 320

TTY teletypewriter, p. 320

TWA time-weighted average, p. 321

TWF Test of Word Finding, p. 321

UCL uncomfortable loudness level, p. 325

UHF ultrahigh frequency, p.325

ULCL upper level of comfortable loudness, p. 325

ULL uncomfortable loudness level, p. 325

UOCRT University of Oklahoma Closed-Response Speech Test, p. 326

V volt, p. 328

VC volume control; vowel-consonant, p. 329

VCN ventral cochlear nucleus, p. 329

VCV vowel-consonant-vowel, p. 329

VEP visual evoked potential, p. 330

VIOLA visual input/output locator algorithm, p. 333

VOR vestibulo-ocular reflex, p. 335

VOT voice-onset time, p. 335

VRA visual reinforcement audiometry, p. 336

VROCA visual reinforcement operant conditioning audiometry, p. 336

VU volume unit meter, p. 336

VVV variable venting valve, p. 336

W watt, p. 337

W-1 CID W-1 test, p. 337

W-2 CID W-2 test, p. 337

W-22 CID W-22 test, p. 337

WDRC wide-dynamic range compression, p. 339

WIPI Word Intelligibility by Picture Identification, p. 340

WIS word-identification score, p. 340

WISC Wechsler Intelligence Scale for Children, p. 340

WN white noise, p. 341

WNL within normal limits, p. 341

WRS word-recognition score, p. 342

WT warble tone, p. 342

X acoustic reactance, p. 343

Y admittance, p. 344

Z impedance , p. 345

APPENDIX

B

Topic Categories

All terms are categorized by general topic area in this appendix. In the beginning of this appendix, a list of the 123 different categories is provided in alphabetical order along with the page number of the appendix where that category of terms begins. If interested in all the terms related to a particular topic area, the reader should locate the appropriate topic/category at the beginning of the appendix and then turn to the corresponding page number for that category. A list of all the terms related to that topic will be found along with specific page numbers where the definitions for each of the terms in that category can be located in the text.

Individual Terms by Topic Categories

Acoustic Modifications in Hearing Aids

Acoustic Reflex

Acoustics

acoustic, 3
acoustic coupler, 4
acoustic distortion, 4
acoustic signature, 5
acoustics, 6
amplitude, 14
amplitude distortion, 14
amplitude modulation (AM), 14
antinode, 17
aperiodic wave, 17
attenuation, 21
aural harmonic, 30
band, 35
bandwidth, 35
body baffle effect, 42
characteristic frequency (CF), 55
combination tone, 64
complex aperiodic, 66
complex periodic, 66
complex tone, 66
complex waveform, 66
compression, 67
concha-related Helmholtz
    resonance, 68
continuous spectrum, 71
crest factor, 77
critical ratio, 77
crossover frequency, 78
cubic distortion product, 79
cue, 79
cycle, 80
cycles per second (cps), 80
decay time, 84
deconvolution, 84
dichotic, 87
diotic, 89
discrete Fourier transform, 90
duration, 95
ear canal acoustics, 98
ear canal dynamics, 98

ear canal resonance, 98
elasticity, 102
envelope, 107
external ear acoustics, 112
external ear effects (EEE), 112
fall time, 114
fast Fourier transform (FFT), 115
force (F), 121
forced vibration, 121
Fourier analysis, 122
Fourier's theorem, 122
free vibration, 122
frequency (f), 122
frequency band, 123
frequency modulation (FM), 123
frequency range, 123
frequency resolution, 123
frequency response, 123
frequency shifting, 124
graphic equalizer, 129
half wavelength resonators, 131
half-wave rectified average, 131
harmonic, 132
harmonic distortion, 132
harmonic motion, 132
harmonic series, 132
head baffle effect, 132
head shadow effect, 133
Helmholtz resonator, 141
inertia, 154
instantaneous amplitude, 156
intensity, 157
interstimulus interval (ISI), 159
line spectrum, 176
linear, 176
mode, 196
natural resonant frequency, 205
node, 210
noise interference level, 212
octave, 218
octave band, 218

Assistive Devices

Audiology Terms, General

Auditory Development

Auditory Late Response

Auditory (Re)habilitation

diagnosis, 86
diagnostic audiology, 86
differential diagnosis, 88
fistula test, 119
Glycerol test, 109
light reflex, 151
neuroaudiology, 208
neurodiagnosis, 208
site of lesion (SOL), 282

Disorders, General

acquired immunodeficiency
    syndrome (AIDS), 6
adenoma, 7
adrenoleukodystrophy (ALS), 8
agnosia, 9
Alzheimer's disease, 12
aneurysm, 15
angioma, 15
anoxia, 16
apnea, 18
arachnoiditis, 18
attention deficit and hyperactivity
    disorder (ADHD), 21
attention deficit disorder (ADD), 21
autism, 31
autoimmune disease, 31
bacterial meningitis, 34
brachycephaly, 44
brain abscess, 44
brain attack, 44
cerebrovascular accident (CVA), 54
CHARGE syndrome, 55
cleft lip, 59
cleft palate, 59
coloboma, 64
coloboma lobuli, 64
cough reflex, 74
degenerative disease, 85
developmental delay, 86
diabetic, 86

diplacusis, 89
dysplasia, 96
ear infection, 98
encephalopathy, 106
endemic, 106
endosteal hyperostosis, 106
epidemic, 107
epidemiology, 107
erythroblastosis fetalis, 109
esotropia/exotropia, 109
exudate, 112
genetic disorder, 127
German measles, 127
head trauma, 133
hearing disorder, 137
human immunodeficiency virus
    (HIV), 143
hyaline membrane disease, 143
hypoplasia, 147
iatrogenic, 149
icterus, 150
idiopathic, 150
incidence, 152
learning disability (LD), 172
lentigenes, 172
leukodystrophy, 173
luetic, 180
macroencephaly, 181
malformation, 182
malignant tumor, 182
mandibulofacial dysostosis, 182
micrognathia, 190
mucopolysaccharidoses, 200
multiple sclerosis (MS), 201
mumps, 201
myasthenia gravis, 202
necrosis, 205
neoplasia, 206
neoplasm, 206
nephritis, 206
neuropathy, 209

Electroacoustic Characteristics of Hearing Aids

Electrocochleography

Filters

adaptive filtering, 7
band-pass filter, 35
band-reject filter, 35
center frequency (CF), 51
cutoff frequency, 80
filter, 118
filter skirt, 118
high-cut filter, 143
high-pass filter, 144
inverse filtering, 160
low-cut filter, 179
low-pass filter, 179
noise floor, 212
notch filter, 214
octave band filter, 218
passband, 231
passive filter, 231
roll-off rate, 268
skirt, 282
third-octave filter, 309
three-dB rule, 309
upper cutoff frequency, 327

Genetics

ageism, 9
allele, 11
allogenic, 11
autosomal dominant, 32
autosomal recessive, 32
chromosomes, 56
congenital, 70
consanguinity, 70
dysmorphology, 95
gene, 127
genetic hearing loss, 127
genome, 127
genotype, 127
heterozygous, 142
homologous, 145
homozygous, 145
karyotype, 166
penetrance, 233
phenotype, 237
sex-linked inheritance, 277
sporadic inheritance, 293
X-linked inheritance, 343

Head and Neck Anatomical Structures

adenoids, 7
auditory pit, 28
auditory placode, 28
basilar artery, 35
basilar crest, 35
branchial arch, 45
condyle, 69
craniofacial, 76
foramen magnum, 120
jugular bulb, 165
jugular fossa, 165
jugular wall, 165
mandible, 182
nasopharynx, 204
otic capsule, 224
otic placode, 224
otic vesicle, 224
pharynx, 237
postauricular muscle (PAM), 243
stylomastoid foramen, 299
temporal bone, 306
tensor veli palatini muscle, 308
thalamus, 309
zygomatic bone, 345

Hearing Aid Circuitry

bass increase at low levels (BILL), 36
capacitance, 48
capacitor, 48
circuit, 58
circuit noise, 58
class A amplifier, 58

Middle Latency Response

Outer Ear Disorders

Pediatric Audiology

Professionals

Prosody

Prosthetic Devices

Sound Propagation

intelligibility, 157
jargon, 163
minimal pair, 194
modified speech transmission index (MSTI), 196
rapid speech transmission index (RASTI), 256
speech intelligibility index (SII), 290
speech intelligibility rating (SIR), 290
speech perception, 290
speech transmission index (STI), 291
viseme, 333
vowel-consonant (VC), 336
vowel-consonant-vowel (VCV), 336

Speech Perception Tests for Children

Auditory Numbers Test (ANT), 28
Change/No Change Test, 55
Children's Auditory Test, 55
Children's Implant Profile (CHIP), 55
Children's Vowel Perception Test, 55
CID Monster Test, 57
CID Phonetic Inventory, 57
Common Objects Token Test, 65
Common Phrases Test, 65
Discrimination by the Identification of Pictures (DIP) Test, 91
Glendonald Auditory Screening Procedure (GASP), 127
Hoosier Auditory-Visual Enhancement Test, 145
Kindergarten Phonetically Balanced Word List (PB-K), 168
Lexical Neighborhood Test, 174
Meaningful Auditory Integration Scale (MAIS), 187
Minimal Pairs Test, 194

Monosyllable-Trochee-Spondee (MTS) test, 198
Northwestern University Children's Perception of Speech (NU-CHIPS), 214
PB-K Monosyllabic Word Lists, 232
Pediatric Speech Intelligibility (PSI) Test, 233
Phonetic Task Evaluation (PTE), 238
Picture Identification Task, 238
Screening Inventory of Perceptual Skills (SCIPS), 273
Word Intelligibility by Picture Identification (WIPI), 341

Speech-Language Pathology

acoustic phonetics, 5
aphasia, 17
aphonia, 18
apraxia, 18
articulation, 19
ataxia, 20
auditory agnosia, 25
Bernoulli principle, 38
coarticulation, 61
communicative competence, 65
dispraxia, 91
dysarthria, 95
dysphagia, 95
dysphasia, 95
dysphonia, 96
fluency, 120
fluent speech, 120
fricative, 124
grapheme-phoneme conversion, 129
hyponasality, 147
International Phonetic Alphabet (IPA), 158
jitter, 164
laminar flow, 170
language, 170
language delay, 170

Treatment for Disorders of the Ear

Tuning Fork Tests

APPENDIX

C

A Poor Man's Tour of Physical Quantities and Units[1]

Michael R. Chial, Ph.D.

Professor, Department of Communicative Disorders
Professor, Department of Professional Development and Applied Studies
University of Wisconsin-Madison

INTRODUCTION

Physical quantities are objective events that can assume numerical values. *Basic quantities* are limited to mass, time, displacement (or length) and electric charge. *Derived quantities* are generated through algebraic combination of basic quantities and other derived quantities. These include velocity, acceleration, pressure, force, work, power, and temperature, as well as the quantities of electricity and electronics (except for electric charge). *Units of measurement*, on the other hand, are standardized amounts of quantities. In most cases, units are named in honor of the individuals whose scientific ef-

---

[1]Reprinted courtesy of M. R. Chial

417

forts clarified our understanding of the respective phenomenon. Finally, *values* are specific amounts of units. In the expression, "she was 5 feet, 4 inches tall," feet and inches are units, the numbers 5 and 4 are values, and "tall" denotes the quantity of vertical length.

QUANTITIES AND UNITS

Quantities differ from units. For example, the basic quantity length is defined as the distance between two points. Any particular length can be expressed by a host of units, including inches, centimeters, feet, meters, rods, furlongs, miles, kilometers, etc. Similarly, the derived quantity force (F) is defined by Newton's second law of motion as mass (M) times acceleration (a), whereas, the metric unit for force is defined as the newton (N).

Force (quantity): $F = M * a$
Force (MKS unit): $1 \text{ N} = 1 \text{ kg} * 1 \text{ m} / \text{sec}^2$

Although physical quantities are well-standardized, the symbols and abbreviations used to represent them are not. Indeed, they differ considerably among authors, scholarly journals, and scientific or professional disciplines. Symbols for units are formally defined by international standards bodies and are even the subject of treaties among nations. Generally, honorific units (those named in honor of individuals) are written without capitalization (to distinguish the unit from the person); when abbreviated, honorific units are capitalized.

MEASUREMENT SYSTEMS

Physical measurement always requires specification of both a value (i.e., a number representing "how much") and a unit (i.e., "of what"). *Systems of measurement* are formal strategies for indexing amounts of specified physical quantities. Such systems include (1) definitions of quantities, (2) units of measurement—the names we give quantities when we want to be specific, (3) standards of measurement—formally defined reference values for units, and (4) procedures (rules) of measurement for applying standards to specific things or events.

Units of measurement and the physical standards underpinning them become progressively more precise as science and technology develop. In other words, newer standards are capable of accommodating smaller *differences* in the amounts of the quantities measured. Standard units (e.g., the standard second and the standard meter) also are periodically redefined in pursuit of greater objectivity and repeatability. The second originally was standardized as the duration between heartbeats (problem: whose heart and after what activity?). Today, the standard second is defined in terms of atomic events, allowing resolution of time to 10^{-12} seconds (one trillionth of a second, or 1 picosecond).

The most common systems of units are the English system (foot-pound-second or FPS), the early metric system (centimeter-gram-second or CGS), and the *Systeme International d'Unites* (meter-kilogram-second or MKS). All three systems use the same units for the basic quantities of time (the second) and electric charge (the coloumb). Different units are employed for mass. The CGS system uses the gram, the MKS system uses the kilogram, and the FPS system uses the *slug* or *poundal*. The more familiar *pound* is a unit of weight (a force), not a unit of mass. Both metric systems employ a powers-of-ten (decimal) number scheme, whereas the English system is based on doublings, triplings, or other multiples (e.g., 2 cups = 1 pint, 2 pints = 1 quart; 3 feet = 1 yard). Confusions related to the inconsistencies of the English FPS system are among the reasons it is seldom used in science and engineering.

The *Systeme International d'Unites* (abbreviated SI) is the contemporary version of the metric system originally developed by the French Academy of Science in 1791. The SI also is referred to as the *rationalized MKS system*, so-called because both basic and derived units are defined as having unity (1) values, even though derived units may be given new names. *Basic units* and *basic quantities* are not the same (see above). Basic units (see Table 1) are required in the SI to accomplish the goal of unity value for derived units. Note that two of the basic units of the SI are honorific. Those for displacement, mass, time, light intensity and molecular substance are not.

The quantities in Table 1 define the MKS system and also underpin the FPS and CGS systems. Many everyday quantities are missing from Table 1, for example, area, volume, velocity (or speed), and power. These and other *derived quantities* are defined as combinations of the quantities listed in Table 1. The methods by which basic quantities are combined to form derived quantities (and, for that matter, by which derived quantities may be

Table 1. Base units of measurement in the *Systeme International d'Unites* (also called the "rationalized MKS system"). Asterisks in the left-hand column designate basic quantities. All other quantities are derived.

Quantity	Unit	Symbol	Physical Definition
*Displacement (Length)	meter	m	distance traveled by light in a vacuum in 1 / 299 792 458 of a second
*Mass	kilogram	kg	mass equal to that of a prototype platinum-iridium cylinder kept in Paris, France
*Time	second	s	duration of 9 192 631 770 periods of radiation of the cesium 133 atom in transition between two states
Electric current	ampere	A	coulomb / s
Temperature	kelvin	K	1 / 273.2 of the triple point of water
Light intensity	candela	cd	directional radiant intensity of 1 / 683 watt per steradian at a monochrome frequency of 540×1012 hertz
Molecular substance	mole	mol	amount of substance equal to that of 0.012 kg of carbon-12

combined to define still other derived quantities) are inherently algebraic. These mathematical methods are based upon known lawful relations of the physical universe and generally are quite simple. Thus, formal systems of measurement constitute a world-view about how the universe and everything in it works. Table 2 lists commonly used derived SI units.

Table 2. Some derived units of measurement in the *Systeme International d'Unites*. Many additional derived units are in common use. Basic and derived units of measurement (including those honoring individuals) always are given in lower-case letters when written out in full. Thus, people can be distinguished from the physical units named after them. When abbreviated, units named to honor people are capitalized. Asterisks in the right-hand column designate multiplication.

Quantity	Unit	Symbol	Other Definition	
Area		m^2	displacement squared	
Volume		m^3	displacement cubed	
Density		kg / m^3	mass / unit volume	
Velocity		m / s	Δ displacement / unit time	
Acceleration		m / s^2	Δ velocity / unit time	
Plane angle	radian	rad	2π rad $= 360°$	
Angular velocity	rad / s	ω	2π rad / s $= 360° / s$	
Solid angle	steradian	sr	(complex)	
Energy	joule	J	$kg * m^2 / s^2$	$= N * m$
Force	newton	N	$kg * m / s^2$	$= J / m$
Pressure or stress	pascal	Pa	$(kg * m / s^2) / m^2$	$= N / m^2$
Power	watt	W	$kg * m^2 / s^3$	$= J / s$
Electric charge	coulomb	C	$A * s$	
Electric potential (emf)	volt	V	$kg * m^2 / s^3 * A = J / A * s$	$= W / A$
Electric resistance	ohm	Ω	$kg * m^2 / s^3 * A^2$	$= V / A$
Electric capacitance	farad	F	$A^2 * s^4 / kg * m^2$	$= A * s / V$
Electric inductance	henry	H	$kg * m^2 / s^2 * A^2$	$= V * s / A$
Frequency	hertz	Hz	cycle / s	$= s^{-1}$
Magnetic flux	weber	Wb	$kg * m^2 / s^2 * A$	$= V * s$
Magnetic flux density	telsa	T	$kg / s^2 * A$	$= Wb / m^2$
Luminous flux	lumen	lm	$cd * sr$	
Customary temperature	degree Celsius	°C	$K - 273.15$	

METRIC PREFIXES

A distinct advantage of the SI system is a set of prefixes that can be applied to units to indicate scale of measurement, i.e., to overall size or magnitude of a measured quantity. The most commonly used prefixes are noted in Table 3. Note that prefixes employ a base-10 exponential progression such that prefixes close to the <unit> (i.e., from milli to kilo) are based upon small differences in exponents, while extremely large and extremely small magnitudes are based upon numerically greater differences in exponents. Table 4 gives instructions for converting values expressed with one common prefix to identical values expressed with another common prefix.

STANDARDS ORGANIZATIONS

The SI is but one part of a larger process by which scientific, technical, and professional communities strive to standardize measurements. In the Unit-

Table 3. Metric prefixes. Note the use of capital letters to distinguish among abbreviations for prefixes.

Prefix	Symbol	Power of 10	Numerical Value
exa	E	10^{18}	1 000 000 000 000 000 000
peta	P	10^{15}	1 000 000 000 000 000
tera	T	10^{12}	1 000 000 000 000
giga	G	10^9	1 000 000 000
mega	M	10^6	1 000 000
kilo	k	10^3	1 000
hecto	h	10^2	100
deka	da	10^1	10
—<unit>—	(none)	10^0	1
deci	d	10^{-1}	0.1
centi	c	10^{-2}	0.01
milli	m	10^{-3}	0.001
micro	μ	10^{-6}	0.000 001
nano	n	10^{-9}	0.000 000 001
pico	p	10^{-12}	0.000 000 000 001
femto	f	10^{-15}	0.000 000 000 000 001
atto	a	10^{-18}	0.000 000 000 000 000 001

Table 4. Metric conversions. To convert a unit of measurement expressed with an original value prefix to the same unit expressed with a different value prefix, start by finding the correct cell in the table below. Then move the decimal point of the original value the number of places indicated by the digit in the direction indicated by the arrow. For example, 5 kilometers equals 500,000 centimeters (5⇒ move the decimal 5 spaces to the right); 12.5 milliseconds equals 0.0125 seconds (⇐3 move the decimal 3 spaces to the left).

Original Prefix ⇒	Desired Prefix ⇒								
	giga	mega	kilo	—(unit)—	centi	milli	micro	nano	pico
giga	⇐0⇒	3⇒	6⇒	9⇒	11⇒	12⇒	15⇒	18⇒	21⇒
mega	⇐3	⇐0⇒	3⇒	6⇒	8⇒	9⇒	12⇒	15⇒	18⇒
kilo	⇐6	⇐3	⇐0⇒	3⇒	5⇒	6⇒	9⇒	12⇒	15⇒
—(unit)—	⇐9	⇐6	⇐3	⇐0⇒	2⇒	3⇒	6⇒	9⇒	12⇒
centi	⇐11	⇐8	⇐5	⇐2	⇐0⇒	1⇒	4⇒	7⇒	10⇒
milli	⇐12	⇐9	⇐6	⇐3	⇐1	⇐0⇒	3⇒	6⇒	9⇒
micro	⇐15	⇐12	⇐9	⇐6	⇐4	⇐3	⇐0⇒	3⇒	6⇒
nano	⇐18	⇐15	⇐12	⇐9	⇐7	⇐6	⇐3	⇐0⇒	3⇒
pico	⇐21	⇐18	⇐15	⇐12	⇐10	⇐9	⇐6	⇐3	⇐0⇒

ed States, the National Technical Institute (NTI—formerly called the National Bureau of Standards) is responsible for defining and increasing the precision of the physical standards that underpin scientific and commercial measurement. A branch of the US Department of Commerce, the NTI was originally formed to insure that materials and equipment purchased by the federal government (including the military) conformed to consistent standards of measurement.

Other national groups, such as the American National Standards Institute (ANSI) and international groups, such as the International Standards Organization (ISO) and the International Electrotechnical Commission (IEC), are voluntary organizations that exist for the purpose of documenting generally accepted practices for making and reporting measurements. A major goal of these groups is to facilitate communication among scientists, technical workers, and various professionals so as to insure that differences in measurement practices do not cause differences in the meaning of reported data.

Standards published by standards organizations fall into four distinct categories.

(1) **Definition standards** which formally define physical quantities, units, and related concepts,
(2) **Data standards** which precisely define reference quantities for units, for technical instruments, or for technical procedures,
(3) **Instrument standards** which specify the tolerances of devices used to make measurements for different purposes, and
(4) **Procedure standards** which detail the steps to be taken in making measurements of interest to the public or particular scientific, technical, or professional groups.

Five groups currently active within ANSI are highly relevant to scientists and clinicians who work with persons who have disorders of speech, language, or hearing. These are designated as ANSI Committee S1-Acoustics (dealing with the physical measurement of sound), ANSI Committee S2-Vibration (dealing with physical measurement of mechanical events), ANSI Committee S3-Bioacoustics (dealing with the measurement of hearing), ANSI Committee S12-Noise (dealing with the physical measurement of generally unwanted acoustical signals, as well as ways to assess and prevent unwanted effects of such sounds), and ANSI Committee S14-Electroacoustics (dealing with sound recording and reproduction).

Hundreds of other industry, government, and professional groups exist to standardize everything from the size of photographic film, to computer languages, to audiogram symbols, to envelope sizes, to screw threads and wire gauges, to the dimensions of the cardboard cores found in toilet paper, to the speed of audio tapes, to the capacity of CD-audio disks. Some of these eventually become standards endorsed by ANSI, ISO, or both. Others do not. In France, for example, a government agency requires that common baked goods such as croissants be prepared using specified recipes. Nonstandardized industries include shoe and clothing manufacturing. If such products were more rigorously standardized, we would have little use for phrases such as "if the shoe fits. . . ."

REFERENCES

Adams, H. (1974). *SI metric units: An introduction* (rev. ed.) Toronto, ON: McGraw-Hill Ryerson, Limited.

Anderson, H. (Ed.). (1989). *A physicist's desk reference: The physics vade mecum* (2nd ed.). New York, NY: American Institute of Physics.

Klein, H. (1974). *The science of measurement: A historical survey.* New York, NY: Simon & Schuster, Inc. Republished (1988) by Dover Publications, Inc.

SELECTED CONVERSION FACTORS

The following material is not intended to encourage you to translate metric measures into the arguably more familiar foot-pound-second (FPS) measures in common use in the United States, but instead to illustrate the complexity of the FPS system and the simplicity of the *Systeme International d'Unites*, even for routine measurement. The superiority of the SI system is particularly evident for dry and liquid volume measurements. The English FPS system employs two entirely different sets of units for such measurements, while the SI uses only one. It is noteworthy that the English FPS system is no longer used in England, or in any of the nations of the former British Commonwealth.

Linear Measure

1 inch = 2.54 centimeters
1 foot = 12 inches = 30.48 centimeters
1 yard = 3 feet = 36 inches = 0.914 4 meters

1 rod = 5.25 yards = 5.029 meters
1 furlong = 40 rods = 201.17 meters
1 statute mile = 5280 feet = 1760 yards = 8 furlongs = 1 609.344 meters
1 league = 3 miles = 4.83 kilometers

1 meter = 39.370 08 inches = 3.280 840 feet = 1.093 613 yards

1 meter = 100 centimeters = 1 000 millimeters = 0.001 kilometers

Square Measure

1 square inch = 6.452 square centimeters
1 square foot = 144 square inches = 929 square centimeters
1 square yard = 9 square feet = 0.836 1 square meters
1 square rod = 30.25 square yards = 25.29 square meters
1 acre = 4 840 square yards = 0.404 7 hectacres
1 square mile = 640 acres = 2.59 square kilometers

1 square meter = 10.763 91 square feet = 1.195 990 square yards

1 square meter = 10 000 square centimeters = 0.000 1 hectacre

Cubic Measure

1 cubic inch = 16.387 cubic centimeters
1 cubic foot = 1 728 cubic inches = 0.028 3 cubic meters
1 cubic yard = 27 cubic feet = 0.764 6 cubic meters
1 cord = 128 cubic feet = 3.625 cubic meters

1 cubic meter = 1 000 liters

Volume or Capacity (Dry Measure)

1 bushel = 4 pecks = 32 dry quarts = 64 dry pints = 2 150.42 cubic inches
= 35.239 07 liters = 0.035 239 07 cubic meters

1 liter = 1.816 166 dry pints

1 liter = 1 000 milliliters = 0.001 cubic meters

Volume or Capacity (Liquid Measure)

1 gallon = 4 liquid quarts = 8 liquid pints = 32 gills = 128 liquid ounces = 728 teaspoons

    = 61 440 minims = 3.785 411 784 liters = 0.003 785 411 784 cubic meters

1 liter = 202.884 136 211 teaspoons = 2.113 376 liquid pints = 0.264 172 05 gallons

1 liter = 1 000 milliliters = 0.001 cubic meters

Nautical Measure

1 fathom = 6 feet = 2 yards = 1.829 meters
1 nautical mile = 1.508 statute miles
60 nautical miles = 1 degree of a great circle of the earth
1 knot = 1 nautical mile per hour (a measure of speed)

1 kilometer = 1 000 meters

Weight

1 avoirdupois pound = 16 avoirdupois ounces = 12 troy ounces
    = 0.000 5 short tons = 0.000 446 428 6 long tons
      = 256 avoirdupois drams = 7 000 grains
        = 0.453 592 37 kilograms
1 kilogram = 15, 432.36 grains = 35.273 96 avoirdupois ounces = 32.150 75 troy ounces = 0.001 102 31 short tons =
      0.000 984 2 long tons = 2.204 623 avoirdupois pounds
        = 2.679 229 troy pounds

1 kilogram = 1 000 grams = 0.001 metric tons

REFERENCES

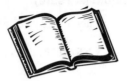

Alford, B., & Jerger, S. (1993). *Clinical audiology: The Jerger perspective.* San Diego, CA: Singular Publishing Group, Inc.

Allum, D. J. (Ed.). (1996). *Cochlear implant rehabilitation in children and adults.* San Diego, CA: Singular Publishing Group, Inc.

Anderson, K. N., Anderson, L. E., & Glanze, W.D. (1998). *Mosby's medical, nursing, and allied health dictionary* (5th ed.). St. Louis, MO: Mosby-Year Book, Inc.

Ballachanda, B. B. (1995). *The human ear canal.* San Diego, CA: Singular Publishing Group, Inc.

Ballantyne, J., Martin, M. C., & Martin, A. (1994). *Deafness* (5th ed.). San Diego, CA: Singular Publishing Group, Inc.

Bamford, J., & Saunders, J. (1994). *Hearing impairment, auditory perception, and language disability* (2nd ed.). London: Whurr Publishers, Ltd.

Beck, D. L. (1994). *Handbook of intraoperative monitoring.* San Diego, CA: Singular Publishing Group, Inc.

Bellis, T. J. (1996). *Assessment and management of central auditory processing disorders in the educational setting.* San Diego, CA: Singular Publishing Group, Inc.

Bench, R. J. (1992). *Communication skills in hearing-impaired children.* San Diego, CA: Singular Publishing Group, Inc.

Berg, F. S. (1993). *Acoustics and sound systems in schools.* San Diego, CA: Singular Publishing Group, Inc.

Berlin C. I. (Ed.). (1996). *Hair cells and hearing aids.* San Diego, CA: Singular Publishing Group, Inc.

Berlin, C. I. (Ed.). (1997). *Neurotransmission and hearing loss: Basic science, diagnosis, and management.* San Diego, CA: Singular Publishing Group, Inc.

Berlin, C. I. (Ed.). (1998). *Otoacoustic emissions: Basic science and clinical applications*. San Diego, CA: Singular Publishing Group, Inc.

Campbell, K. (1998). *Essential audiology for physicians*. San Diego, CA: Singular Publishing Group, Inc.

Chasin, M. (1996). *Musicians and the prevention of hearing loss*. San Diego, CA: Singular Publishing Group, Inc.

Chasin, M. (1997). *CIC handbook*. San Diego, CA: Singular Publishing Group, Inc.

Chermak, G. D., & Musiek, F. E. (1997). *Central auditory processing disorders: New perspectives*. San Diego, CA: Singular Publishing Group, Inc.

Clark, G. M., Cowan, R. S. C., & Dowell, R. C. (1997). *Cochlear implantation for infants and children*. San Diego, CA: Singular Publishing Group, Inc.

Cooper, H. (1993). *Cochlear implants*. San Diego, CA: Singular Publishing Group, Inc.

Crandell, C. C., Smaldino, J. J., & Flexer, C. (1995). *Sound-field FM amplification*. San Diego, CA: Singular Publishing Group, Inc.

DeConde Johnson, C., Benson, P.B., & Seaton, J. B. (1997). *Educational audiology handbook*. San Diego, CA: Singular Publishing Group, Inc.

Ferraro, J. A. (1997). *Laboratory exercises in auditory evoked potentials*. San Diego, CA: Singular Publishing Group, Inc.

Flexer, C. (1999). *Facilitating hearing and listening in young children*. (2nd ed.). San Diego, CA: Singular Publishing Group, Inc.

Gerber, S. E. (1998). *Etiology and prevention of communicative disorders* (2nd ed.). San Diego, CA: Singular Publishing Group, Inc.

Hall, J. W., III, & Mueller, H. G., III. (1997). *Audiologists' desk reference Vol. I: Diagnostic audiology—principles, procedures, and practices*. San Diego, CA: Singular Publishing Group, Inc.

Hayes, D. & Northern, J. L. (1996). *Infants and hearing*. San Diego, CA: Singular Publishing Group, Inc.

Hood, L. J. (1998). *Clinical applications of the auditory brainstem response*. San Diego, CA: Singular Publishing Group, Inc.

Hosford-Dunn, H., Dunn, D. R., & Harford, E. R. (1995). *Audiology business and practice management*. San Diego, CA: Singular Publishing Group, Inc.

House, W. F., Luetje, C. M., & Doyle, K. J. (1997). *Acoustic tumors: Diagnosis and management* (2nd ed.). San Diego, CA: Singular Publishing Group, Inc.

Hull, R. H. (1995). *Hearing in aging*. San Diego, CA: Singular Publishing Group, Inc.

Hull, R. H. (1997). *Aural rehabilitation: Serving children and adults*

(3rd ed.). San Diego, CA: Singular Publishing Group, Inc.

Kelly, B. R., Davis, D., & Hegde, M. N. (1994). *Clinical methods and practicum in audiology.* San Diego, CA: Singular Publishing Group, Inc.

Lipscomb, D. M. (1994). *Hearing conservation.* San Diego, CA: Singular Publishing Group, Inc.

Lubinski, R., & Frattali, C. (1994). *Professional issues in speech-language pathology and audiology.* San Diego, CA: Singular Publishing Group, Inc.

Lynas, W. (1995). *Communication options in the education of deaf children.* London: Whurr Publishers, Ltd.

Martini, A., Read, A., & Stephens, D. (1996). *Genetics and hearing impairment.* San Diego, CA: Singular Publishing Group, Inc.

McCormick, B. (1994). *Practical aspects of audiology: Pediatric audiology 0–5 years* (2nd ed.). San Diego, CA: Singular Publishing Group, Inc.

McCormick, B., Archbold, S., Sheppard, M., & Sheppard, S. (Eds.). (1997). *Cochlear implants for young children.* San Diego, CA: Singular Publishing Group, Inc.

McPherson, D. L. (1996). *Late potentials of the auditory system.* San Diego, CA: Singular Publishing Group, Inc.

Mendel, L. L., & Danhauer, J. L. (1996). *Audiologic evaluation and management and speech perception assessment.* San Diego, CA: Singular Publishing Group, Inc.

Mueller, H. G., III., & Hall, J. W., III. (1998). *Audiologists' desk reference Vol II: Audiologic management, rehabilitation, and terminology.* San Diego, CA: Singular Publishing Group, Inc.

Mueller, H. G., Hawkins, D. B., & Northern, J. L. (1992). *Probe microphone measurements: Hearing aid selection and assessment.* San Diego, CA: Singular Publishing Group, Inc.

Nevins, M. E., & Chute, P. M. (1996). *Children with cochlear implants in educational settings.* San Diego, CA: Singular Publishing Group, Inc.

Orlans, H. (Ed.). (1991). *Adjustment to adult hearing loss.* San Diego, CA: Singular Publishing Group, Inc.

Pappas, D. G. (1998). *Diagnosis and treatment of hearing impairment in children* (2nd ed.). San Diego, CA: Singular Publishing Group, Inc.

Paul, P. V., & Quigley, S. P. (1994). *Language and deafness* (2nd ed.). San Diego, CA: Singular Publishing Group, Inc.

Plant, G., & Spens, K. (1995). *Profound deafness and speech communication.* San Diego, CA: Singular Publishing Group, Inc.

Resnick, D. M. (1993). *Professional ethics for audiologists and speech-language pathologists.* San Diego,

CA: Singular Publishing Group, Inc.

Rizzo, S. R. Jr., & Trudeau, M.D. (Eds.). (1994). *Clinical administration in audiology and speech-language pathology.* San Diego, CA: Singular Publishing Group, Inc.

Sahley, T. L., Nodar, R. H., & Musiek, F. E. (1997). *Efferent auditory system: Structure and function.* San Diego, CA: Singular Publishing Group, Inc.

Sandlin, R. E. (1988). *Handbook of hearing aid amplification, Volume I: Theoretical and technical considerations.* San Diego, CA: Singular Publishing Group, Inc.

Sandlin, R. E. (1990). *Handbook of hearing aid amplification, Volume II: Clinical considerations and fitting practices.* San Diego, CA: Singular Publishing Group, Inc.

Seikel, J. A., King, D. W., & Drumright, D. G. (1997). *Anatomy and physiology for speech, language, and hearing (Exp. ed., Instructor's copy).* San Diego, CA: Singular Publishing Group, Inc.

Shepard, N. T., & Telian, S. A. (1996). *Practical management of the balance disorder patient.* San Diego, CA: Singular Publishing Group, Inc.

Shimon, D. A. (1992). *Coping with hearing loss and hearing aids.* San Diego, CA: Singular Publishing Group, Inc.

Shprintzen, R. J. (1997). *Genetics, syndromes, and communication disorders.* San Diego, CA: Singular Publishing Group, Inc.

Shulman, A., Aran, J., Tonndorf, J., Feldmann, H., & Vernon, J. A. (1997). *Tinnitus: Diagnosis/ treatment.* San Diego, CA: Singular Publishing Group, Inc.

Speaks, C. E. (1999). *Introduction to sound* (3rd ed.). San Diego, CA: Singular Publishing Group, Inc.

Spray, M., & Randolph, E. (1995). *Stedman's medical dictionary* (26th ed.). Baltimore, MD: Williams & Wilkins.

Stach, B. A. (1998). *Clinical audiology.* San Diego, CA: Singular Publishing Group, Inc.

Tye-Murray, N. (1998). *Foundations of aural rehabilitation: Children, adults, and their family members.* San Diego, CA: Singular Publishing Group, Inc.

Tyler, R. S. (1993). *Cochlear implants.* San Diego, CA: Singular Publishing Group, Inc.

Vonlanthen, A. (1995). *Hearing instrument technology.* San Diego, CA: Singular Publishing Group, Inc.

Wiley, T. L., & Fowler, C. G. (1997). *Acoustic immittance measures in clinical audiology.* San Diego, CA: Singular Publishing Group, Inc.

Willott, J. F. (1991). *Aging and the auditory system.* San Diego, CA: Singular Publishing Group, Inc.